Atlas of Oral and Maxillofacial Histopathology

Atlas of Oral and Maxillofacial Histopathology

Harry S. Lumerman, DDS
Professorial Lecturer and formerly Clinical Professor of Pathology and Dentistry
and Director of the Oral and Maxillofacial Pathology Division
The Mount Sinai School of Medicine
New York, New York

Robert B. Bowe, DDS
Clinical Assistant Professor
Department of Pathology
SUNY Downstate Medical Center
Brooklyn, New York

Wolters Kluwer | Lippincott Williams & Wilkins
Health

Philadelphia • Baltimore • New York • London
Buenos Aires • Hong Kong • Sydney • Tokyo

Senior Executive Editor: Jonathan W. Pine, Jr.
Product Manager: Marian Bellus
Vendor Manager: Bridgett Dougherty
Senior Manufacturing Manager: Benjamin Rivera
Senior Marketing Manager: Angela Panetta
Creative Director: Doug Smock
Production Service: Integra Software Services

Two Commerce Square
2001 Market Street
Philadelphia, PA 19103

Printed in China

Library of Congress Cataloging-in-Publication Data

Lumerman, Harry.
Atlas of oral and maxillofacial histopathology / Harry S. Lumerman, Robert B. Bowe.
p. ; cm.
ISBN-13: 978-1-4511-4314-0 (alk. paper)
ISBN-10: 1-4511-4314-1 (alk. paper)
Includes bibliographical references and index.
I. Bowe, Robert B. II. Title.
[DNLM: 1. Mouth Diseases–pathology–Atlases. 2. Diagnostic Techniques, Surgical–Atlases. 3. Jaw Diseases–pathology–Atlases. 4. Jaw Diseases–surgery–Atlases. 5. Mouth Diseases–surgery–Atlases. WU 17]
LC classification not assigned

616.310710022'2–dc23 2011039960

9 8 7 6 5 4 3 2 1

RRS1111

To Harriet Edith, my wife; Larry and Elisa, my son and daughter-in-law; Brandon and Jason, my wonderful grandchildren.

With gratitude to my teachers and coworkers of yesteryear:
Dr. Charles Darlington and Dr. Gregory N. Brown, my first teachers of Pathology at NYU College of Dentistry.
Dr. Paul Scheman, who was my mentor in oral cytology and oral surgery.

Dr. Paterno Remigio, director of pathology at Mary Immaculate Hospital, Dr. Henry Grinvalsky, chairman of pathology at the Catholic Medical Center, and Dr. Raymond Zambito, chairman of oral and maxillofacial surgery at the Catholic Medical Center. These individuals were in charge of the departments I worked in, in the 1970s and 1980s, and gave me an opportunity to start a biopsy service and a residency program in oral and maxillofacial pathology.

Dr. Nasser Said-Al-Naif and Dr. Adham Fahmy past fellows who worked with me in the Advanced Oral Maxillofacial and ENT Pathology Fellowship at Mount Sinai School of Medicine and who are carrying on successful teaching, research and diagnostic services at their Universities.

In memoriam of Dr. Ruth Spiegel, who came to me in 1971 and insisted that I start an oral and maxillofacial pathology residency program at the Catholic Medical Center, a specialty she was interested in studying. Dr. Spiegel was the first of more than three dozen residents who have completed the program to date.

Harry S. Lumerman, DDS

Foreword

Oral and maxillofacial diseases are entities that involve multiple surgical and medical specialists, including otolaryngologists, oral and maxillofacial surgeons, general dentists and other dental specialists, head and neck surgeons, dermatologists, and oncologists. In addition, the complex anatomy of this region usually requires subspecialty training for radiologists to be able to interpret the radiographic appearance and biologic behavior of the lesions. The pathology is often enigmatic for most pathologists since they see few cases and many of these cases are often referred to oral pathologists. So there is clearly a need for a text written primarily for general pathologists, dermatopathologists, and ENT pathologists regarding oral and maxillofacial disorders. We are indeed fortunate that Harry Lumerman, DDS, has assembled just such a text in the form of a practical atlas.

Dr. Lumerman has been reviewing oral and maxillofacial pathology cases for over 40 years. He has examined and/or supervised the sign-out of over 150,000 cases during his professional lifetime and is well known amongst the nation's surgical oral and maxillofacial pathologists. He is a gifted writer and teacher and has made a complex subject simpler for us to comprehend. His text, *Atlas of Oral and Maxillofacial Histopathology*, has beautiful and well-organized color illustrations, which come from his vast collection of microscopic slides, clinical photographs, and radiographs.

With 40 years spent at three major medical centers in New York City, Dr. Lumerman's career has culminated with his professorship in pathology, dentistry and dermatology at The Mount Sinai School of Medicine for the last 16 years. In 1970, he founded what later would become the largest oral biopsy service in the United States. He also started the first residency program in oral and maxillofacial pathology in 1972 in the New York metropolitan area, which is still active.

The *Atlas of Oral and Maxillofacial Histopathology* consists of six compact chapters, each containing the most common and also unusual entities that are submitted by surgeons working in this anatomic area. Dr. Lumerman presents the defining diagnostic histopathology by means of carefully selected images and captions, in addition to a brief outline of the demographic information and histopathologic differential diagnoses. Pitfall problems in diagnosis are also discussed and resolved.

In the three chapters dealing with the lesions arising within the mandibular and maxillary bones, each entity has a brief description of the radiographic appearance as it may be written on the specimen examination request form submitted by the surgeon. This information is needed to correlate the diagnostic radiographic features with the clinical features and histopathology and arrive at a more accurate diagnosis.

In our discussion on the utilization of this atlas, Dr. Lumerman respectfully suggests the following approach to the diagnosis of the oral and maxillofacial biopsy material: The pathologist, after examining the specimen and reviewing the examination request sheet, decides which group of lesions covered in the six chapters the specimen belongs to. This should direct the pathologist to the appropriate images and outlines in the atlas. Comparing the atlas images with the slide material should help the pathologist to arrive more quickly at a correct diagnosis after carefully considering the histopathologic differential for the lesion in question.

It has been a privilege for me to work with Harry Lumerman for over 25 years as a colleague and friend. This atlas is a wonderful capstone to Harry's distinguished career and innovative initiatives. Enjoy this *Atlas of Oral and Maxillofacial Histopathology* written by the "master" with the fine editorial collaboration of Dr. Robert B. Bowe.

Alan Schiller, MD
Irene Heinz Given and John Laporte Given
Professor and Chairman Emeritus of Pathology
Mount Sinai School of Medicine
New York, New York.

Preface

The Atlas of Oral and Maxillofacial Histopathology is designed to offer a practical and user-friendly guide to surgical pathologists in the interpretation of oral biopsy specimens.

Several events and ideas led to the evolution of this text. Working alongside general and specialty surgical pathologists over a period of 40 years, I recognized the need for a concise atlas of oral and maxillofacial pathology, especially for pathologists in hospitals without an oral and maxillofacial specialist on staff. I was also inspired by Stelow and Mills's *Biopsy Interpretation of the Upper Aerodigestive Tract and Ear*. In the preface to this excellent text, the authors mention that because of the complexity of the region, they had been forced to exclude primary tumors of jaws as well as odontogenic lesions. This gave me additional impetus to create a companion text.

Over the past 15 years, I worked at Mount Sinai Medical Center with Dr. Naomi Ramer, Dr. Hope Wettan, and Dr. Adham Fahmy, oral and maxillofacial pathologists, and we developed a large oral biopsy service, accounting for a total of over 75,000 cases by 2010. From these cases, I collected hundreds of slides and built dozens of PowerPoint presentations that I have used to instruct pathology and oral and maxillofacial surgery residents at various hospitals and that I have now gathered in this atlas.

In 2008, I began to sort through the microscopic slide collection and photograph utilizing the Nikon Coolscope, cases for the atlas. Just as I was on the verge of finishing this project, a colleague called to ask whether I would be willing to assist a fellow oral and maxillofacial pathologist, Robert Bowe, in preparing for his specialty boards. When I met Dr. Bowe in March of 2009, I discovered that he had taken time off after his residency to work in the field of publishing. I invited him to join me in my project. Together we reviewed and selected images from my collection and carefully revised and edited the text for this atlas. I am indebted to Dr. Bowe's ability to combine his editorial skills and knowledge of oral and maxillofacial pathology in the preparation of this atlas.

Harry S. Lumerman, DDS
New York
August 9, 2011

Acknowledgments

It is with great appreciation that I acknowledge the individuals mentioned below. The atlas was made possible only with their contributions and cooperation.

First and foremost, the oral and maxillofacial pathology staff members who worked with me over the years at Mount Sinai Department of Pathology and who were in many cases the first to review some of the interesting tumors presented in the atlas: Dr. Naomi Ramer, currently the director of the division of oral and maxillofacial pathology, and Dr. Hope Wettan and Dr. Adham Fahmy, who also functioned as oral biopsy service coordinators.

My heartfelt thanks go to Dr. Alan Schiller, chairman emeritus of pathology at Mount Sinai, under whom I worked for over 25 years, both at Mount Sinai and, previously, at Booth Memorial Medical Center in Queens. His encouragement and support were instrumental in the continued development of the oral pathology specialty and residency program in the New York Metropolitan area and the biopsy service at Booth and Mount Sinai.

I am grateful to Dr. Robert Poppiti, chairman of pathology at Mount Sinai Medical Center in Miami Beach, for allowing me for the past 7 years to present an annual tutorial to his pathology residents. It was in these tutorials that I was able to work out the method of teaching oral pathology to general pathology residents and where I first presented the material that culminated in the atlas.

Dr. Michael Siegel, professor and chairman of diagnostic sciences at Nova College of Dental Medicine in Fort Lauderdale, Florida, Dr. Ines Velez, professor and director of the division of oral and maxillofacial pathology, and Dr. Steven Kaltman, professor and chair of oral and maxillofacial surgery at Nova, have helped greatly by affording me a forum to present sessions of oral pathology to the residents in oral and maxillofacial surgery.

My thanks go to Dr. Daniel Buchbinder and Dr. Andre Montazem, former chiefs of oral and maxillofacial surgery and Dr. Gregory Chotokowski, chief of oral and maxillofacial surgery, Dr. John Pfail, chairman department of dentistry at Mount Sinai, whose residents I taught for 15 years and who, over the years, operated on many cases used in the atlas.

Special thanks go to Dr. Carlos Cordon-Cardo, MD, PhD, chairman of the department of pathology, Mount Sinai School of Medicine and Dr. Mark Lebwohl, professor and chairman of dermatology in whose department I established and conducted an oral medicine clinic.

The advantage of working in a large department of pathology is the availability of the numerous consultants, all experts in their field. Dr. James Strauchen, for lymphomas and soft tissue tumors; Dr. Michael Rivera, for head and neck and ENT pathology; Dr. Roberto Garcia, for bone/soft tissue; Dr. Ira Bleiweiss, for breast pathology; Dr. Noam Harpaz, for Gastrointestinal; Dr. Pamela Unger, for Genitourinary; Dr. Liane Deligdisch and Dr. Tamara Kalir, for gynecology; Dr. Michael Klein, for bone pathology; Dr. George Kleinman and Dr. Mary Fowkes, for neuropathology; Dr. Mary Beasly, for pulmonary pathology; Dr. Robert Phelps, Dr. Miriam

Birge, and Dr. Helen Shim, for dermatopathology; Dr. Arnold Szporn, for cytology; and Dr. Ronald Gordon, for electron microscopy.

In the past 3 years, Joseph Samet, chief medical photographer, has processed and organized hundreds of the images I shot while Irwin Magnayon was laboring over my handwritten notes and helping in constructing tables and charts.

I am grateful to the following individuals in our Histology department who processed the tissues and prepared the microscopic slides with care and precision: Lily Antonio and Jonathan Truong, managers, Wei Chen and Ghanchand Chanderdatt, supervisors and all the wonderful histotechnicians, Roma Rosario, pathologist assistants supervisor and Sabino Senosin, grossing supervisor.

My thanks also go to Ms. Gloria Turner, Histotechnician at New York University college of dentistry who showed me in the dawn of my pathology career what great histologic preparations should look like.

Thanks also go to the secretarial staff of the pathology department: Ida White, Rosemarie Lewis, and Laura Stanganelli, who greatly facilitated my work with their preparation of the pathology reports and some of the material for the atlas.

Finally, my thanks go to the oral and maxillofacial surgeons and ENT surgeons for the confidence they had in sending us their biopsies and whose cases appear in the atlas.

Because of space limitations I can acknowledge only some of the hundreds of the professionals with whom I had the pleasure to work with over the past 40 years: Dr. Arthur Adamo, Dr. Stanley Berman, Dr. Nathan Bryks, Dr. Barry Elbaum, Dr. Brian Krost, Dr. Jeffrey Elbaum, Dr. George Anastassov, Dr. Larry Brookner, Dr. Vito Cardo, Jr., Dr. Gregory Chotkowski, Dr. Harrison G. Linsky, Dr. Jeffrey Berkley, Dr. Jason Diamond, Dr. Marc Bienstock, Dr. Jeffrey Burkes, Dr. Paul Calat, Dr. Suchie Chawla, Dr. Mike Costello, Dr. Moses Datson, Dr. Hamlet Garabadian, Dr. Gerald Geldzhaler, Dr. Norman Gold, Dr. Claudia Kaplan, Dr. Martina Laifook, Dr. Ho Lee, Dr. Olumide Olawaye, Dr. Zvi Osterweil, Dr. Lynn Pierri, Dr. Zev Shulhoff, Dr. Jerome Friedman, Dr. Sam Straus, Dr. Steven Cho, Dr. Michael Chan, Dr. Scott Cohen, Dr. Leon Cheris, Dr. Antonio del Valle, Dr. Todd Eggleston, Dr. Mathew Eichen, Drs. Arthur and Richard Elias, Dr. Keith Fisher, Dr. William Friedel, Dr. Gerald Friedman, Dr. Eric Genden, Dr. Jay Goldsmith, Dr. Alex Greenberg, Dr. Harvey Grossman, Dr. Andrew Catania, Dr. William Rakower, Dr. Gregory Hatzis, Dr. Eugene Herman, Dr. Dwight Hershman, Dr. Andrew Horowitz, Dr. David Hoffman, Dr. Ean James, Dr. Andrew D. Kim, Dr. Andrew K. Kim, Dr. Lloyd Klausner, Dr. Stephen Klein, Dr. Gary Kolinsky, Dr. William Kopp, Dr. Michael Kremer, Dr. Harold Kresberg, Dr. J Phillip Kurtz, Dr. William Lawson, Dr. Alvaro Marin, Dr. Andrei Mark, Dr. Michael Marshall, Dr. David Mashadian, Dr. Vincent Novelli, Dr. Brian ONeill, Dr. Daniel Pompa, Dr. Arlene Rodriguez, Dr. Martin Rosencrans, Dr. Clifford Salm, Dr. Jonathan Sasportas, Dr. Leonard Schiffman, Dr. Joseph Sciarrino, Dr. Larry Shemen, Dr. Shahab Soleymani, Dr. Norman Snyder, Dr. Jay Sonnenshein, Dr. Mark Stein, Dr. Ira Sturman, Dr. David Tabaroki, Dr. Dmitry Tokar, Dr. Yan Trokel, Dr. Mark Urken, Dr. David Valauri, Dr. Desmond Ward, Dr. Steven Wasserman, Dr. William D. Weber, Dr. Howard Weitzman, Dr. Steven Wettan, Dr. Ben Recant, and Dr. Boris Zats.

Finally my appreciation goes to Jonathan Pine, Editor in Chief, Marian Bellus, Pathology Product Manager and Tintu Thomas of Integra India, for expediting and managing this difficult project.

Harry S. Lumerman, DDS

Contents

CHAPTER

1

Odontogenic Cysts

Radicular (periapical) cyst
Dentigerous cyst
Odontogenic keratocyst
Orthokeratinized odontogenic cyst
Lateral periodontal cyst
Calcifying odontogenic cyst
Glandular odontogenic cyst

Introduction

Cysts of the jaws are common, and most are related to the presence of teeth and their embryologic precursors; that is, they are odontogenic.

For the frequently encountered radicular cyst, the inciting factor is inflammation, generally due to caries (dental decay), while the not-so frequently encountered cysts are thought to be developmental and are related to the proliferation of various epithelial residues left over from normal tooth formation.

The most important entity in this chapter is the odontogenic keratocyst (OKC). It is a common lesion, unique to the jaws, and often misdiagnosed. To ensure correct diagnosis and adequate treatment of this aggressive cyst/tumor, the pathologist must recognize the characteristics of its distinctive epithelial lining. The keratocyst can also appear as the initial manifestation of the nevoid basal cell carcinoma syndrome (Gorlin syndrome).

The glandular odontogenic cyst, while a much rarer entity, is also aggressive and frequently recurrent. In addition, its histopathology can sometimes be confused with that of a true malignancy—mucoepidermoid carcinoma.

1.1 Radicular (Periapical) Cyst

Definition

The common inflammatory cyst associated with the root apex of an infected tooth

Presentation

Swelling and pain. Mostly in adults.

Radiographic Appearance

Radiolucency at the apex of a nonvital tooth

Microscopic Findings

- Fibrous cyst wall containing a mixture of inflammatory cells—lymphocytes, plasma cells, and neutrophils. The cyst wall can also contain cholesterol clefts, foreign body giant cells, and corrugated, eosinophilic hyaline bodies. Hyaline bodies are thought to be a cellular reaction to extravasated serum and can be seen in other types of odontogenic cysts as well.
- Nonkeratinizing stratified squamous lining, often destroyed by intense inflammation. The lining can contain mucous cells and curvilinear, brightly eosinophilic Rushton bodies.

Histopathologic Differential

Dental granuloma (see Additional, below)

Treatment and Prognosis

Extraction of tooth or root canal therapy in addition to curettage of cyst

Additional

When the pulp inside a tooth becomes necrotic, usually due to extensive caries (decay), the inflammatory response spreads into bone, producing a mass of granulation tissue known as a *dental granuloma.* Adjacent or entrapped odontogenic epithelial rests proliferate, eventually outgrowing their blood supply and becoming cystic. The result is a radicular cyst.

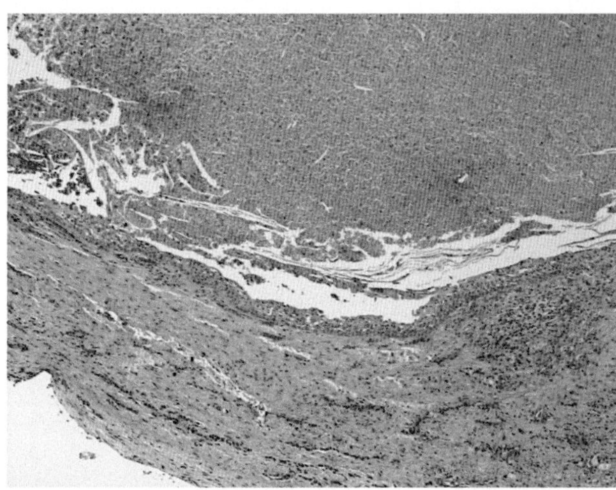

Figure 1.1.1.
Radicular cyst. Stratified squamous epithelium lines an inflamed, thick-walled fibrous cystic structure filled with necrotic debris. If the cyst remains after tooth extraction, it is known as a *residual cyst.*

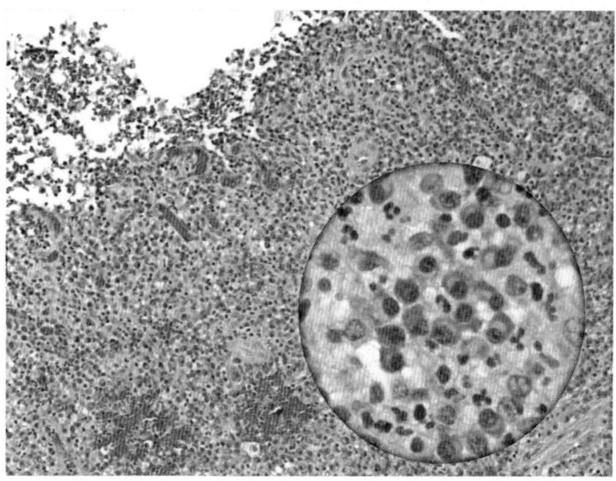

Figure 1.1.2.
Radicular cyst. This cystic mass of granulation tissue without an epithelial lining resembles a *dental granuloma.* Inset: The inflammatory infiltrate consists of lymphocytes, neutrophils, and abundant plasma cells.

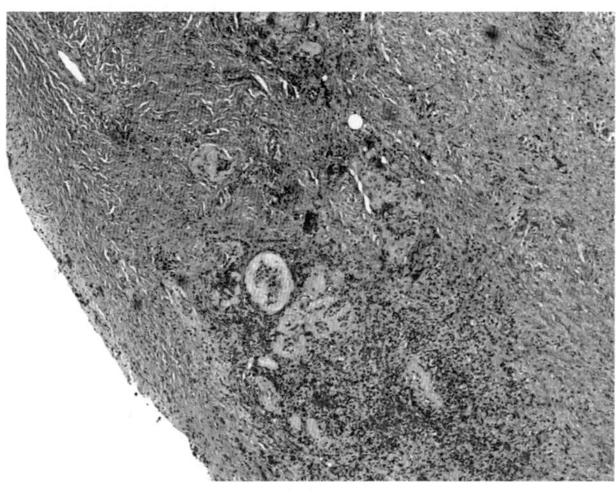

Figure 1.1.3.
Radicular cyst. Hyaline bodies are sometimes encountered within the wall of radicular cysts. Epithelial lining has been destroyed by the intense inflammation.

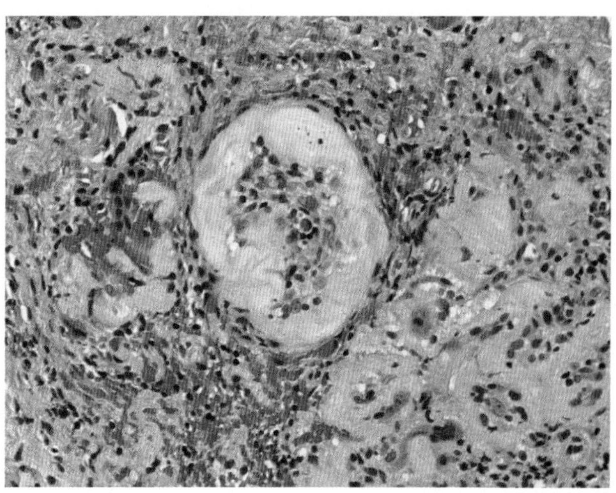

Figure 1.1.4.
Radicular cyst. Hyaline bodies can be in the form of pools of exudate, as at lower right, or glassy, pink corrugated rings surrounding clusters of lymphocytes, plasma cells, and erythrocytes. Foreign body giant cells often accompany these structures.

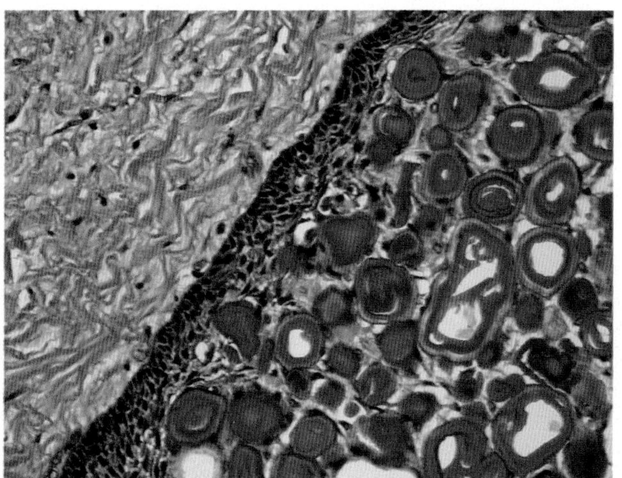

Figure 1.1.5.
Radicular cyst. Curvilinear, brightly eosinophilic Rushton bodies occur almost exclusively within the epithelial lining of odontogenic cysts. They are thought to be a secretory product of odontogenic epithelium deposited on cell debris or other particulate matter.

1.2 Dentigerous Cyst

Definition

The common developmental cyst found in association with the crown of an impacted tooth

Presentation

Usually an asymptomatic radiographic finding. If the cyst becomes infected, pain and swelling can result. Most commonly found around the third molars of the mandible. Generally in teenagers and young adults.

Radiographic Appearance

Well-defined radiolucency around the crown of an impacted tooth

Microscopic Findings

- Well-developed fibrous connective tissue wall.
- Thin, nonkeratinizing stratified squamous or cuboidal lining that may also contain ciliated, columnar, or mucous cells.
- If the lining becomes inflamed, it often proliferates, creating elongated, interconnected rete ridges.

Histopathologic Differential

- Extensive proliferation of the lining into the cyst lumen can be mistaken for *unicystic ameloblastoma.* An inflammatory background supports the diagnosis of inflamed dentigerous cyst; the absence of hyperchromatic, palisaded cells effectively rules out ameloblastoma.

Treatment and Prognosis

Enucleation of cyst and extraction of tooth

Additional

Dentigerous cysts are among the most common lesions received by the pathology laboratory. Usually they are submitted following a surgical procedure for the removal of the third molars (wisdom teeth).

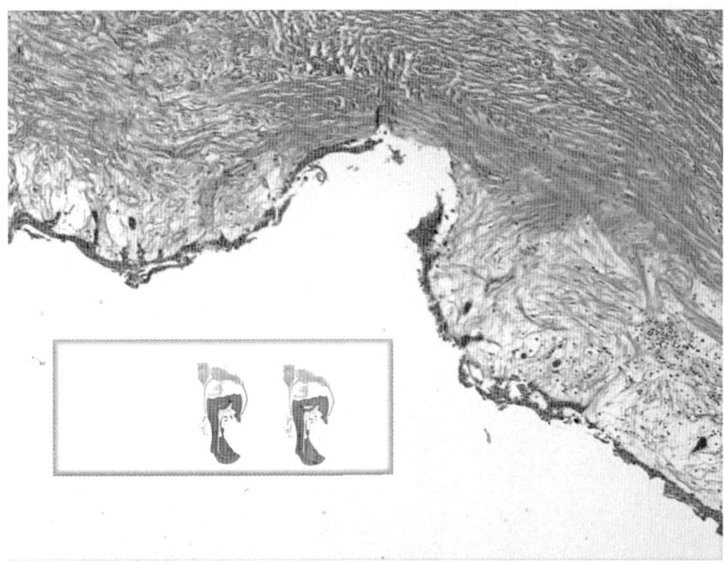

Figure 1.2.1.
Dentigerous cyst. The wall is typically thick and fibrocollagenous. Inflammatory cells are absent or minimal. The whole mount shows a dilated cystic structure surrounding the crown of a tooth above the space created by decalcified enamel.

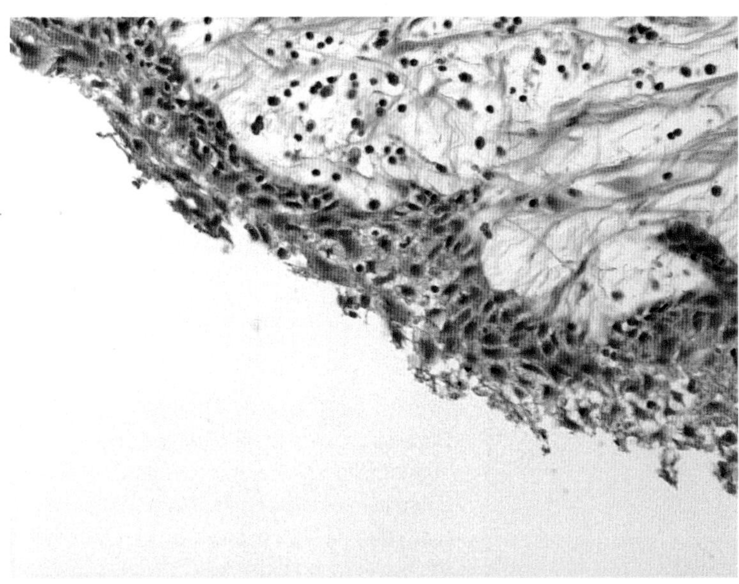

Figure 1.2.2.
Dentigerous cyst. The lining typically consists of several layers of nonkeratinizing stratified squamous epithelium with rete ridge formation.

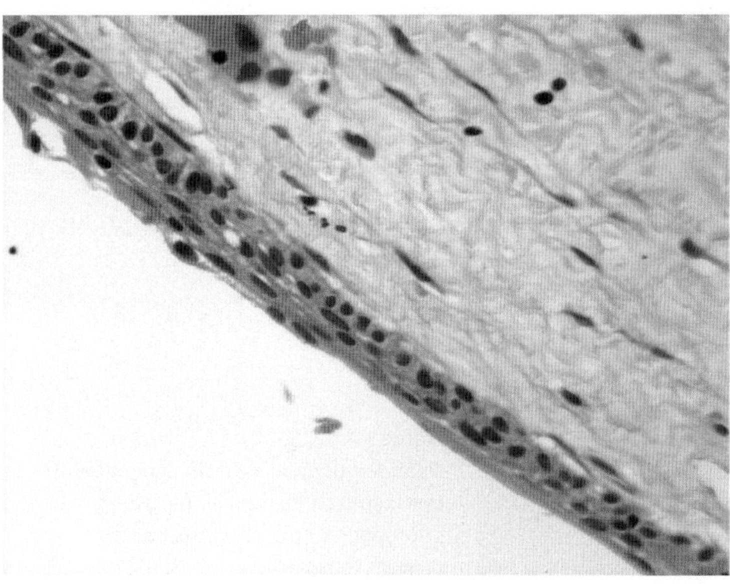

Figure 1.2.3.
Dentigerous cyst. Multilayered compressed epithelium lines this example.

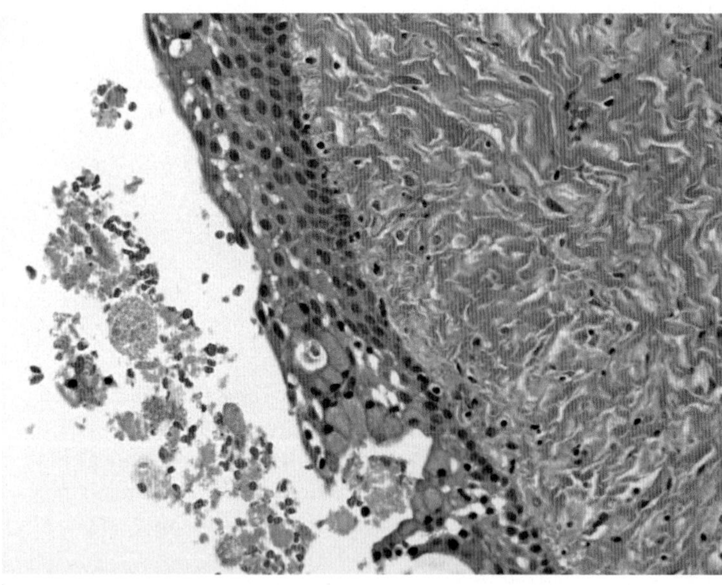

Figure 1.2.4.
Dentigerous cyst. The stratified squamous lining can also contain mucous cells.

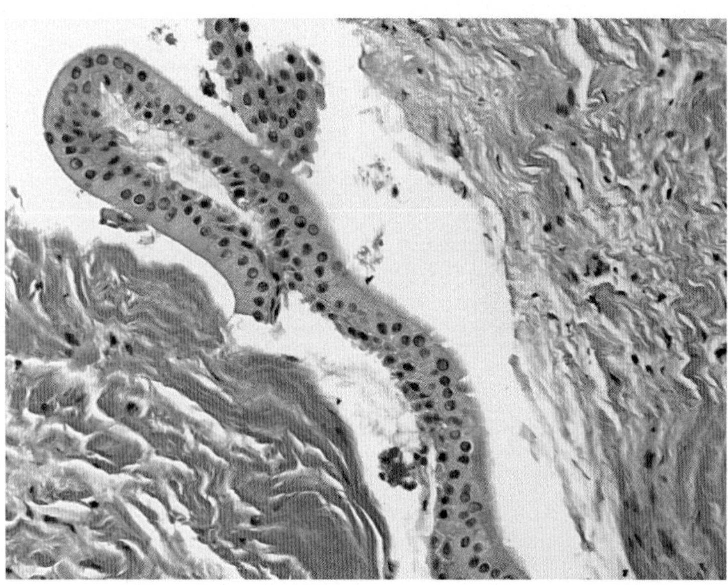

Figure 1.2.5.
Dentigerous cyst. These bilayered columnar eosinophilic cells represent the reduced enamel epithelium, a normal part of the embryologic tooth bud. Rarely, a dentigerous cyst forms with these cells as its lining.

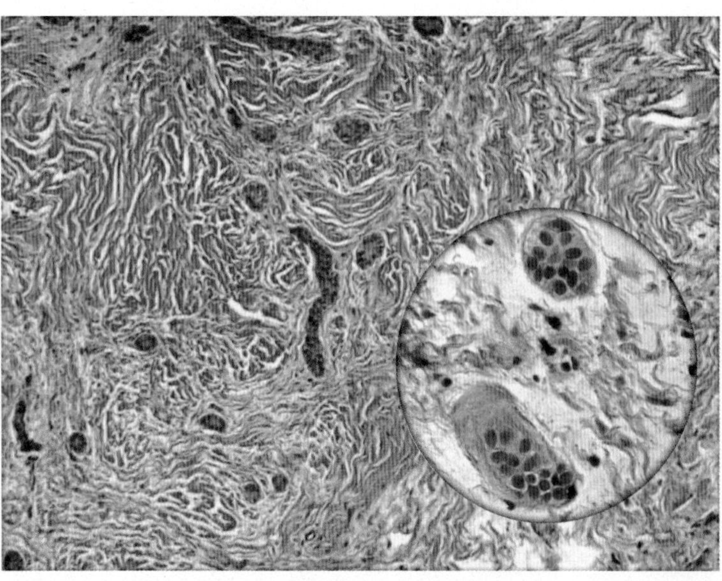

Figure 1.2.6.
Dentigerous cyst. The walls of dentigerous cysts often contain small, inactive odontogenic epithelial rests, remnants of tooth formation.

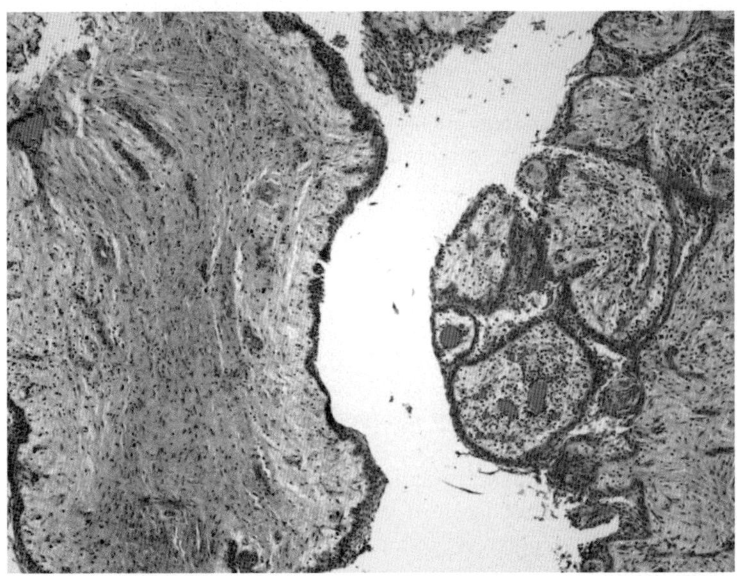

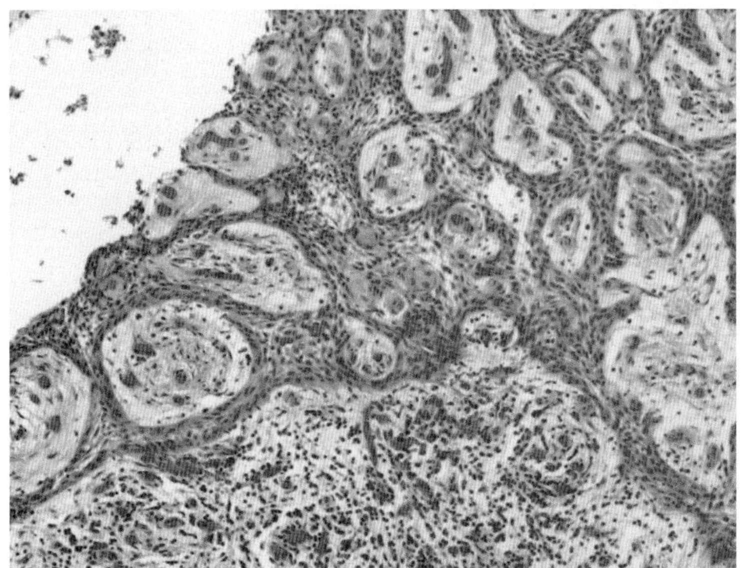

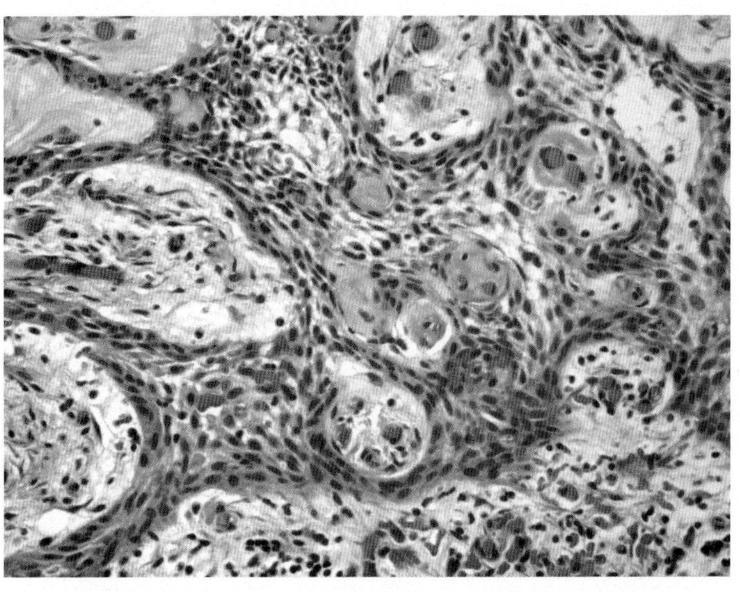

Figures 1.2.7–1.2.9.
Dentigerous cyst. Areas of epithelial proliferation in an inflamed odontogenic cyst can be cause for concern. In these examples, all from a dentigerous cyst, a plexiform growth pattern mimics ameloblastoma. The presence of hypervascularity and a robust inflammatory infiltrate supports a reactive process; the absence of hyperchromatic, peripheral, palisaded epithelial cells rules out ameloblastoma.

1.3 Odontogenic Keratocysts

Presentation

Frequently an incidental radiographic finding, often in the posterior body and ramus of the mandible. OKCs grow in an anteroposterior direction and can become large before producing jaw swelling. Any age, but most patients are between 10 and 40. Multiple OKCs are encountered in the nevoid basal cell carcinoma syndrome (Gorlin syndrome).

Radiographic Appearance

Unilocular, well-defined radiolucency frequently associated with an impacted tooth

Microscopic Findings

- Uniform, thin, six- to eight-layer-thick stratified squamous epithelium.
- Corrugated, parakeratotic surface.
- Basal cells with prominent, hyperchromatic, palisaded nuclei.
- Flat epithelial–connective tissue interface devoid of rete ridges. The lining is often artifactually separated from the underlying fibrous cyst wall.
- Abundant keratin scales within the lumen.
- Epithelial buds and microcysts within the fibrous cyst wall.

Note: When inflamed, the epithelial lining of the OKC, proliferates, rete ridges form, and many of the above diagnostic histologic features are lost.

Histopathologic Differential

- The lining of a *dentigerous cyst* lacks the OKC's uniform thickness, prominent palisading basal cell layer, and parakeratotic surface.
- The lining of an *orthokeratinized odontogenic cyst* has a prominent granular cell layer and an orthokeratinized surface.

Treatment and Prognosis

Enucleation followed by removal of peripheral bone, either surgically with a bur (peripheral ostectomy) or by means of chemical cautery (Carnoy's solution). The recurrence rate is high—about 30%.

Additional

Since 2005, the World Health Organization(WHO) has referred to the OKC as the keratocystic odontogenic tumor, a unique odontogenic "cyst" with a distinctive histopathology and aggressive clinical behavior.

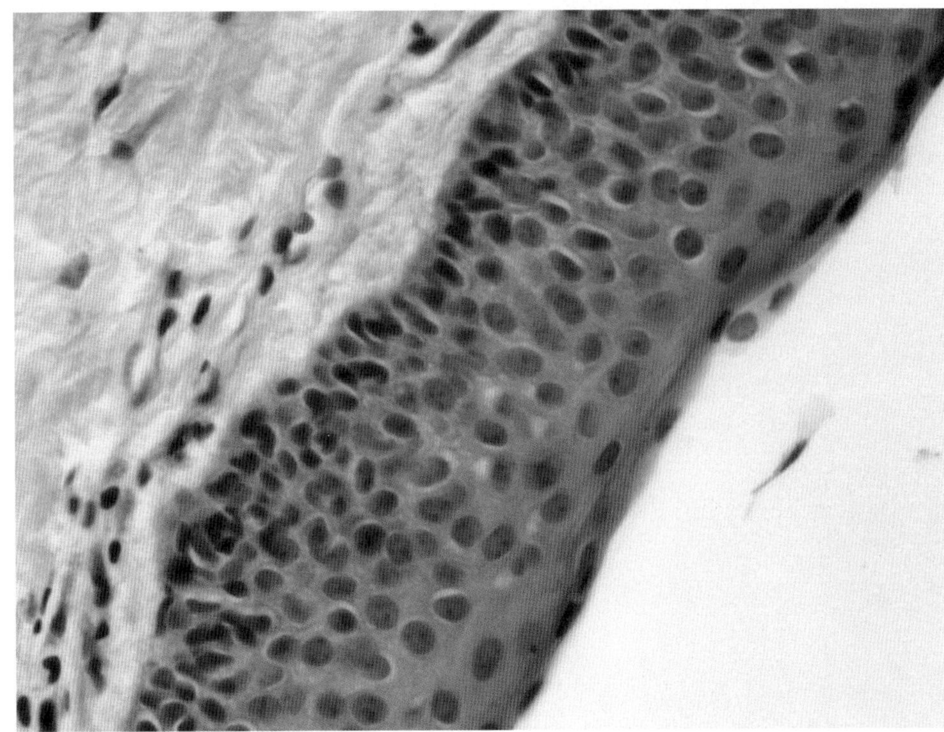

Figure 1.3.1.
Odontogenic keratocyst. The lining consists of parakeratotic stratified squamous epithelium six to eight cells thick. The basal cells are prominent and palisaded. The connective tissue interface is usually flat, but it can also be gently undulating, as here.

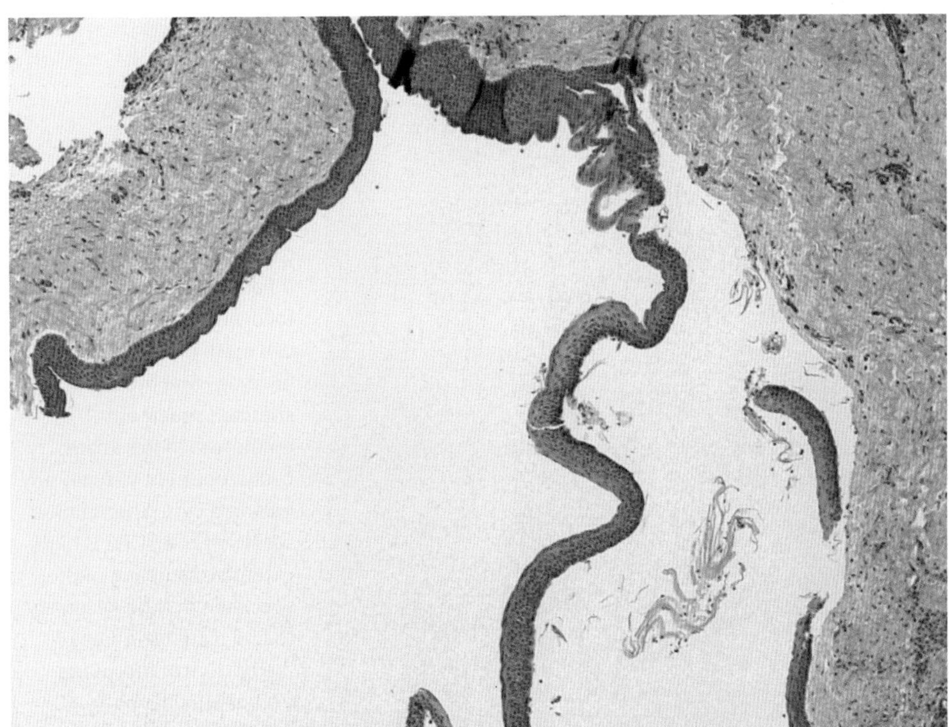

Figure 1.3.2.
Odontogenic keratocyst. Artifactual separation of the lining from the cyst wall is often seen.

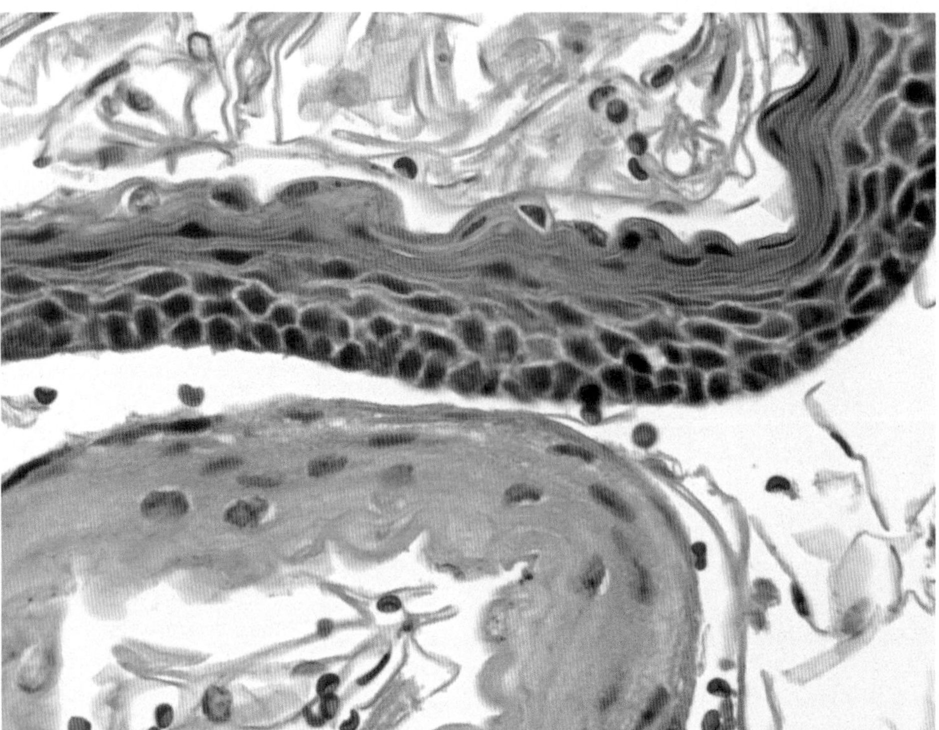

Figure 1.3.3. Odontogenic keratocyst. These two strips of detached epithelial lining are producing keratin. Keratinaceous debris in the lumen can be abundant and obvious at the time of gross inspection.

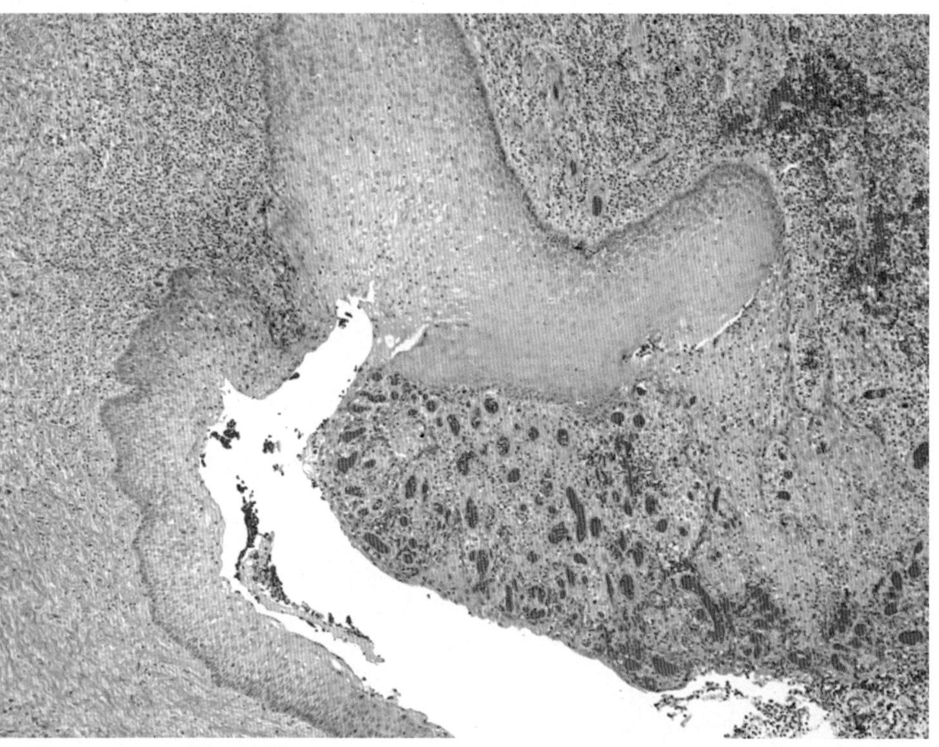

Figure 1.3.4. Odontogenic keratocyst. Inflammation, frequently following incisional biopsy, can mask the OKC's specific histology. The hyperplastic stratified squamous epithelium in this image could represent virtually any inflamed cyst. When clinical suspicion of an OKC is high, extensive sampling of the specimen may be necessary to find diagnostic areas. At the bottom of the image, residual, uninflamed OKC lining is seen.

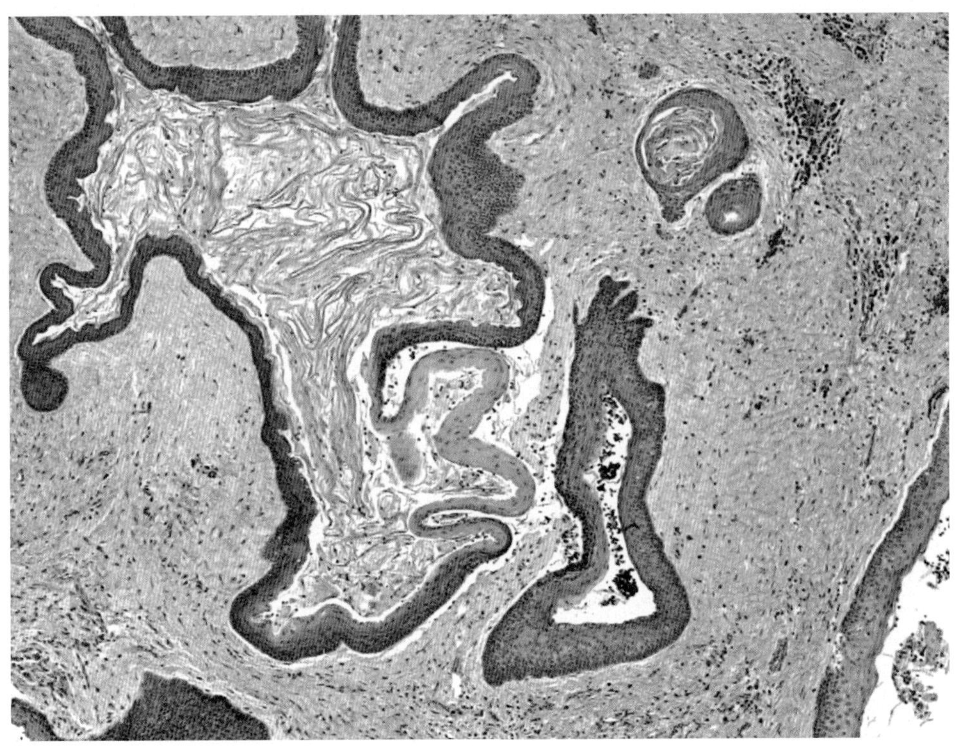

Figure 1.3.5.
Odontogenic keratocyst. Small satellite, or daughter, cysts can also be present within the cyst wall.

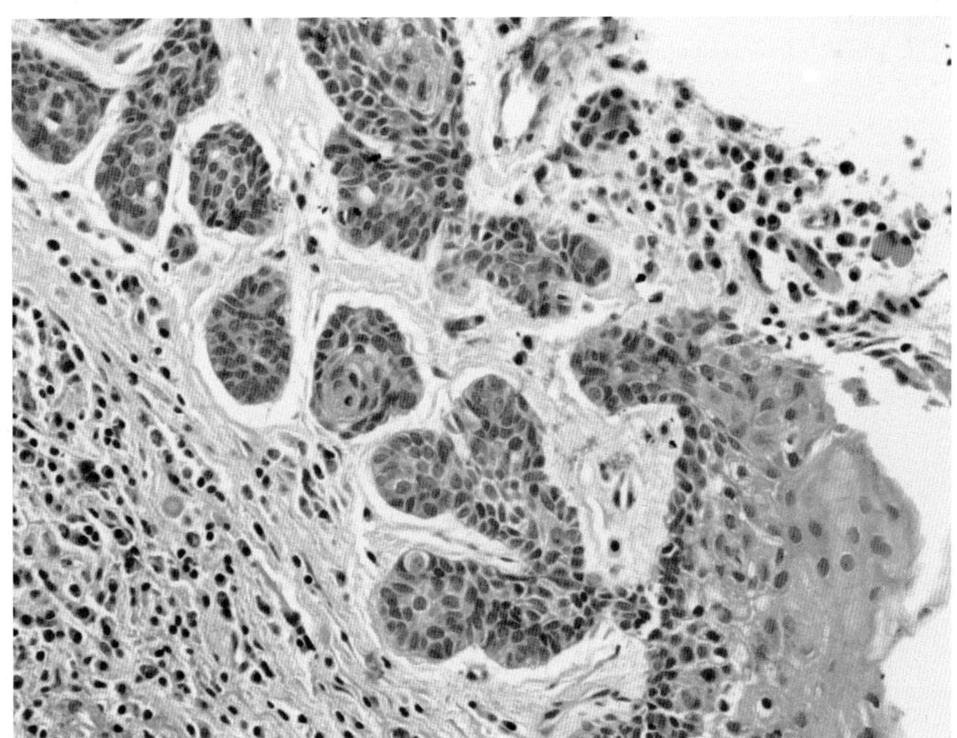

Figure 1.3.6.
Odontogenic keratocyst. Buds of basaloid epithelial cells proliferate into the underlying fibrous stroma.

1.4 Orthokeratinized Odontogenic Cyst

Definition

A rare odontogenic cyst whose histology is sometimes mistaken for that of the more aggressive OKC

Presentation

Usually an incidental radiographic finding. Most common in the posterior mandible. In young adults.

Radiographic Appearance

Unilocular, well-defined radiolucency. Frequently associated with the crown of an unerupted third molar.

Microscopic Findings

- Stratified squamous epithelial lining overlying a fibrous connecting tissue wall
- Prominent granular cell layer
- Orthokeratinized surface

Histopathologic Differential

- The lining of an OKC has a basal cell layer with prominent, hyperchromatic, palisaded nuclei. The surface is corrugated and parakeratotic. There is no granular cell layer.

Treatment and Prognosis

Enucleation and curettage of cyst cavity. Recurrence rare.

Additional

The orthokeratinized odontogenic cyst is not seen in the gorlin syndrome, unlike the OKC.

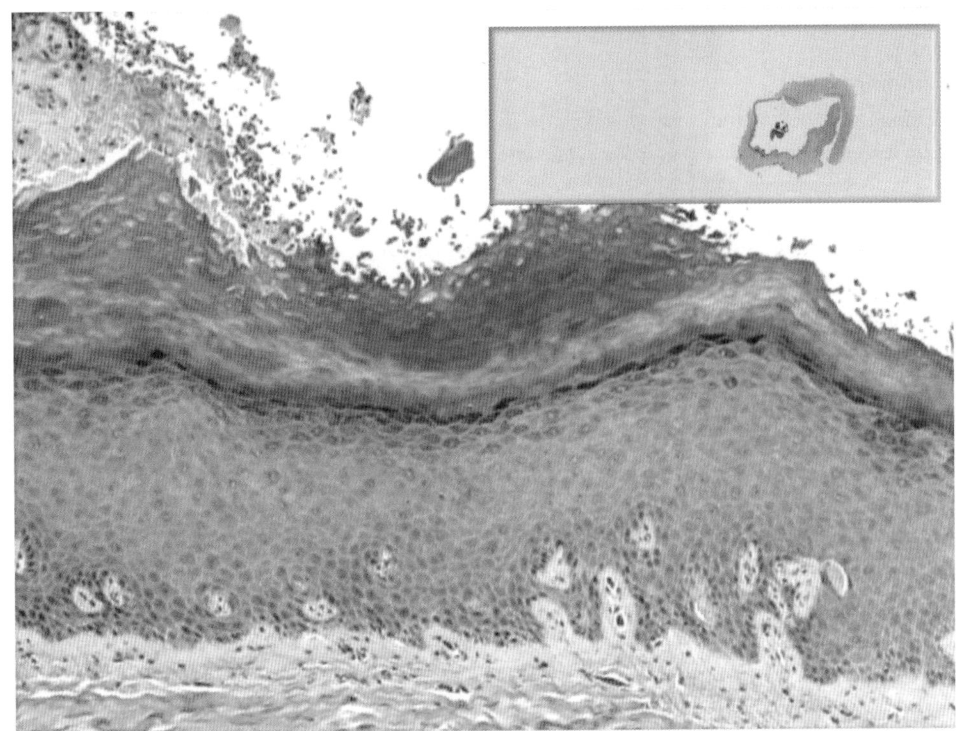

Figure 1.4.1. Orthokeratinized odontogenic cyst. Orthokeratin, not parakeratin, is produced and the basal epithelial cells are neither prominent nor palisaded. The whole mount shows a thick-walled, uninflamed fibrous cystic structure lined by epithelium.

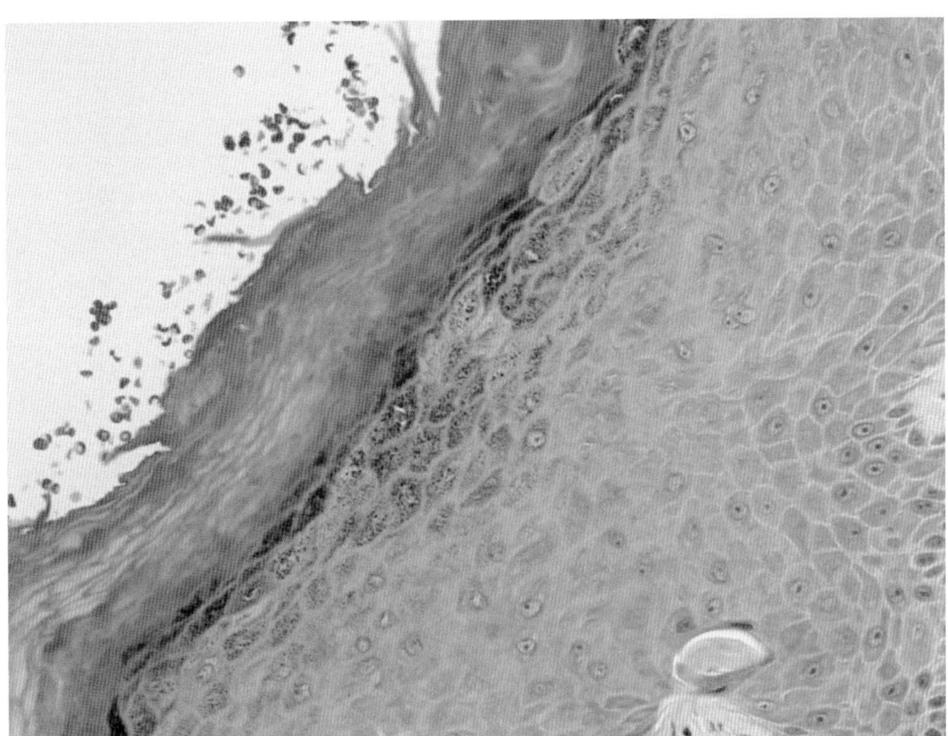

Figure 1.4.2. Orthokeratinized odontogenic cyst. A well-developed granular cell layer lies below the cap of orthokeratin.

1.5 Lateral Periodontal Cyst

Definition

A small, developmental cyst that occurs in the bone between the roots of healthy teeth. The larger, polycystic variant is known as the *botryoid odontogenic cyst*.

Presentation

Incidental radiographic finding, mostly in the premolar area of the mandible. Usually in adults.

Radiographic Appearance

A small (under 1 cm) radiolucency between the roots of healthy teeth. The botryoid variant can reach a large size.

Microscopic Findings

- Nonkeratinizing stratified squamous epithelial lining one to two cell(s) thick, overlying a fibrous wall.
- The lining contains oval to triangular nodular thickenings (thèques, plaques) containing glycogen-rich clear cells.

Special Stains/Immunopathology

The glycogen-containing clear cells are PAS-positive, diastase-labile.

Histopathologic Differential

The *glandular odontogenic cyst* features duct-like structures and mucous cells within the lining and eosinophilic hobnail cells and cilia on its surface.

Treatment and Prognosis

Complete excision

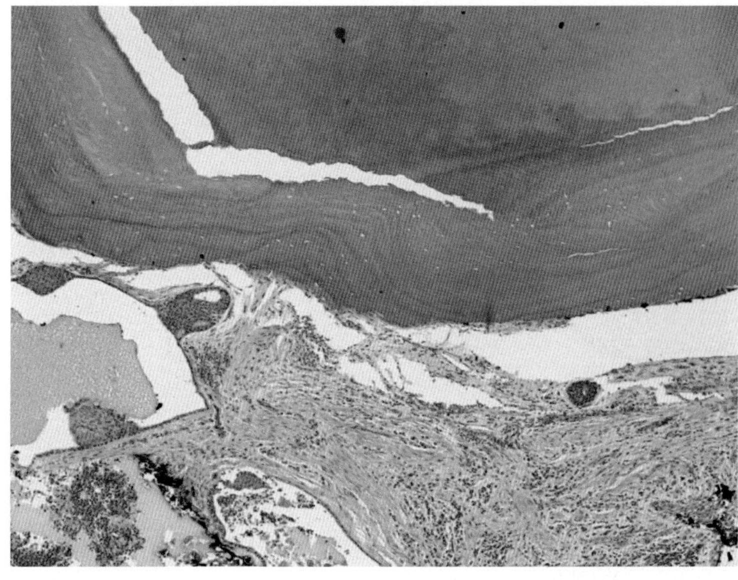

Figure 1.5.1.
Lateral periodontal cyst, botryoid variant. A portion of tooth root is surrounded by a multicystic proliferation lined by a thinned epithelium.

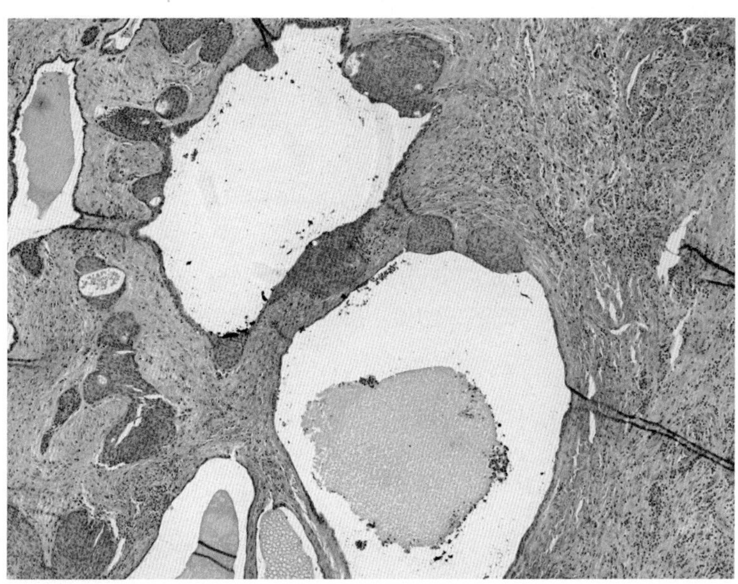

Figure 1.5.2.
Lateral periodontal cyst, botryoid variant. Abundant cystic spaces with an attenuated lining containing ovoid, nodular thickenings (thèques) of squamous epithelium.

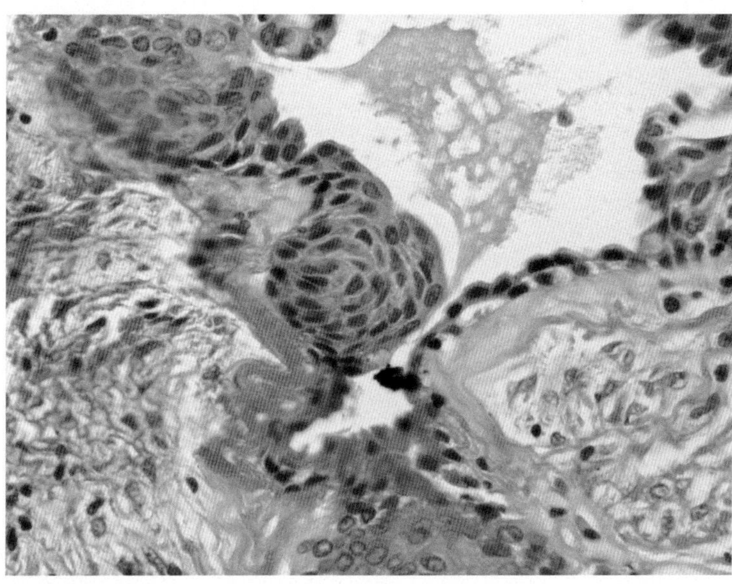

Figure 1.5.3.
Lateral periodontal cyst, botryoid variant. The nodular thickenings are composed of whorls of bland squamous epithelium often containing glycogen-rich clear cells (not seen in this case).

1.6 Calcifying Odontogenic Cyst

Definition

A developmental odontogenic cyst whose proliferating lining resembles, in areas, an ameloblastoma

Presentation

Incidental radiographic finding or firm expansion of buccal cortical plate. In young adults. Anterior location.

Radiographic Appearance

Unilocular radiolucency. Calcifications are seen in about half of the cases.

Microscopic Findings

- Stratified squamous epithelium and ameloblastomatous lining (peripheral palisading, hyperchromasia, and reverse polarization).
- The lining contains aggregates of ghost cells (epithelial cells with a pale, swollen cytoplasm and spaces where nuclei once stood).
- Possible dystrophic calcifications within ghost cell aggregates.
- Fibrous connective tissue wall.

Histopathologic Differential

Masses of ghost cells are absent in an *ameloblastoma.*

Treatment and Prognosis

Enucleation. Prognosis is good.

Additional

Since 2005, the World Health Organization (WHO) has referred to the "calcifying odontogenic cyst" as the "calcifying cystic odontogenic tumor". It is also known as *Gorlin cyst.*

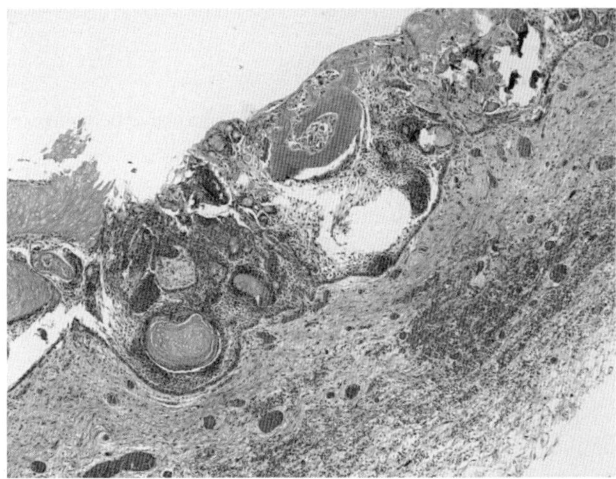

Figure 1.6.1.
Calcifying odontogenic cyst. The cyst has areas in which the stratified squamous lining becomes exuberant and hyperchromatic. Eosinophilic masses are present within the lining.

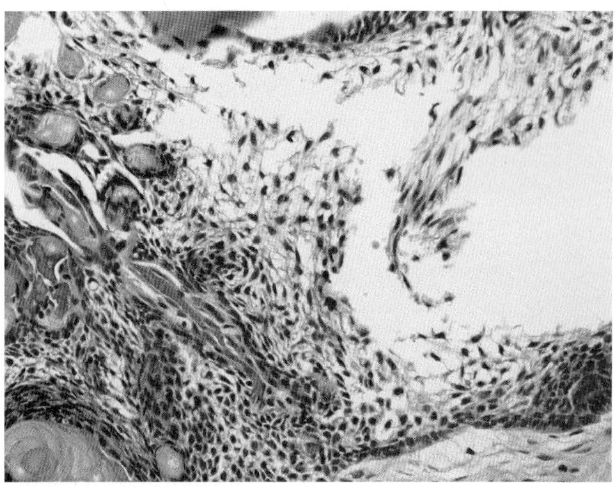

Figure 1.6.2.
Calcifying odontogenic cyst. At higher power, the ameloblastic nature of this epithelium becomes clear. Nuclei are hyperchromatic and palisaded; other areas resemble the stellate reticulum of the enamel organ.

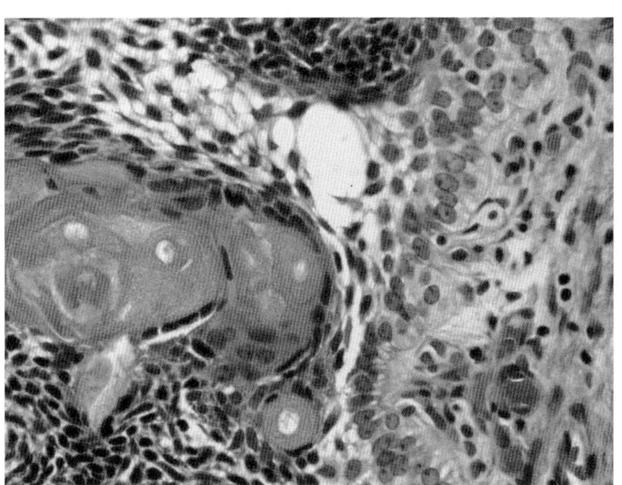

Figure 1.6.3.
Calcifying odontogenic cyst. The eosinophilic masses are actually clusters of ghost cells, epithelial cells with spaces where nuclei once stood. Aggregates of ghost cells are a diagnostic feature of the calcifying odontogenic cyst.

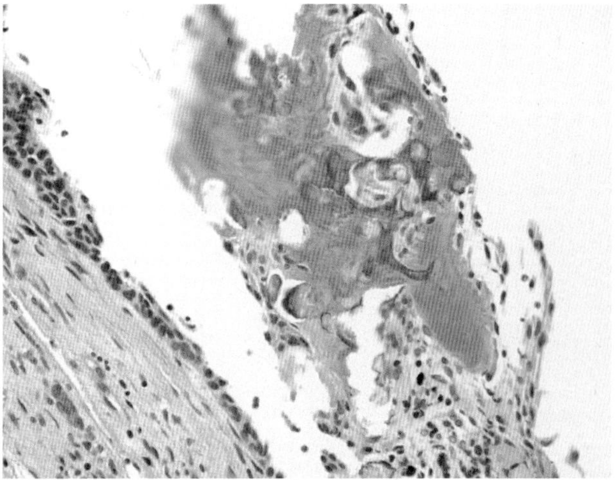

Figure 1.6.4.
Calcifying odontogenic cyst. In this example, the ghost cells are undergoing calcification. When extensive, these calcifications are evident radiographically.

1.7 Glandular Odontogenic Cyst

Definition

An uncommon developmental jaw cyst with unpredictable, potentially aggressive behavior

Presentation

Slow-growing swelling of the anterior mandible. Generally asymptomatic but can be associated with pain or paresthesia. In adults. Rare under the age of 30 years.

Radiographic Appearance

Large expansile radiolucency of the anterior mandible, often crossing the midline

Microscopic Findings

- Complex, nonkeratinizing stratified squamous epithelial lining containing heaped up, thickened areas and mucin-filled, duct-like spaces.
- Mucous, ciliated, and hobnail cells are in the superficial portion of the lining.
- Fibrous connective tissue wall.

Histopathologic Differential

- There is considerable similarity between the histology of the glandular odontogenic cyst and the histology of low-grade intraosseous *mucoepidermoid carcinoma.* Ciliated and hobnail cells, epithelial plaques, and a relatively uniform lining with only occasional mucous cells favor the diagnosis of glandular odontogenic cyst. An invasive, cystic tumor with extensive epithelial proliferation containing epidermoid, mucous, and intermediate cells favors the diagnosis of mucoepidermoid carcinoma.
- The botryoid variant of *lateral periodontal cyst* lacks glandular structures as well as hobnail cells and cilia but contains abundant epithelial thèques.

Treatment and Prognosis

Enucleation or marginal resection. A 30% recurrence rate has been reported.

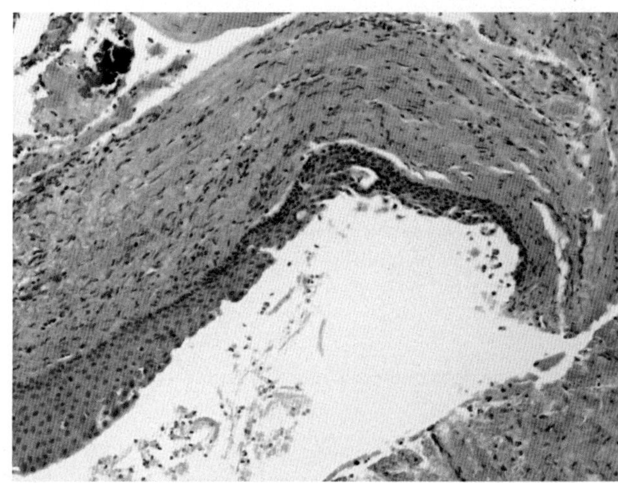

Figure 1.7.1.
Glandular odontogenic cyst. The stratified squamous epithelium is of variable thickness, containing microcystic intraepithelial spaces and heaped-up projections lined with ciliated and hobnail cells.

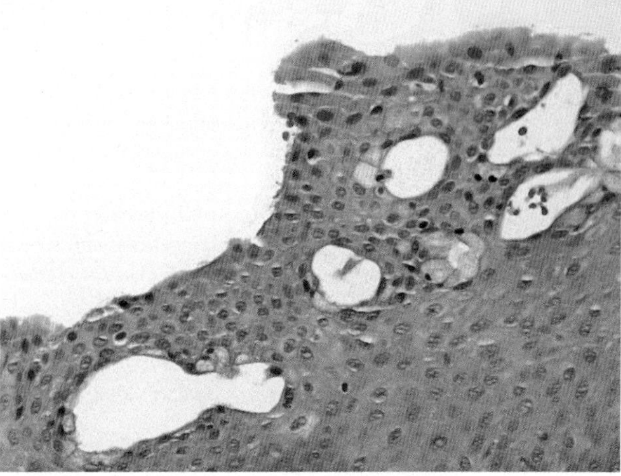

Figure 1.7.2.
Glandular odontogenic cyst. The epithelial lining contains mucous cells and microcystic spaces. Hobnail and ciliated cells are present on the surface.

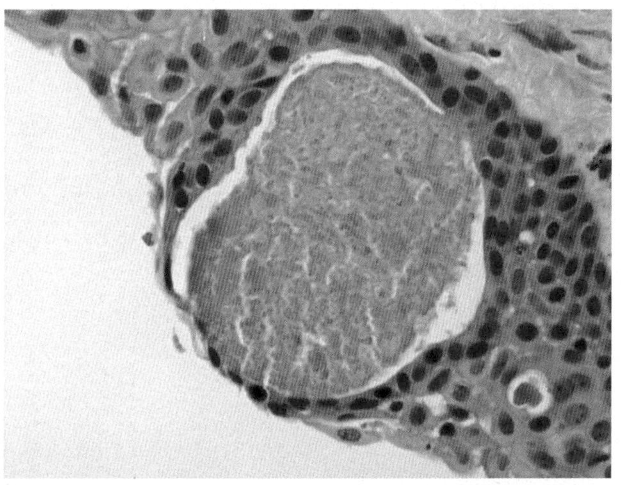

Figure 1.7.3.
Glandular odontogenic cyst. A mucin-filled, intraepithelial duct-like structure.

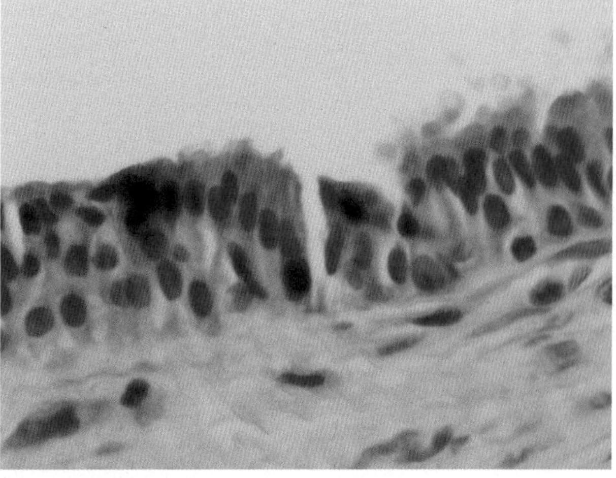

Figure 1.7.4.
Glandular odontogenic cyst. Higher power of ciliated and hobnail cells.

Bibliography and Suggested Reading

1.1

Lin HP, Chen HM, Yu CH, et al. Clinicopathological study of 252 jaw bone periapical lesions from a private pathology laboratory. *J Formos Med Assoc.* 2010;109:810–818.

1.2

Philipsen HP, Reichart PA. The development and fate of epithelial residues after completion of the human odontogenesis with special reference to the origins of epithelial odontogenic neoplasms, hamartomas and cysts. *Oral Biosci Med.* 2004;1:171–179.

1.3

González-Alva P, Tanaka A, Oku Y, et al. Keratocystic odontogenic tumor: a retrospective study of 183 cases. *J Oral Sci.* 2008;50:205–212.

1.4

Aragaki T, Michi Y, Katsube K, et al. Comprehensive keratin profiling reveals different histopathogenesis of keratocystic odontogenic tumor and orthokeratinized odontogenic cyst. *Hum Pathol.* 2010;41:1718–1725.

Li TJ, Kitano M, Chen XM, et al. Orthokeratinized odontogenic cyst: a clinicopathological and immunocytochemical study of 15 cases. *Histopathology.* 1998;32:242–251.

1.5

De Andrade Santos PP, Freitas VS, de Almeida Freitas R, et al. Botryoid odontogenic cyst: a clinicopathologic study of 10 cases. *Ann Diagn Pathol.* 2011;15(4):221–4.

1.6

Li TJ, Yu SF. Clinicopathologic spectrum of the so-called calcifying odontogenic cysts: a study of 21 intraosseous cases with reconsideration of the terminology and classification. *Am J Surg Pathol.* 2003;27:372–384.

1.7

Kaplan I, Anavi Y, Hirshberg A. Glandular odontogenic cyst: a challenge in diagnosis and treatment. *Oral Dis.* 2008;14:575–581.

CHAPTER

2

Odontogenic Tumors

Epithelial odontogenic tumors
Solid/multicystic ameloblastoma
Unicystic ameloblastoma
Peripheral ameloblastoma
Ameloblastic carcinoma
Adenomatoid odontogenic tumor
Calcifying epithelial odontogenic tumor (Pindborg tumor)
Calcifying ghost cell odontogenic tumor
Squamous odontogenic tumor

Mixed epithelial and mesenchymal odontogenic tumors
Ameloblastic fibroma
Ameloblastic fibro-odontoma
Ameloblastic fibrosarcoma
Odontoma

Mesenchymal odontogenic tumors
Odontogenic myxoma
Odontogenic fibroma
Cementoblastoma

Introduction

Odontogenic tumors arise from the embryonic epithelial and ectomesenchymal tissue remnants of tooth formation. They are usually found in the alveolar (tooth-bearing) part of the jawbones but can also occur in the gingival tissues outside of bone.

Ameloblastoma is the most common and the most aggressive of the epithelial odontogenic tumors. One variant deserves special mention, the unicystic. Occurring in younger patients, it potentially requires less aggressive treatment and has a better prognosis than does the typical solid/multicystic ameloblastoma. The problem is that the entire cystic structure must be received and examined at multiple levels to make a diagnosis of unicystic ameloblastoma.

Ameloblastic fibroma, a tumor with both epithelial and mesenchymal components, usually occurs in very young patients. Although the prognosis is good if the tumor is completely removed, the surgical procedure is sometimes compromised in an attempt to preserve developing teeth. This strategy carries the risk of recurrences that can undergo malignant transformation.

Of the mesenchymal tumors, the odontogenic myxoma is the most important entity to consider. Its myxoid histology is identical to that of two normal dental soft tissue structures sometimes submitted along with an extracted tooth: papilla and follicle. The dental papilla is the tooth's developing pulp (nerve canal contents), and the follicle is a membranous sac surrounding its crown. Misdiagnosing these normal tissues as an aggressive neoplasm can result in unnecessary surgery.

Epithelial Odontogenic Tumors

2.1a Solid/Multicystic Ameloblastoma

Presentation

Painless expansile swelling. Mostly in the posterior mandible. The average age of the patient is 34 years.

Radiographic Appearance

Unilocular or multilocular radiolucency

Microscopic Findings

Unencapsulated, infiltrative tumor, usually with one of the following two patterns:

FOLLICULAR VARIANT

- Large nests (follicles) of odontogenic epithelium bordered by columnar cells with nuclei oriented toward the center of the follicle (reverse polarity).
- Follicular centers are composed of loose spindle or squamoid cells or, rarely, large cells with a granular, eosinophilic cytoplasm. Follicles can become cystic, and a good portion of the tumor may be composed of large cysts.
- Mature fibrous connective tissue stroma.

PLEXIFORM VARIANT

- Thin, interconnecting cords of cuboidal or columnar cells devoid of stellate reticulum
- Reverse polarity and nuclear hyperchromasia present at least focally
- Cyst formation rare
- Mature fibrous connective tissue stroma

Histopathologic Differential

- An *ameloblastic carcinoma* has hypercellularity, cellular anaplasia, mitotic figures, and tumor necrosis.
- An *ameloblastic fibroma* has a prominent immature mesenchymal component resembling the dental papilla. The ameloblastic portion is in the form of thin epithelial ribbons which lack a prominent follicular component or stellate reticulum.

Treatment and Prognosis

Excision with an adequate margin of uninvolved tissue. Long-term follow-up necessary: The tumor can recur after many years.

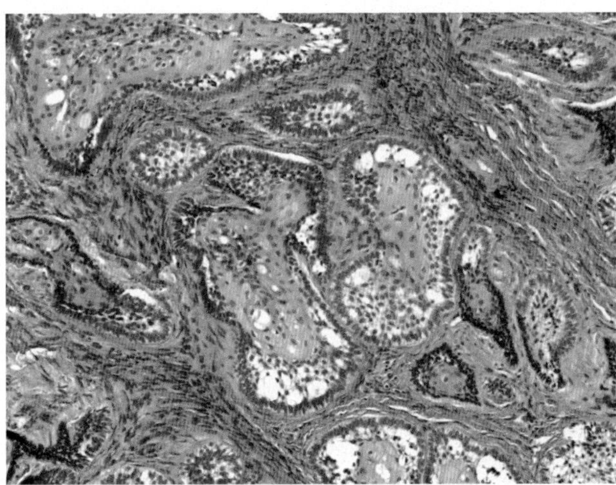

Figure 2.1a.1.
Solid/multicystic ameloblastoma, follicular variant. Multiple islands of ameloblastic epithelium set in a mature fibrous connective tissue stroma.

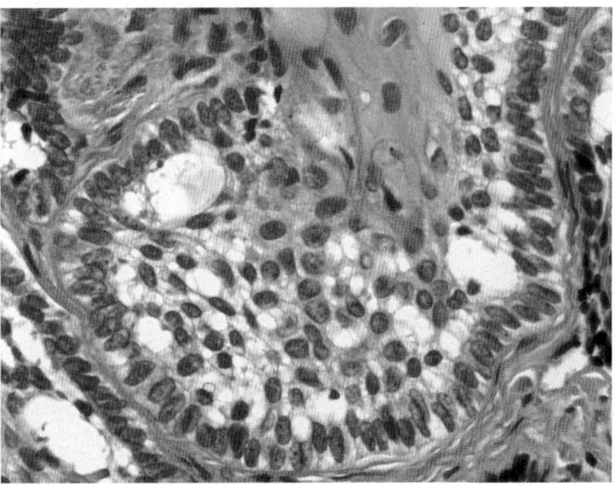

Figure 2.1a.2.
Solid/multicystic ameloblastoma, follicular variant. Follicles consist of a peripheral columnar cell layer exhibiting reverse polarity (nuclei situated away from the basement membrane). The center of the follicle consists of squamous cells and edematous epithelium showing microcyst formation.

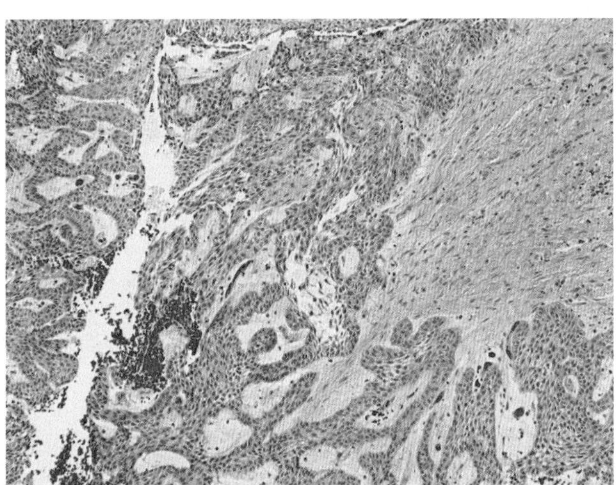

Figure 2.1a.3.
Solid/multicystic ameloblastoma, plexiform variant. Long, anastomosing cords of ameloblastic epithelium.

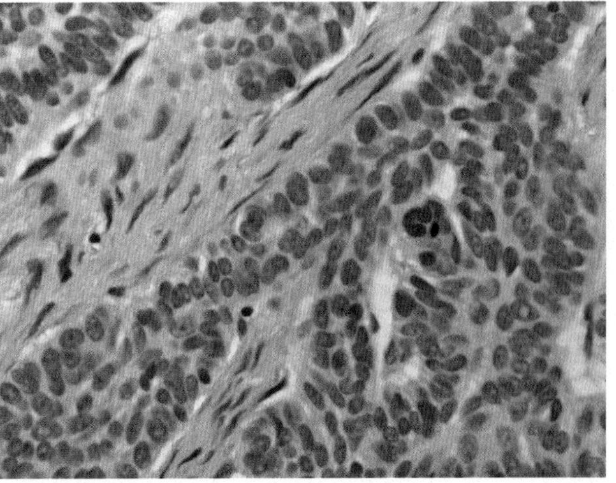

Figure 2.1a.4.
Solid/multicystic ameloblastoma, plexiform variant. The epithelial cords are narrow and lack stellate reticulum. A subtle reverse polarity can be seen in some of the peripheral epithelial cells.

2.1b Unicystic Ameloblastoma

Presentation

Painless swelling. Mostly in the mandible. The average age of the patient is 22 years.

Radiographic Appearance

Large, unilocular radiolucency surrounding the crown of an unerupted tooth, usually a mandibular third molar

Microscopic Findings

Three types are recognized:

LUMINAL VARIANT

Ameloblastic lining only: Overlying a fibrous cyst wall there is a basal layer of polarized columnar epithelial cells with hyperchromatic nuclei covered by edematous, loosely arranged epithelial cells (stellate reticulum) and surfaced by a thin layer of parakeratin.

INTRALUMINAL VARIANT

Lining with plexiform or other ameloblastic epithelial proliferation extending into the lumen.

MURAL VARIANT

Ameloblastic lining with islands of follicular or plexiform ameloblastoma infiltrating the cyst wall.

Histopathologic Differential

- A *dentigerous cyst* does not have a lining of ameloblastic epithelium or ameloblastic nests within the fibrous cystic wall.
- The epithelial proliferations of an inflamed *radicular cyst* are edematous and associated with intense inflammation.

Treatment and Prognosis

For the luminal and intraluminal variants, careful enucleation of the cyst lining. The mural variant is treated by enucleation of the cyst followed by peripheral ostectomy and/or Carnoy's solution. In all cases, close follow-up is necessary to monitor for recurrence.

Additional

A diagnosis of unicystic ameloblastoma should be rendered only upon examination of the entire surgical specimen. Areas of mural infiltration can be easily missed by a small biopsy. All variants may have a portion of unremarkable stratified squamous epithelium within the lining.

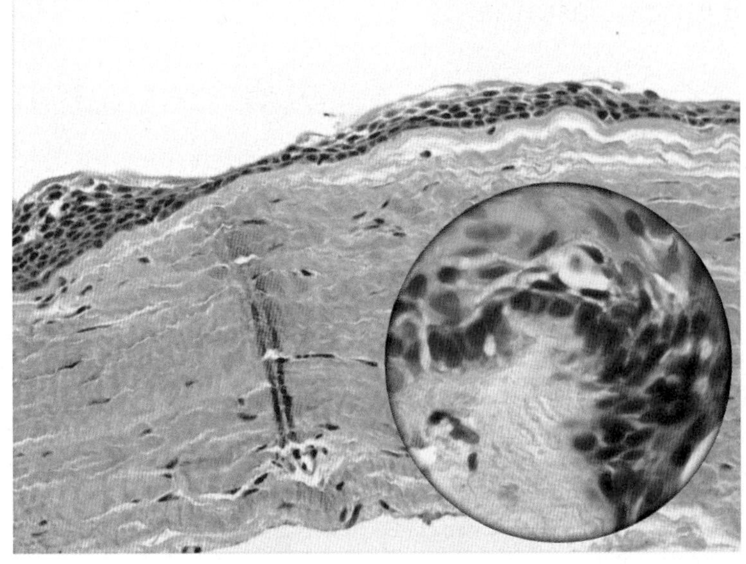

Figure 2.1b.1.
Unicystic ameloblastoma, luminal variant. The fibrous cystic structure is lined by hyperchromatic basaloid cells exhibiting reverse polarity, at least focally (inset).

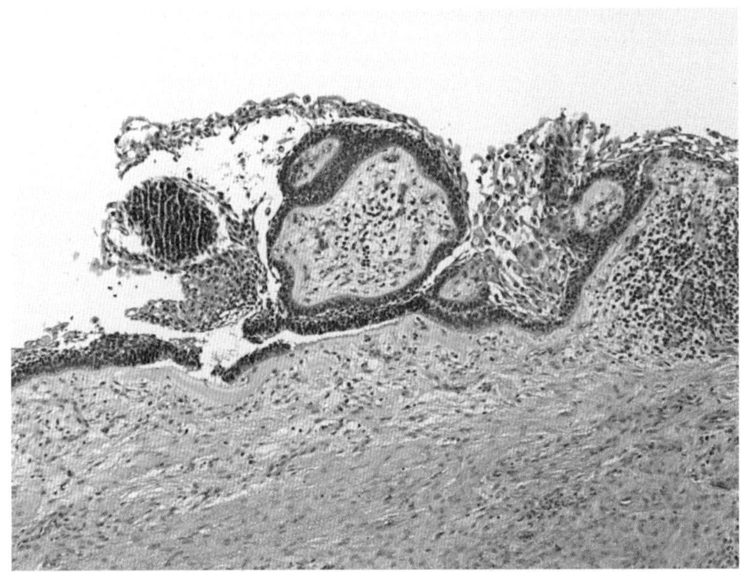

Figure 2.1b.2.
Unicystic ameloblastoma, intraluminal variant. An area of lining containing proliferating ameloblastic epithelium.

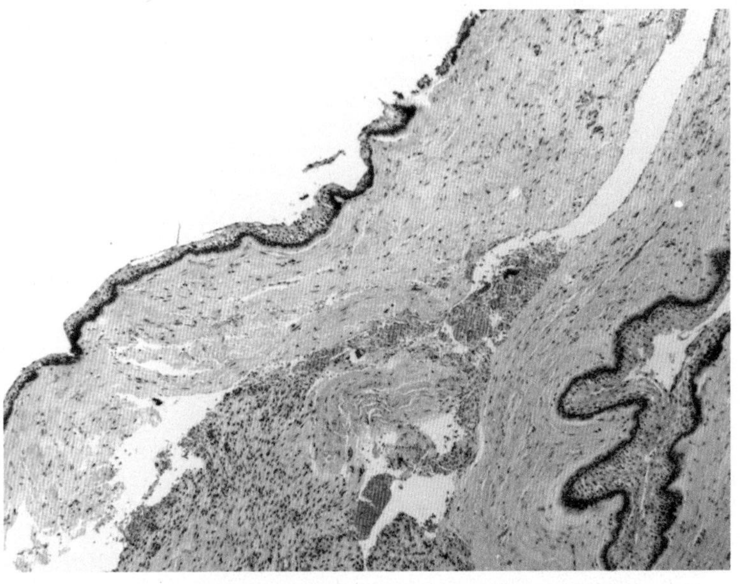

Figure2.1b.3.
Unicystic ameloblastoma, mural variant. The cyst lining consists of ameloblastic epithelium. The fibrous wall contains an ameloblastic "follicle".

2.1c Peripheral Ameloblastoma

Presentation

Painless nodular mass of the tooth-bearing portion of the gingiva, usually in the mandible. The average age of the patient is 52 years.

Radiographic Appearance

Underlying bone is generally not involved.

Microscopic Findings

- Follicular or plexiform ameloblastic nests extending from the basilar portion of the surface epithelium into the fibrous tissue
- No invasion of underlying bone
- Connection to the overlying mucosa not always apparent

Histopathologic Differential

A *peripheral odontogenic fibroma* has small, inactive epithelial rests and lacks ameloblastic nests with columnar cells and reverse polarity.

Treatment and Prognosis

Excision. Unlike its bony counterpart, the peripheral ameloblastoma is an innocuous tumor and is usually cured by simple excision.

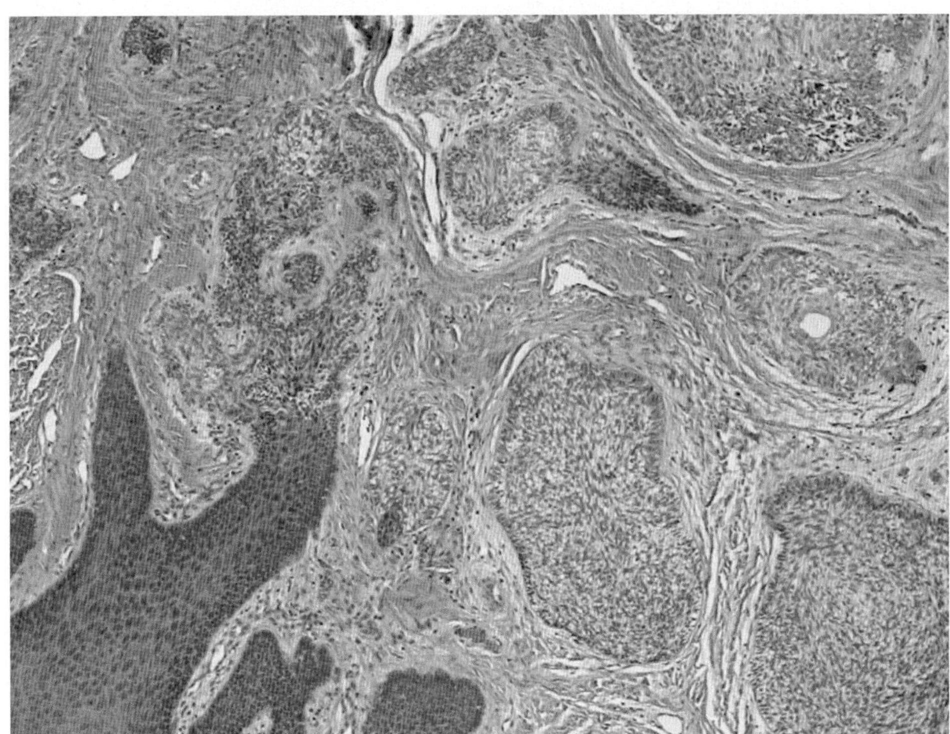

Figure 2.1c.1.
Peripheral ameloblastoma. Nests of ameloblastic epithelium infiltrate dense, fibrous connective tissue. Some tumor nests are contiguous with the overlying mucosa.

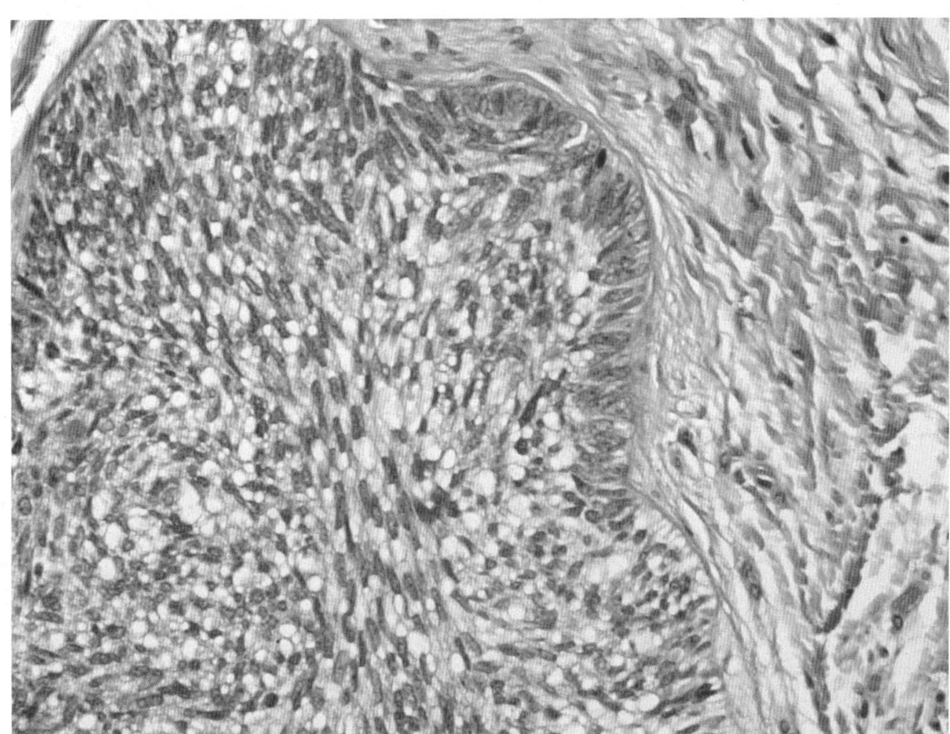

Figure 2.1c.2.
Peripheral ameloblastoma. The ameloblastic nests consist of a polarized peripheral columnar cell layer and centrally spindled, loosely arranged epithelial cells.

2.1d Ameloblastic Carcinoma

Presentation

Aggressive, rapidly growing, painful swelling of the mandible. In adults, especially males.

Radiographic Appearance

Destructive radiolucency

Microscopic Findings

- Sheets of densely packed, hyperchromatic cells with peripheral palisading and reverse polarity, at least focally
- Cellular pleomorphism, nuclear hyperchromasia, and mitoses
- Necrosis of tumor islands
- Fibrous connective tissue stroma

Histopathologic Differential

Ameloblastoma lacks hypercellularity, cellular anaplasia, mitotic figures, and tumor necrosis.

Treatment and Prognosis

Wide local excision with en bloc resection and close follow-up.

The term "malignant ameloblastoma" is given to a histologically well-differentiated, histologically benign ameloblastoma that metastasizes, generally to the lungs, usually after multiple attempts at excision.

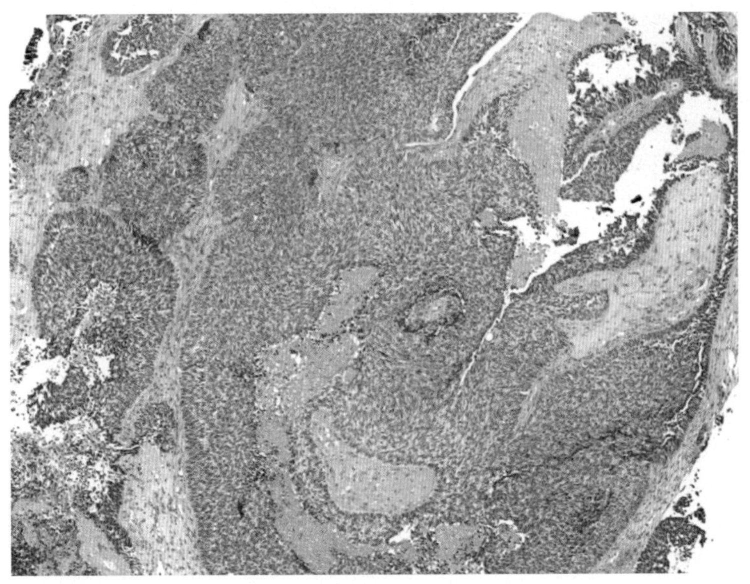

Figure 2.1d.1.
Ameloblastic carcinoma. Hypercellular sheets of atypical ameloblastic epithelium set in a mature fibrous connective tissue stroma.

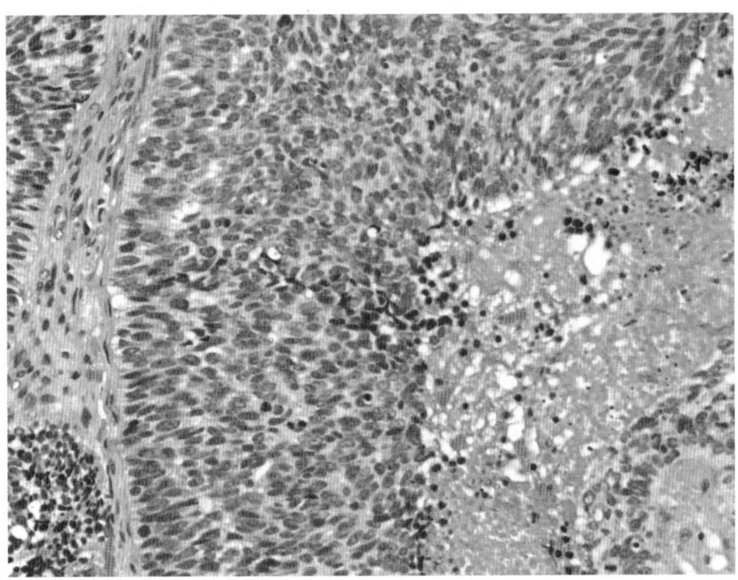

Figure 2.1d.2.
Ameloblastic carcinoma. Hypercellular nest of ameloblastic epithelium. Note the extensive necrosis on the right side of the image.

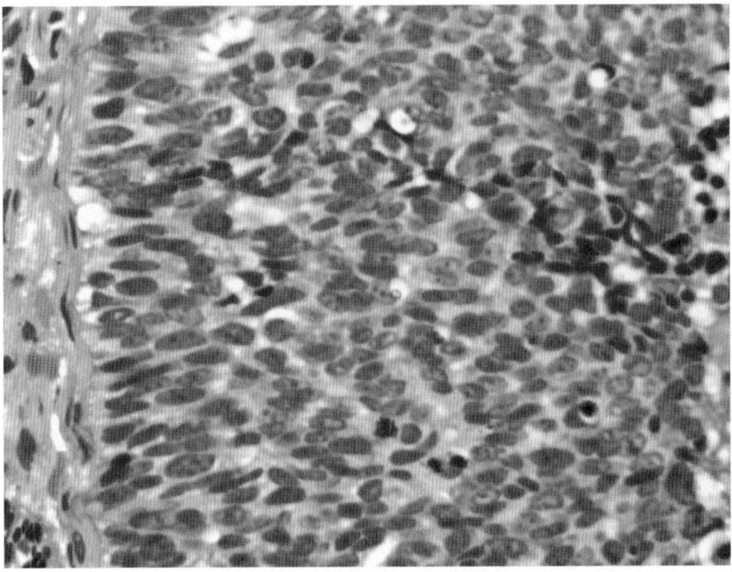

Figure 2.1d.3.
Ameloblastic carcinoma. Tumor cells are tightly packed and have elongated, hyperchromatic nuclei. Some of the peripheral columnar cells exhibit reverse polarization.

2.2 Adenomatoid Odontogenic Tumor

Presentation

Painless swelling. More common in the maxilla, most often associated with an unerupted canine tooth. In children and young adults, especially females.

Radiographic Appearance

Well-circumscribed radiolucency, often around the crown of an unerupted tooth. Radiopaque flecks are sometimes present.

Microscopic Findings

- Well-encapsulated, cystic or solid tumor
- Spherical nodules of swirling, spindled epithelial cells containing small ductal structures
- Lattice-like network of fine, epithelial strands
- Calcifications, sometimes of the Liesegang type
- Scant fibrous stroma

Treatment and Prognosis

Enucleation. Recurrence is very rare. In the past, the adenomatoid odontogenic tumor was mistaken for an *ameloblastoma.* However, the histopathology is generally sufficiently distinctive to not cause confusion.

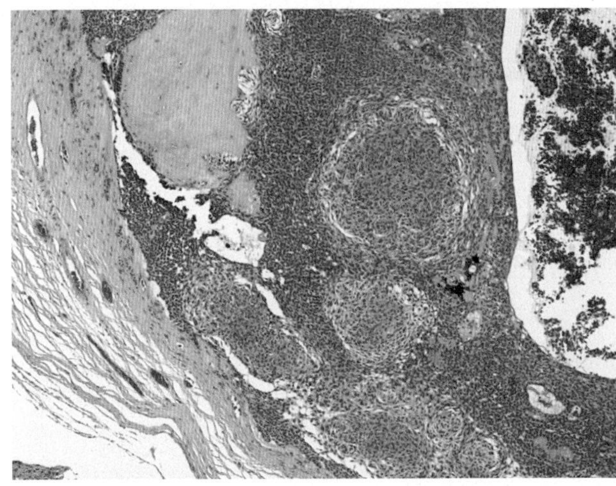

Figure 2.2.1.
Adenomatoid odontogenic tumor. Closely packed epithelial cells surround spherical nodules of more loosely packed cells. The fibrous capsule is thickened.

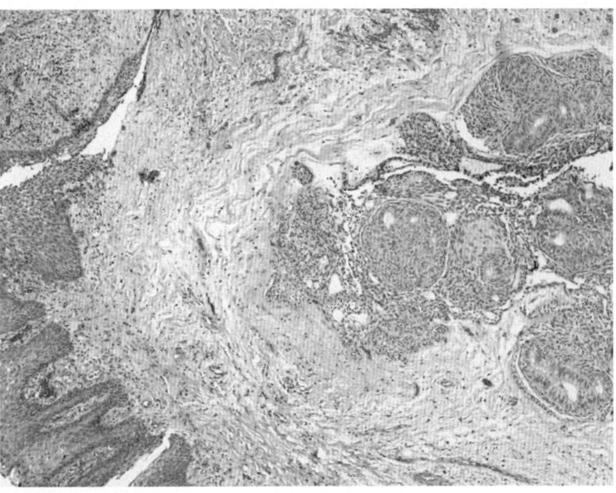

Figure 2.2.2.
Adenomatoid odontogenic tumor. Spherical nests of basaloid epithelial cells containing ductal structures. This tumor is outside of bone (peripheral). The stroma is fibrous connective tissue.

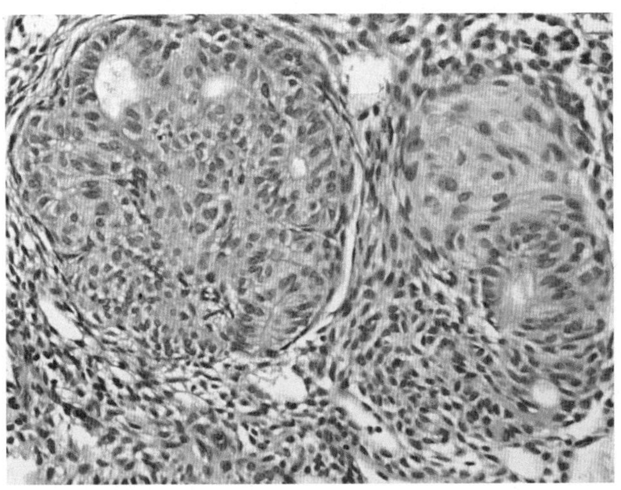

Figure 2.2.3.
Adenomatoid odontogenic tumor. Nodules of whorling, spindled epithelial cells interconnected by a lattice of fine epithelial strands.

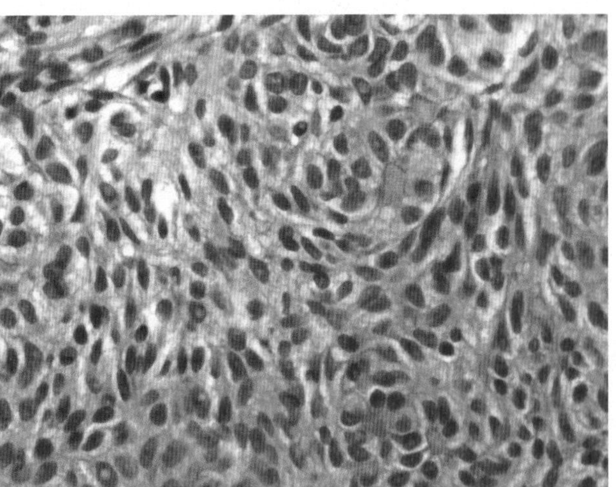

Figure 2.2.4.
Adenomatoid odontogenic tumor. Whorls of spindled basaloid cells form primitive ductal structures containing eosinophilic droplets.

2.3 Calcifying Epithelial Odontogenic Tumor (Pindborg Tumor)

Presentation

Painless swelling. Mostly in the posterior mandible. The average age of the patient is 34 years.

Radiographic Appearance

Unilocular or multilocular radiolucency

Microscopic Findings

- Unencapsulated, infiltrative tumor.
- Large, pink, polygonal epithelial cells with intercellular bridges. Nuclei are pleomorphic and hyperchromatic, but mitotic figures are absent.
- Amyloid-like material within the stroma and tumor cells.
- Fibrous stroma.
- Calcifications, sometimes of the Liesegang type may be seen.

Special Stains/Immunopathology

Amyloid-like material stains with Congo red, exhibiting apple-green birefringence on polarization.

Histopathologic Differential

- An intraosseous *squamous cell carcinoma* has anaplasia, keratin pearl formation, individual-cell keratinization, and mitotic figures. Significantly, it lacks amyloid.
- An *odontogenic fibroma* lacks amyloid.

Treatment and Prognosis

Complete excision. The recurrence rate is 10% to 15%. In the non-calcifying variant, epithelial cells are only minimally pleomorphic and calcifications are absent; amyloid-like material, however, is a constant feature.

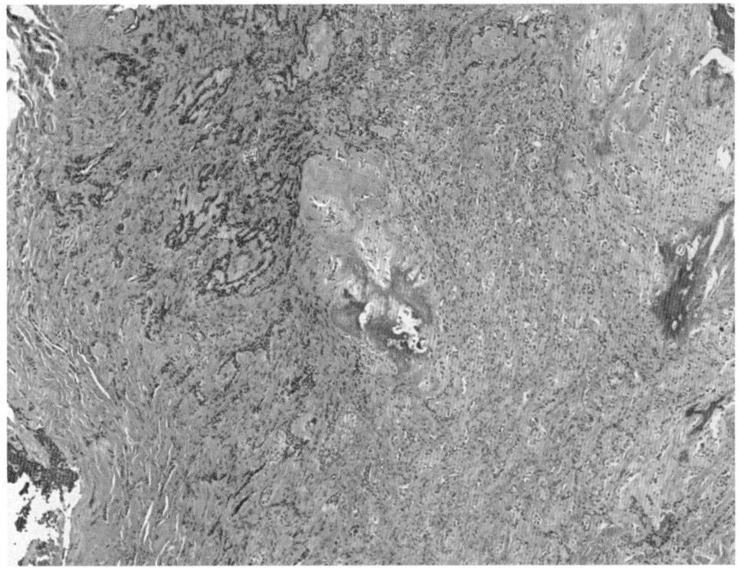

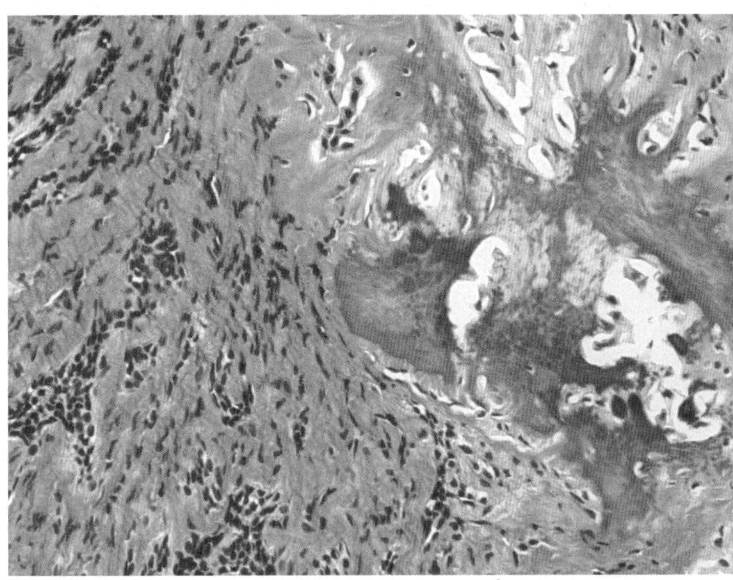

Figures 2.3.1–2.3.2.
Calcifying epithelial odontogenic tumor. Slender nests of epithelium set in a fibrous connective tissue stroma containing amyloid-like material and calcifications.

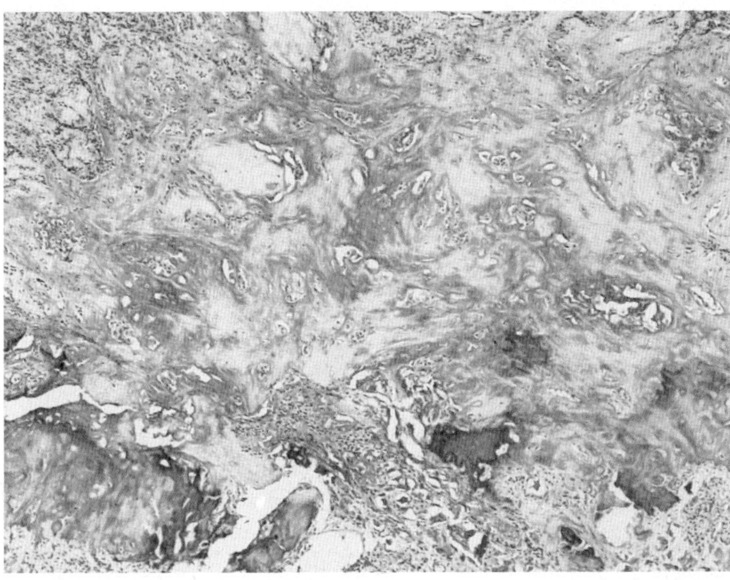

Figure 2.3.3.
Calcifying epithelial odontogenic tumor. Amyloid deposits are highlighted by Congo red stain.

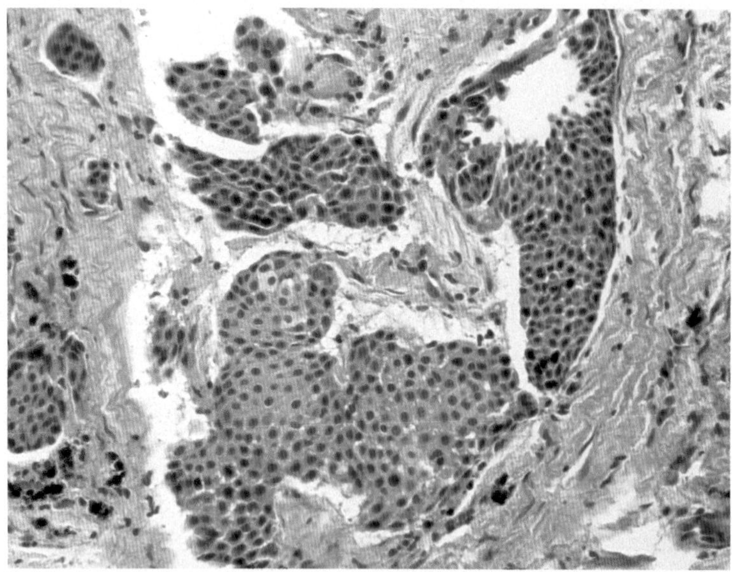

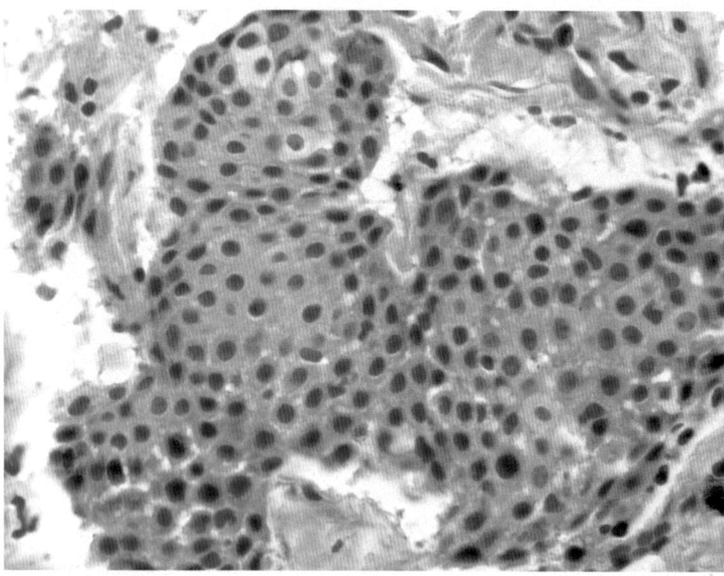

Figures 2.3.4–2.3.5.
Calcifying epithelial odontogenic tumor. These two images illustrate the characteristics of the Pindborg tumor's distinctive epithelium. The cells are polyhedral and have enlarged, hyperchromatic, mildly pleomorphic nuclei. Intercellular bridges are also seen.

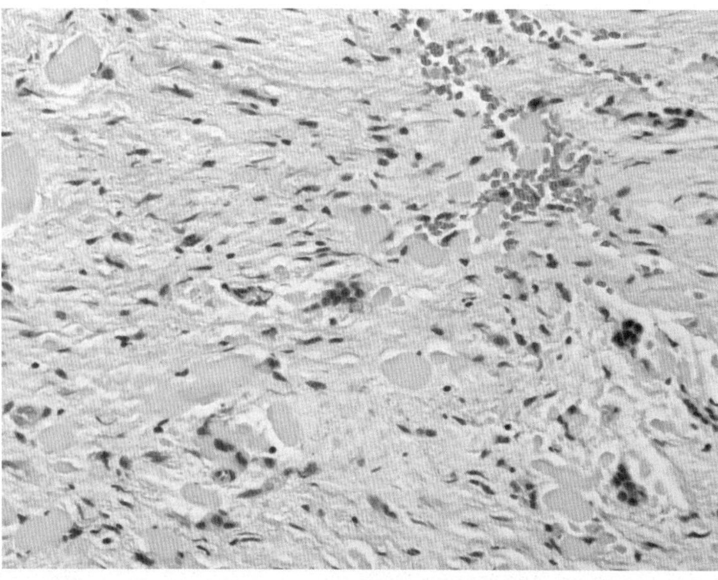

Figure 2.3.6.
Calcifying epithelial odontogenic tumor, noncalcifying variant. Small epithelial nests are scattered throughout a loose, fibrous stroma with abundant amorphous eosinophilic deposits.

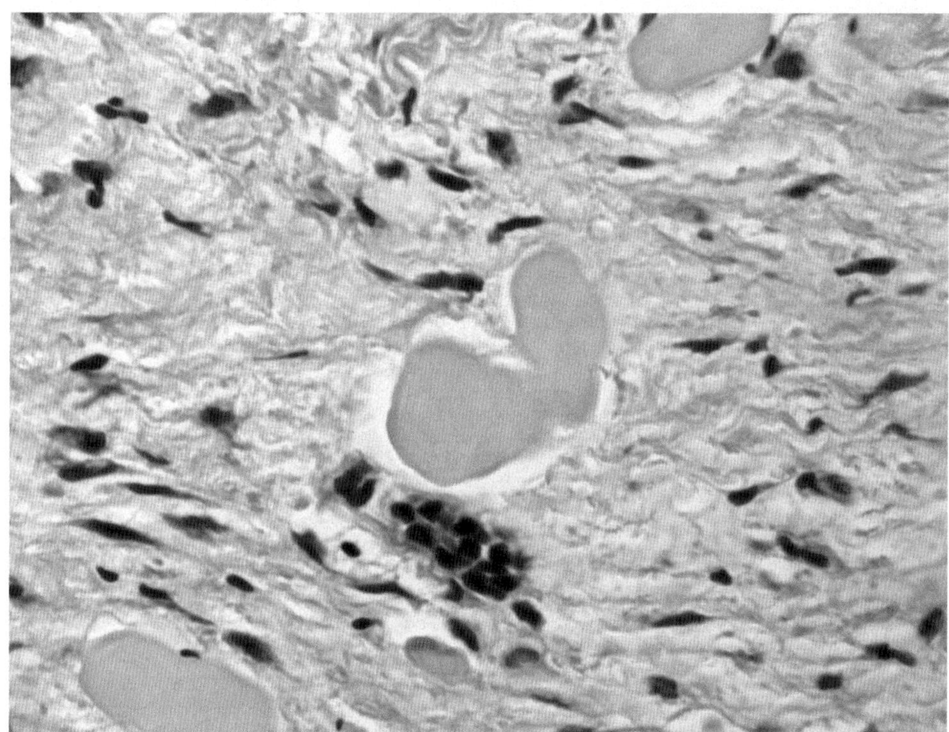

Figure 2.3.7.
Calcifying epithelial odontogenic tumor, noncalcifying variant. Some calcifying epithelial odontogenic tumors are more cellular than others. Amyloid, however, is a constant feature.

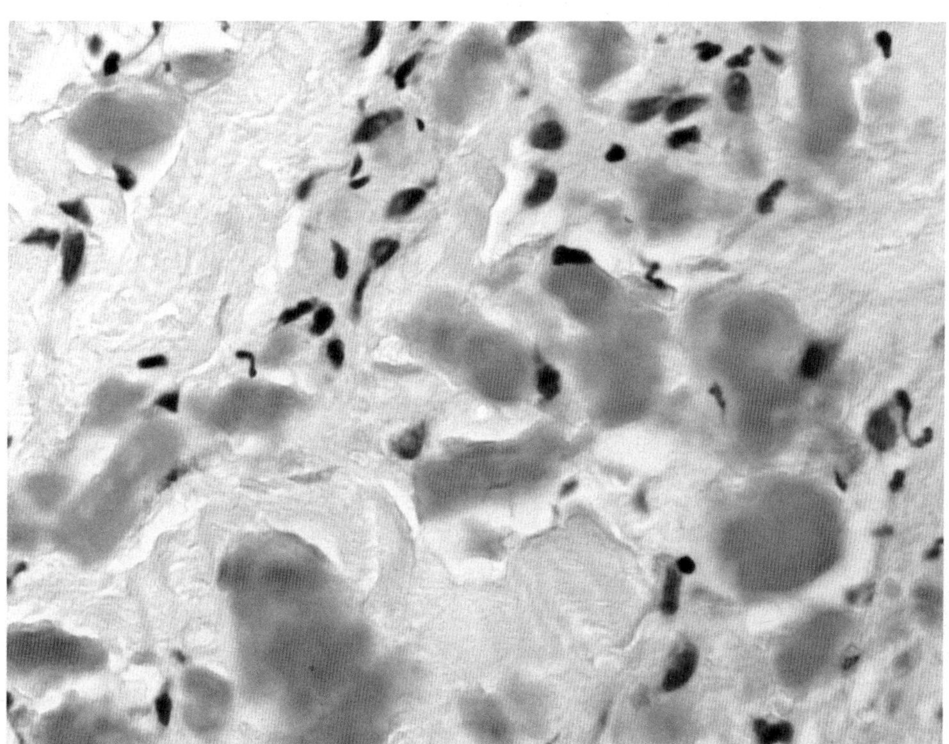

Figure 2.3.8.
Congo red stain is positive in the amyloid deposits and showed green birefringence upon polarization.

2.4 Calcifying Ghost Cell Odontogenic Tumor

Presentation

Painless swelling, either jaw, mostly anterior. The average age of the patient is 33 years.

Radiographic Appearance

Radiolucency, sometimes with radiopaque foci

Microscopic Findings

- Ameloblastic epithelial nests are seen in this mostly solid tumor.
- Abundant sheets of ghost cells.
- Foci of ghost cell calcification may be seen.
- Small cystic areas are sometimes seen.
- Fibrous stroma.

Histopathologic Differential

The *calcifying odontogenic cyst* is cystic and lacks significant epithelial ameloblastic proliferations.

Treatment and Prognosis

Excision with adequate margins and close follow-up

Additional

Ghost cell lesions (calcifying odontogenic cysts, calcifying ghost cell odontogenic tumors) can be cystic, cystic and solid, or, less commonly, entirely solid. They can also be associated with an odontoma and may contain a prominent ameloblastic component. Some ghost cell tumors can become malignant.

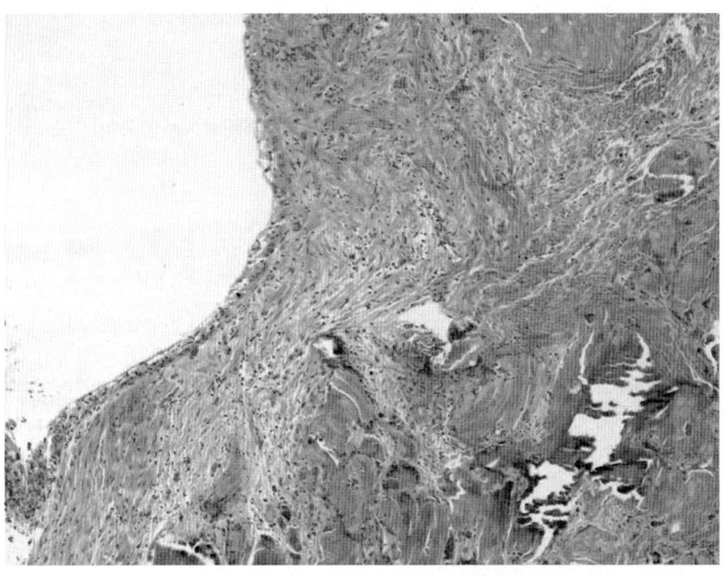

Figure 2.4.1.
Calcifying ghost cell odontogenic tumor. The cystic portion of this mostly solid tumor is lined by stratified squamous epithelium. The fibrous stroma contains masses of focally calcified eosinophilic ghost cells.

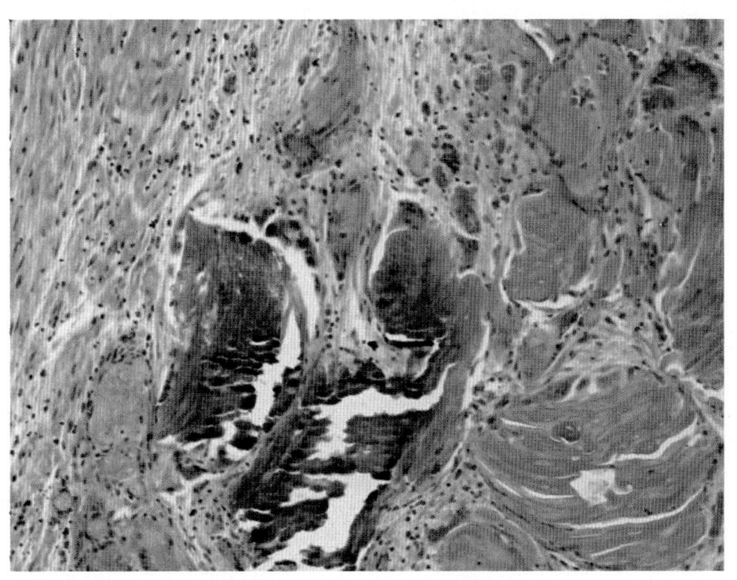

Figure 2.4.2.
Calcifying ghost cell odontogenic tumor. Calcified ghost cell masses.

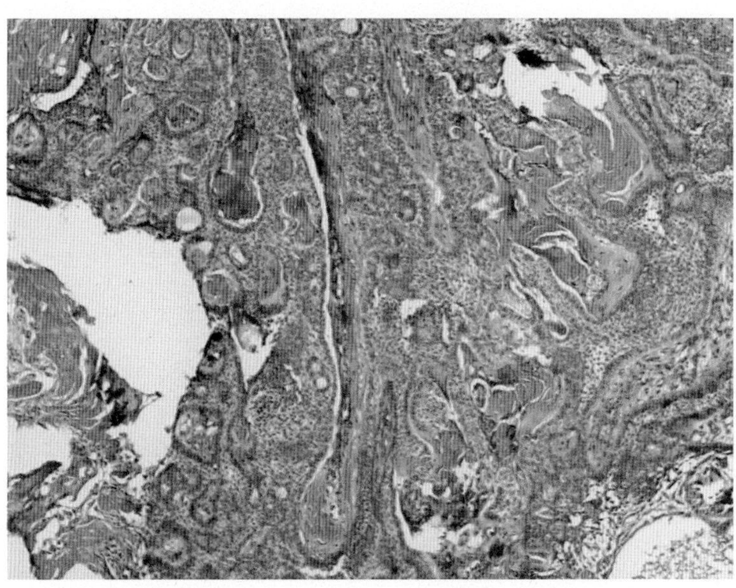

Figure 2.4.3.
Calcifying ghost cell odontogenic tumor. The tumor is solid and composed of interdigitating cords of ameloblastic epithelium. The presence of ghost cells precludes the diagnosis of conventional, solid ameloblastoma.

2.5 Squamous Odontogenic Tumor

Presentation

Gingival and bony swelling, possibly painful. The average age of the patient is 38 years. Tumors are occasionally multiple.

Radiographic Appearance

Irregularly shaped radiolucency around and between tooth roots

Microscopic Findings

- Unencapsulated tumor.
- Nests of mature squamous cells with compressed nuclei at the periphery appearing as a hyperchromatic line at low power.
- Centers of epithelial nests can have central keratinization and microcystic spaces.
- Abundant mature fibrous connective tissue stroma.

Histopathologic Differential

- The epithelial nests of an *ameloblastoma* have peripheral palisading, hyperchromasia, and reverse polarization.
- A *squamous cell carcinoma* has anaplasia, keratin pearl formation, individual-cell keratinization, and mitotic figures.

Treatment and Prognosis

Complete excision. Prognosis is good.

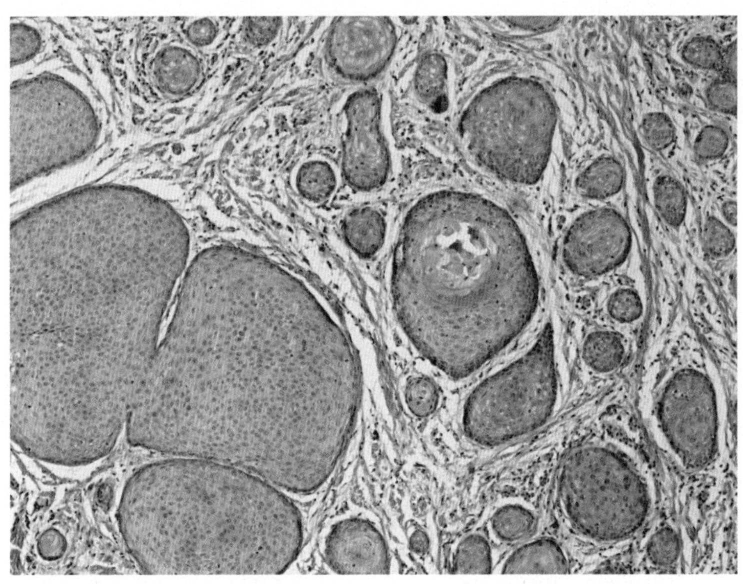

Figure 2.5.1.
Squamous odontogenic tumor. Variably sized nests of normal-appearing squamous cells proliferate in a loose fibrous connective tissue stroma.

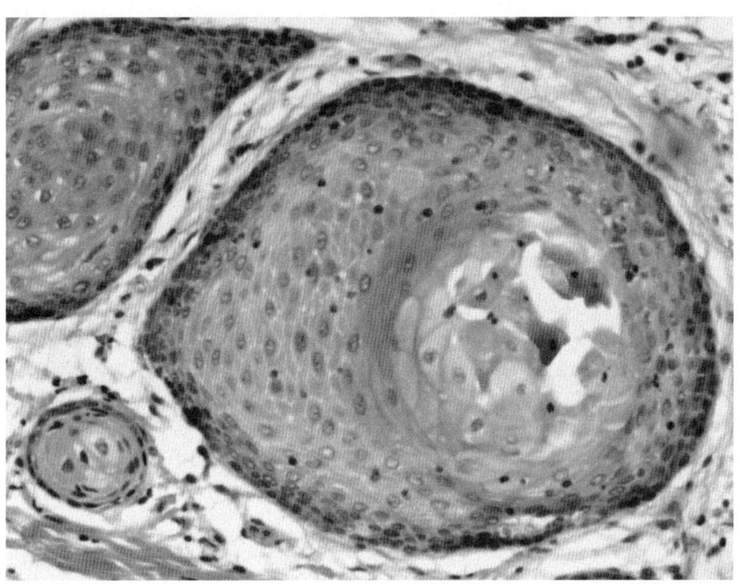

Figure 2.5.2.
Squamous odontogenic tumor. This section shows a tumor nest with compressed, hyperchromatic nuclei at the periphery, central keratinization, and early microcystic change.

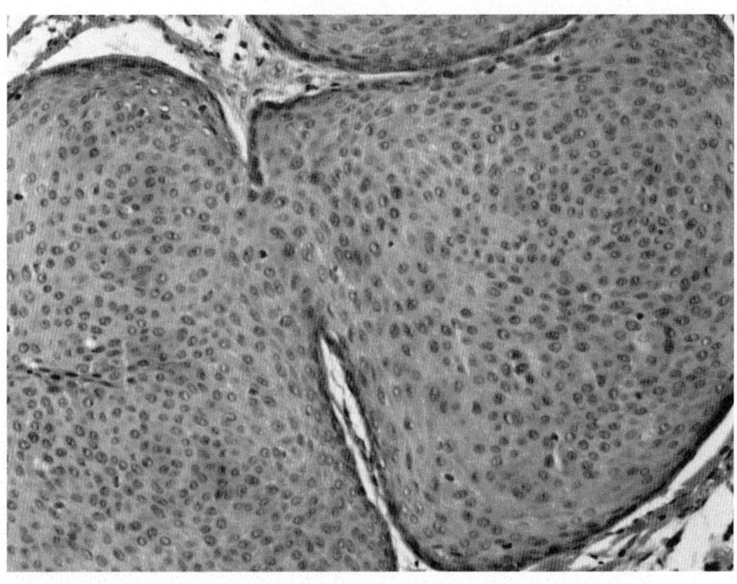

Figure 2.5.3.
Squamous odontogenic tumor. Contiguous nests of mature squamous cells with compressed, hyperchromatic nuclei at the periphery.

Mixed Epithelial and Mesenchymal Odontogenic Tumors

2.6 Ameloblastic Fibroma

Presentation

Slow-growing, painless, expansile tumor. Most common in molar area of the mandible. The average age of the patient is 15 years; most are diagnosed before the age of 20 years.

Radiographic Appearance

Unilocular or multilocular radiolucency with well-defined margins

Microscopic Findings

- Biphasic, benign tumor of ameloblastic and mesenchymal tissue.
- Mass of stellate cells in a loose, primitive mesenchymal matrix resembling the dental papilla.
- Thin, anastomosing cords and nests of epithelium resembling the dental lamina containing, at least focally, areas of ameloblastic change (palisading and reverse polarization).
- Occasionally, the epithelial nests will have follicles resembling ameloblastoma and, rarely, microcyst formation.

Histopathologic Differential

- An *ameloblastoma* lacks the primitive mesenchymal component; its stroma is mature fibrous.
- An *odontogenic fibroma* lacks the extensive epithelial proliferation and the primitive mesenchymal stroma.

Treatment and Prognosis

Complete excision with close follow-up. A considerable percentage of ameloblastic fibrosarcomas occur in patients who have had recurrent ameloblastic fibromas.

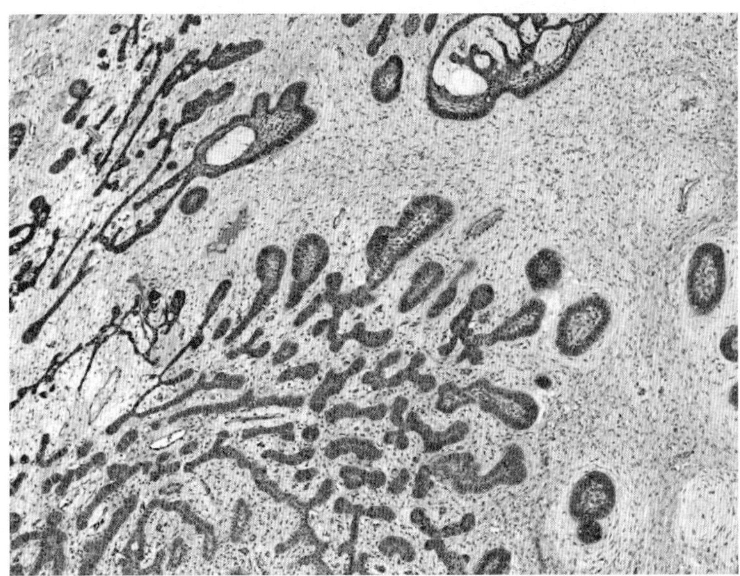

Figure 2.6.1.
Ameloblastic fibroma. Long, narrow cords of ameloblastic epithelium proliferate within a cellular, primitive, mesenchymal stroma.

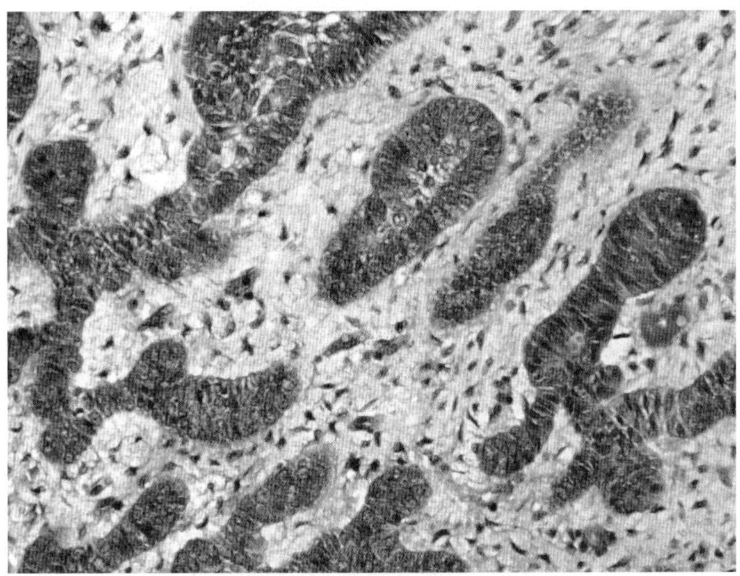

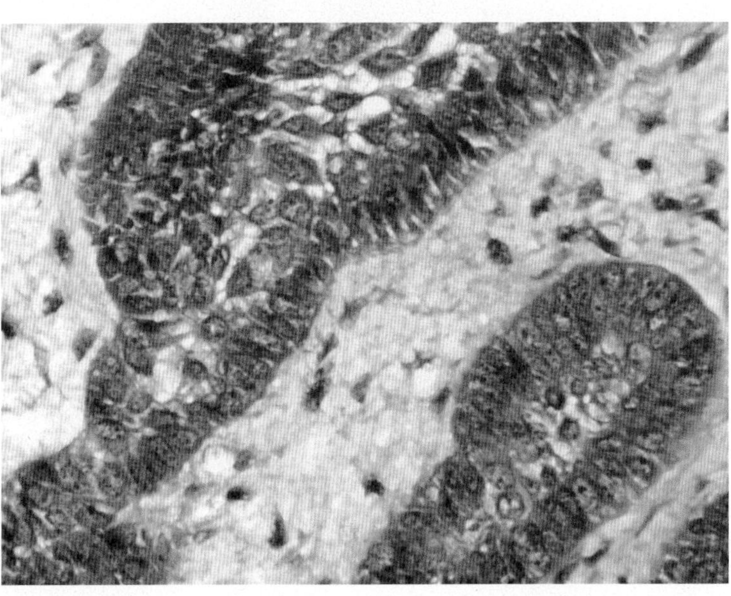

Figures 2.6.2–2.6.3.
Ameloblastic fibroma. The epithelial component is clearly ameloblastic, with nuclear palisading and reverse polarization. The dense fibrous stroma that accompanies ameloblastoma, however, is absent. Instead, the epithelium is surrounded by stellate cells in a myxoid background.

2.7 Ameloblastic Fibro-odontoma

Presentation
Slow-growing, expansile, painless tumor. The average age of the patient is 10 years.

Radiographic Appearance
Radiolucency with calcifications of variable size

Microscopic Findings
Same as those for ameloblastic fibroma, but with the formation of irregular masses of tooth structures composed of dentin and enamel

Histopathologic Differential
The *complex odontoma* consists mainly of dental hard tissues; the epithelial component is scant.

Treatment and Prognosis
Complete excision with close follow-up

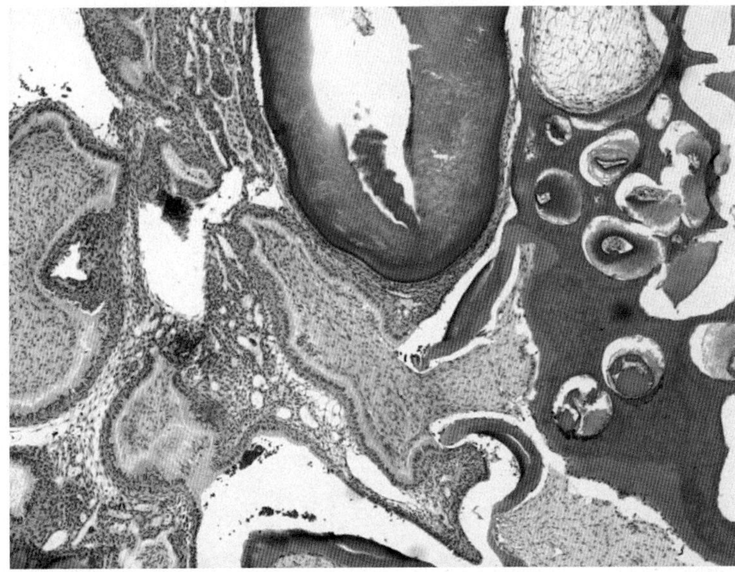

Figure 2.7.1.
Ameloblastic fibro-odontoma. The tumor consists of an ameloblastic fibroma admixed with malformed dental tissues: a tooth root, dentinoid, enamel matrix, and enamel spaces.

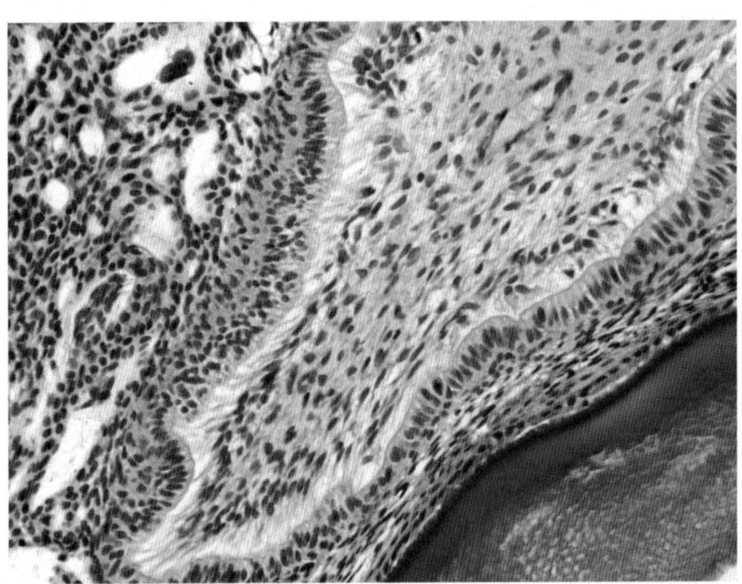

Figure 2.7.2.
Ameloblastic fibro-odontoma. Ameloblastic cords show peripheral palisading and reverse polarity. Tooth root on the right. The stroma consists of cellular, primitive mesenchymal tissue.

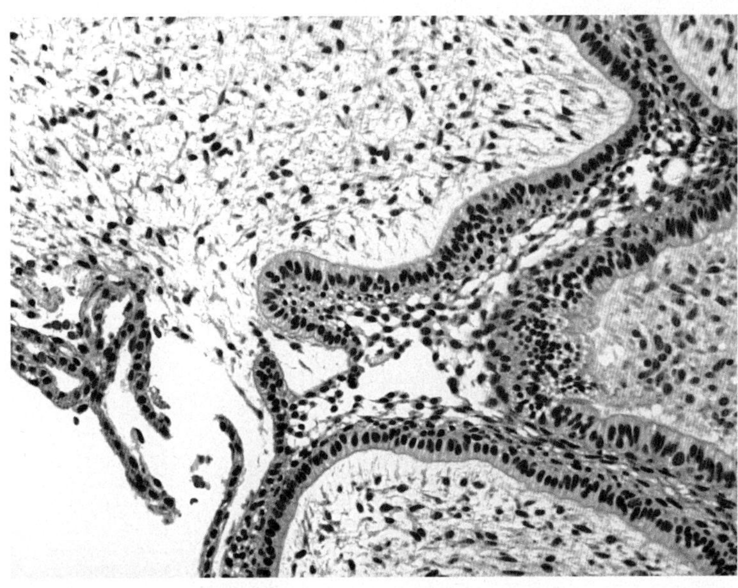

Figure 2.7.3.
Ameloblastic fibro-odontoma. In areas devoid of hard tissues, the histology is identical to that of ameloblastic fibroma.

2.8 Ameloblastic Fibrosarcoma

Presentation

Rapidly growing swelling with pain and paresthesia. In over a third of the patients, there is a history of ameloblastic fibroma. The average age of the patient is 25 years.

Radiographic Appearance

Destructive radiolucency with irregular margins

Microscopic Findings

- Bony invasion
- Cellular mesenchymal component containing pleomorphic spindle cells with hyperchromatic nuclei and, often, abundant mitoses
- Benign-appearing epithelial component resembling that seen in the ameloblastic fibroma, but less abundant

Histopathologic Differential

The mesenchymal component of an *ameloblastic fibroma* is less cellular and lacks the cytomorphologic features of malignancy.

Treatment and Prognosis

Complete excision with adequate margins and close follow-up

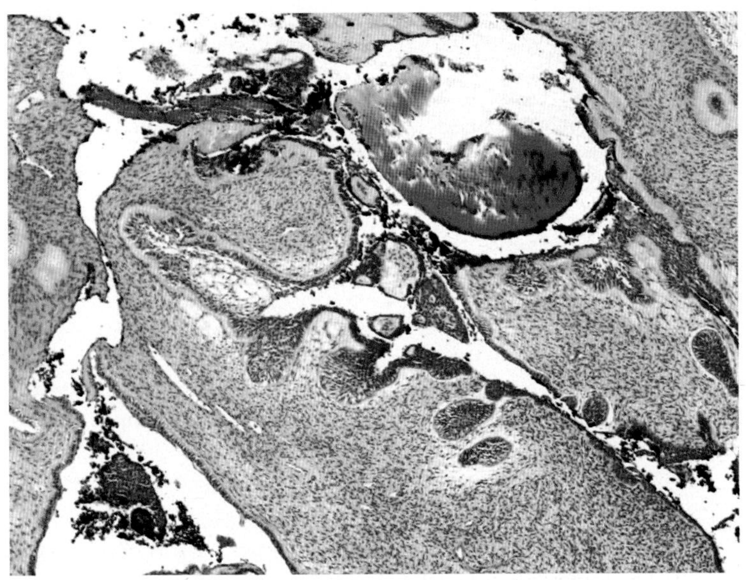

Figure 2.8.1.
A 10-cm destructive radiolucent tumor in a 25-year-old male. Ameloblastic fibrosarcoma. The tumor consists of ameloblastic epithelium with a highly cellular mesenchymal component. The dentinoid material suggests that this tumor has arisen in an ameloblastic fibro-odontoma.

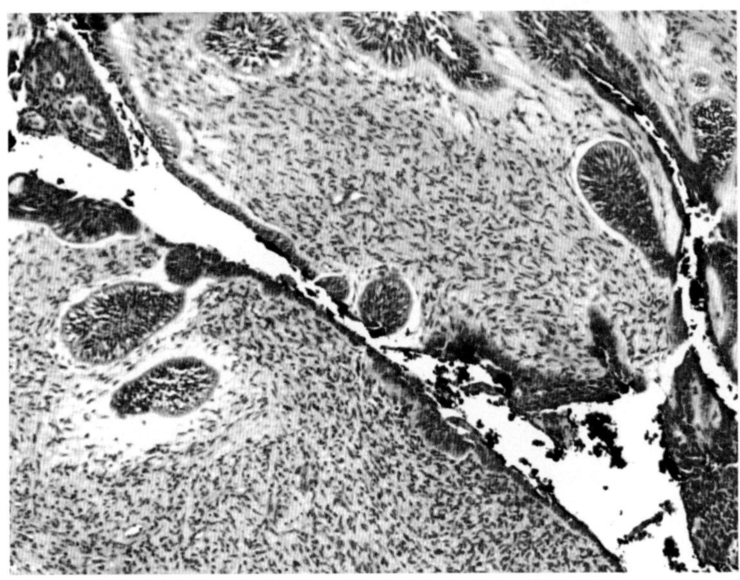

Figure 2.8.2.
Ameloblastic fibrosarcoma. The epithelium resembles that of ameloblastic fibroma, but the surrounding mesenchyme is hypercellular and more spindled.

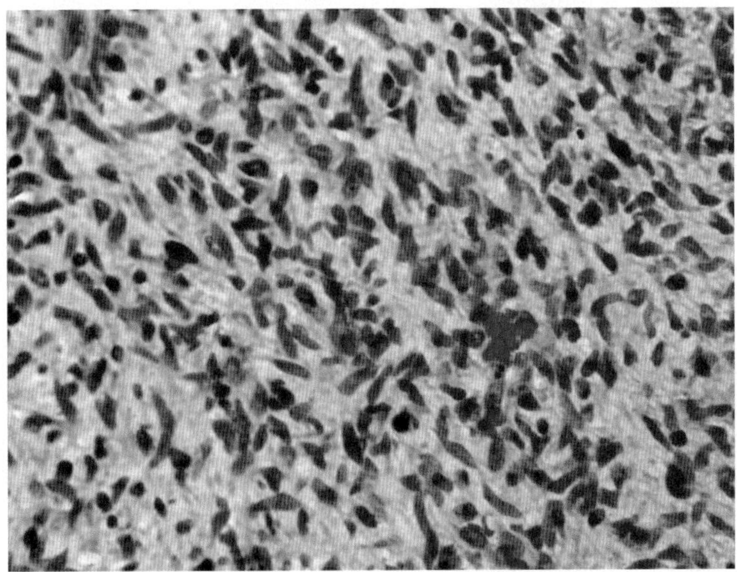

Figure 2.8.3.
Ameloblastic fibrosarcoma. The atypical mesenchymal component is hypercellular and exhibits enlarged, pleomorphic, hyperchromatic nuclei.

2.9 Odontoma

Presentation

Asymptomatic radiographic finding. The average age of the patient is 14 years.

Radiographic Appearance

Irregular radiodense mass with a thin radiolucent rim or tooth-like structures

Microscopic Findings

The *complex odontoma* consists of a haphazard arrangement of dentin and enamel prisms along with clusters of ghost cells and entrapped odontogenic epithelium.

The *compound odontoma* consists of an encapsulated mass of numerous, tiny, single-rooted toothlets admixed with fibrous connective tissue.

Histopathologic Differential

The *ameloblastic fibro-odontoma* and the complex odontoma in an early stage of development can be similar histologically. The former has more of an ameloblastic component.

Treatment and Prognosis

Enucleation. Does not recur.

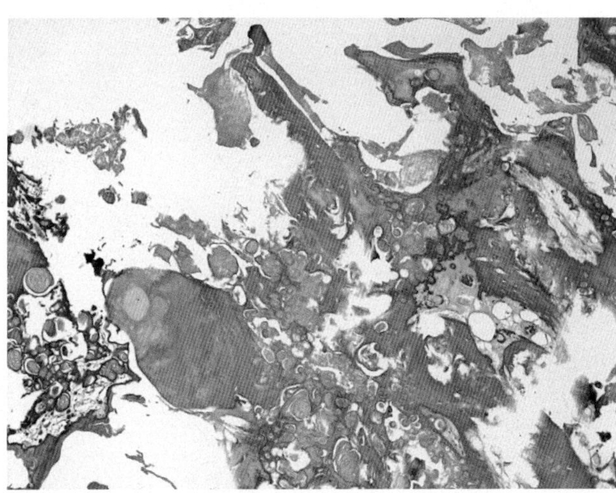

Figure 2.9.1.
Complex odontoma. Organized masses of dentinoid (eosinophilic material) and enamel matrix (basophilic masses).

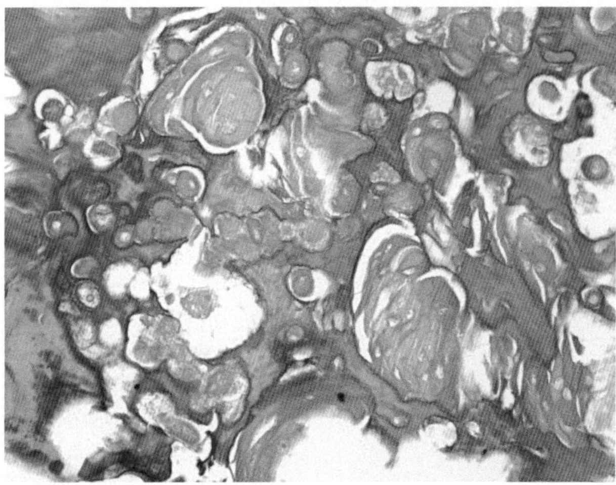

Figure 2.9.2.
Complex odontoma. Disorganized masses of dentinoid and enamel matrix together with ghost cells.

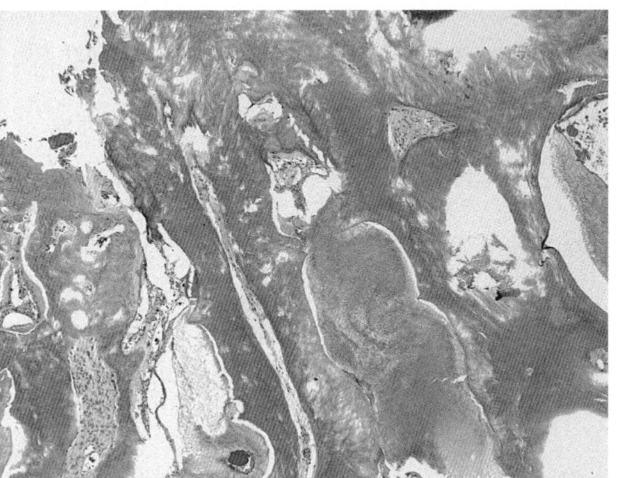

Figure 2.9.3.
Complex odontoma. Disorganized mass of dentinoid material and enamel prisms.

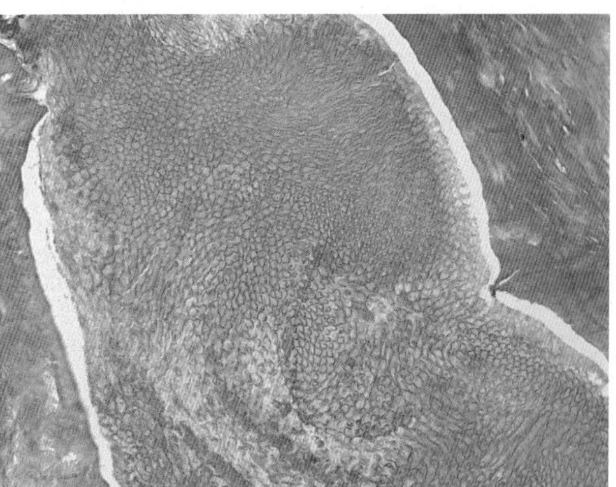

Figure 2.9.4.
Complex odontoma. Enamel prisms enveloped by dentinoid material.

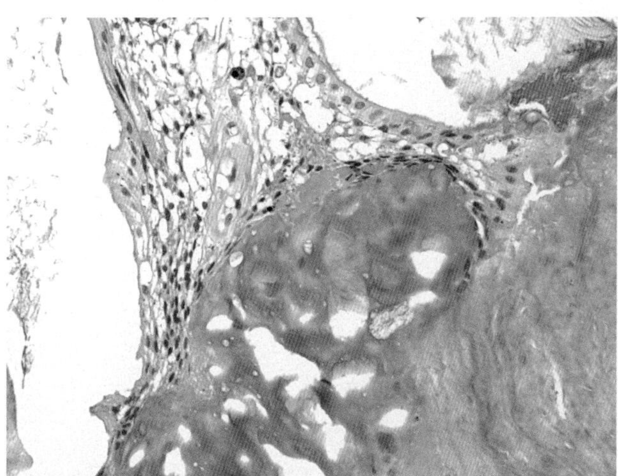

Figure 2.9.5.
Complex odontoma. Odontogenic epithelium from the enamel organ, enamel matrix, and dentinoid material.

Mesenchymal Odontogenic Tumors

2.10 Odontogenic Myxoma

Presentation

Asymptomatic expansion of bone, usually of the posterior mandible. The average age of the patient is 28 years.

Radiographic Appearance

Unilocular or multilocular radiolucency with a fine crisscrossing of bone trabeculae

Microscopic Findings

- Infiltrative, unencapsulated tumor.
- Myxoid tissue consisting of widely dispersed spindle cells with elongated, delicate cytoplasmic processes.
- Denser, fibrous areas may be seen. When considerable fibrous tissue is present, the tumor is sometimes designated as an odontogenic fibromyxoma.
- Odontogenic epithelial nests are rarely seen.

Special Stains/Immunopathology

The tumor is positive for vimentin and focally positive for smooth muscle actin. It is negative for S100.

Histopathologic Differential

- An *enlarged dental follicle,* which is often composed of myxoid tissue, is in close association with a developing tooth.
- A *dislodged dental papilla* is submitted along with an extracted tooth in a young person.
- A *myxoid neurofibroma* is reactive for S100.

Treatment and Prognosis

Excision with safe margin and close follow-up. The microscopic appearance of an odontogenic myxoma is identical to that of the dental follicle and dental papilla, normal structures associated with a developing tooth.

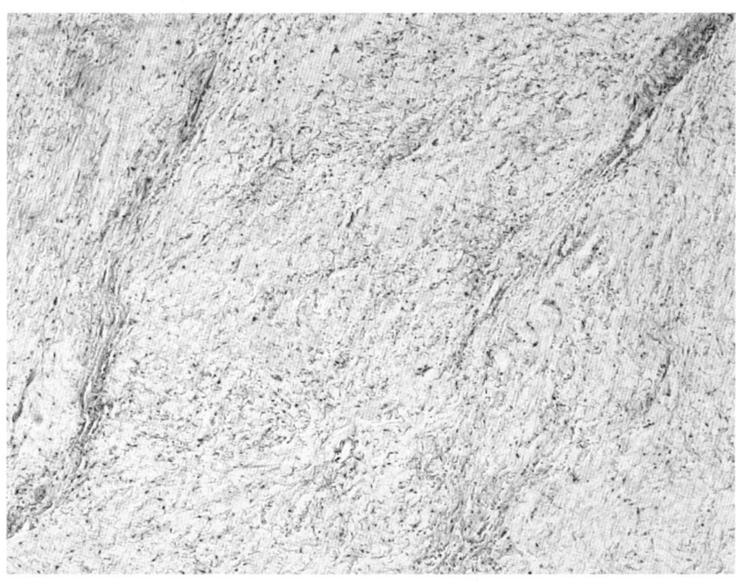

Figure 2.10.1.
Odontogenic myxoma. Stellate-shaped cells and tiny collagen fibers within a myxoid stroma.

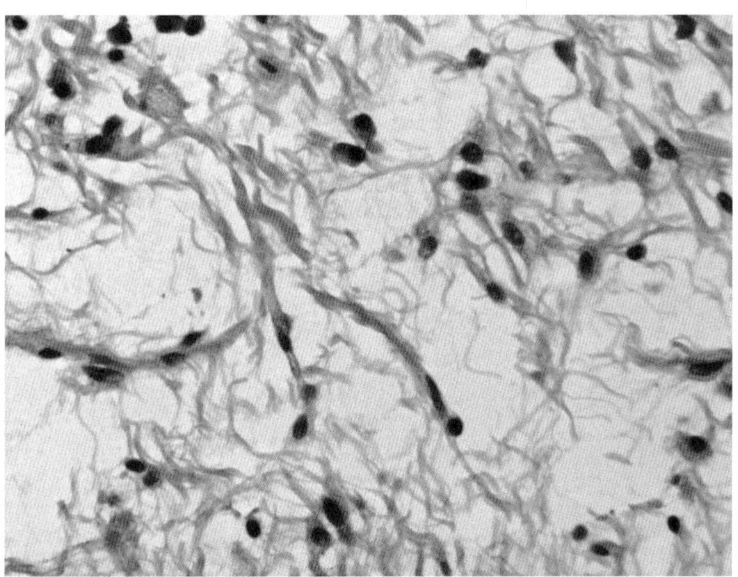

Figure 2.10.2.
Odontogenic myxoma. Stellate-shaped cells and tiny collagen fibrils.

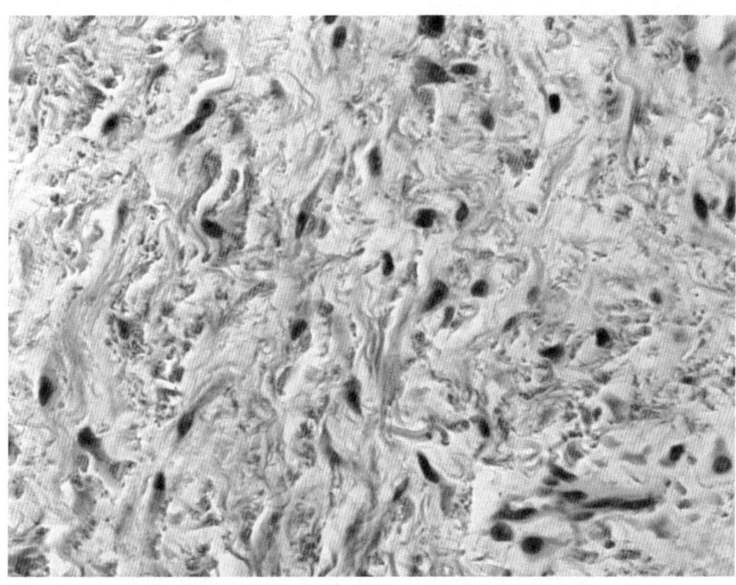

Figure 2.10.3.
Odontogenic myxoma. The tumors containing abundant dense collagen are sometimes referred to as *odontogenic fibromyxomas.*

2.11 Odontogenic Fibroma

Presentation

Expansile, asymptomatic mass. The average age of the patient is 40 years.

Radiographic Appearance

Unilocular or multilocular radiolucency

Microscopic Findings

- Interlacing fascicles of mature fibrous connective tissue.
- Scattered, inactive epithelial odontogenic nests.
- Small, spherical basophilic calcifications may be seen.

Histopathologic Differential

- An *enlarged dental follicle* surrounds a developing tooth.
- A non-*calcifying epithelial odontogenic tumor* will have amyloid.

Treatment and Prognosis

Enucleation. Prognosis favorable.

Additional

The odontogenic fibroma has also been reported in association with a giant cell granuloma and can contain prominent granular cells.

The peripheral odontogenic fibroma is the soft-tissue counterpart of this tumor.

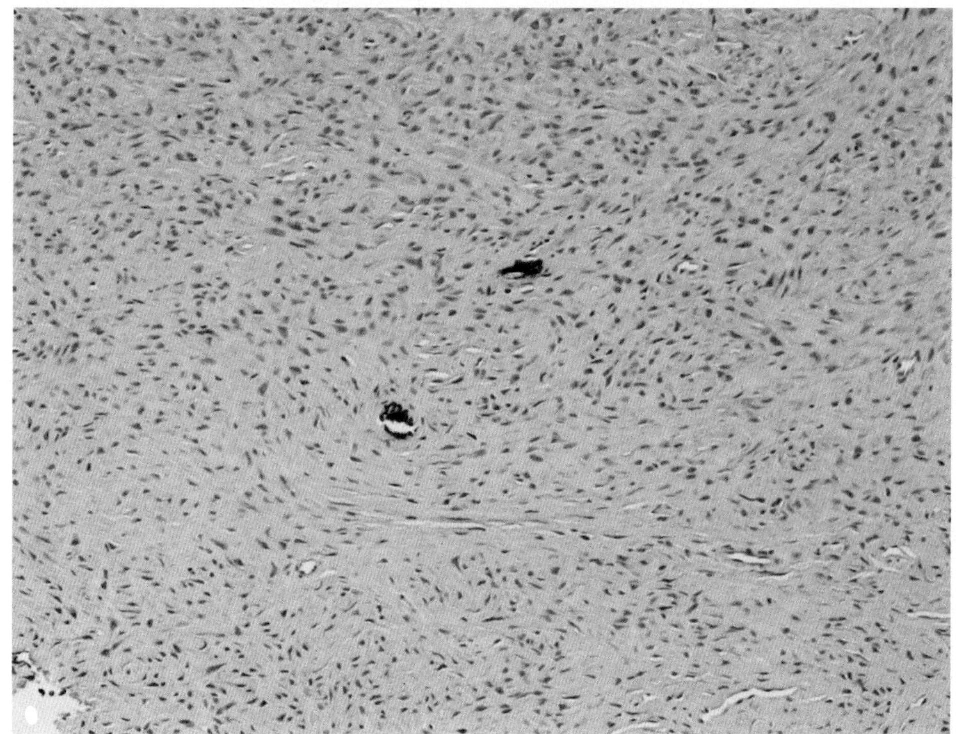

Figure 2.11.1. Odontogenic fibroma. The tumor is composed of cellular fibrous connective tissue containing small, spherical calcifications.

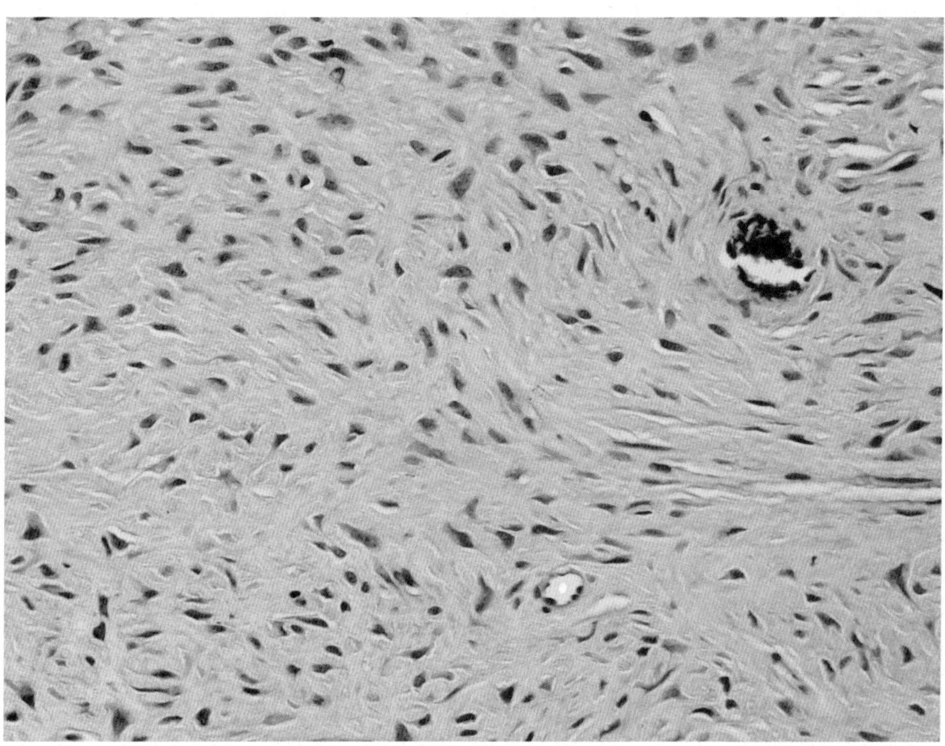

Figure 2.11.2. Odontogenic fibroma. The fibroblasts have variably shaped, plump nuclei. Odontogenic epithelial nests, occasionally seen in this tumor, are absent here.

2.12 Cementoblastoma

Presentation
Pain and swelling, especially of the mandibular first or second molar. In teenagers.

Radiographic Appearance
A calcified mass attached to a tooth root. A fine radiolucent line surrounds the radiopacity.

Microscopic Findings
- Calcified mass attached to a tooth root.
- Large encapsulated mass of bone or cementum-like material containing basophilic, incremental lines.
- Clusters of plump cementoblasts or osteoclasts line the periphery of the mineralized tissue and the trabeculae within.
- Scant well-vascularized fibrous connective tissue stroma separates the hard tissue components.

Histopathologic Differential
An *osteoblastoma* is not attached to the root of a tooth. The histology is otherwise identical.

Treatment and Prognosis
Removal of tooth and enucleation of tumor

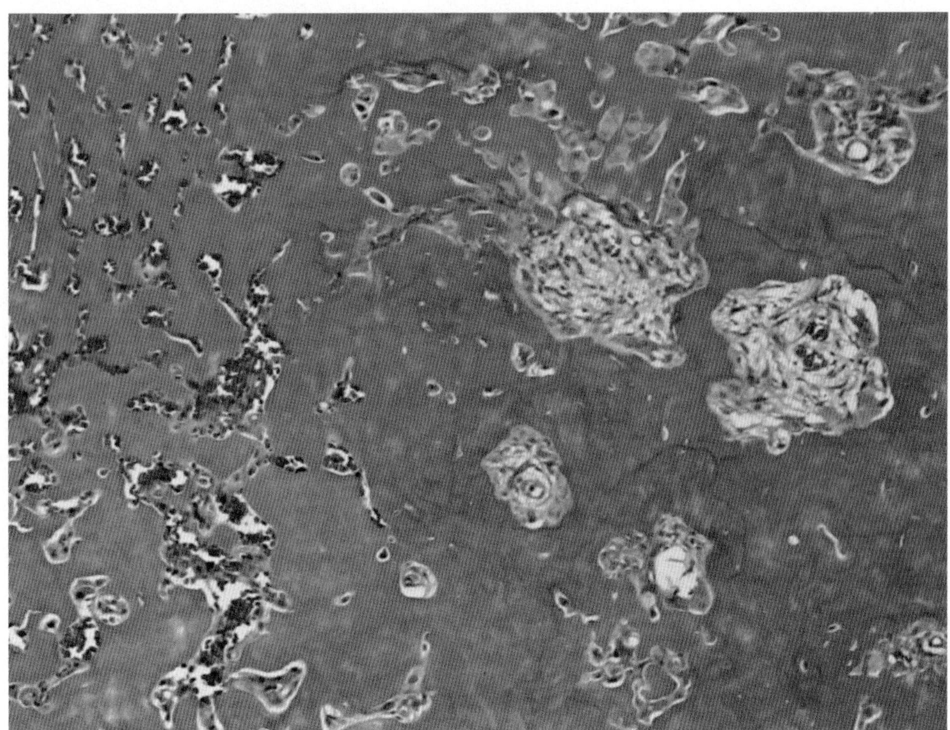

Figure 2.12.1. Cementoblastoma. The tumor is usually seen attached to the root of a molar tooth. It consists of a dense mass of calcified material resembling woven bone or cementum. Basophilic appositional lines are seen.

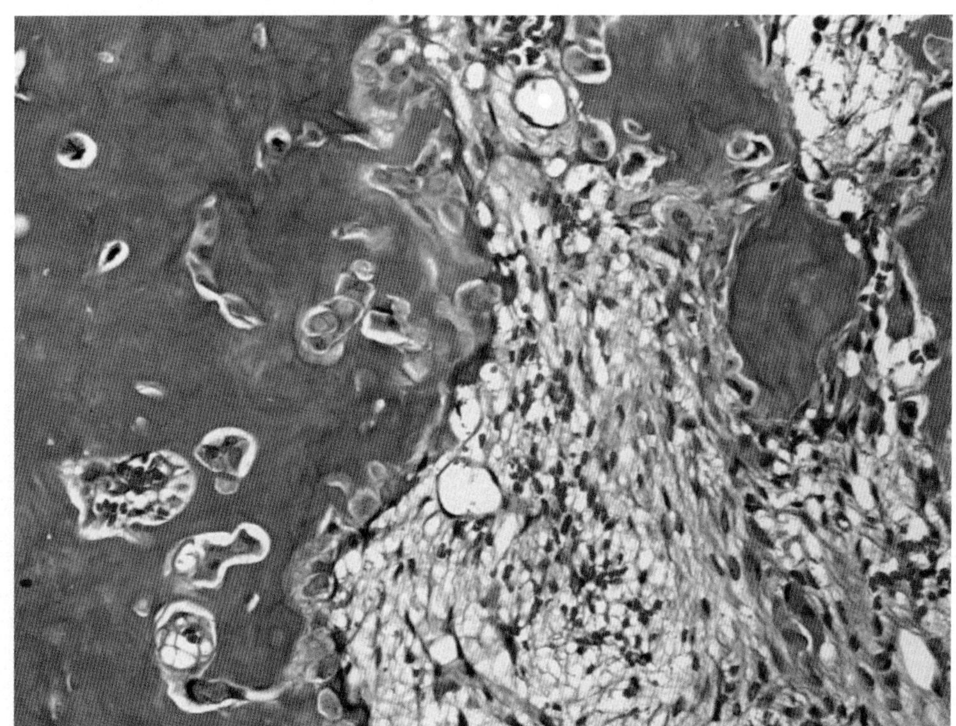

Figure 2.12.2. Cementoblastoma. Clusters of cementoblasts abut the cementum and are also entrapped within. The stroma is a loose, well-vascularized fibrous connective tissue.

Bibliography and Suggested Reading

2.1a

Reichart PA, Philipsen HP, Sonner S. Ameloblastoma: biological profile of 3677 cases. *Oral Oncol Eur J Cancer.* 1995;31:86–99.

Hertog D, Schulten EA, Leemans CR, Winters HA, Van der Waal I. Management of recurrent ameloblastoma of the jaws; a 40-year single institution experience. *Oral Oncol.* 2011;47(2):145-6. Epub 2010 Dec 14.

2.1b

Lau SL, Samman N. Recurrence related to treatment modalities of unicystic ameloblastoma: a systematic review. *Int J Oral Maxillofac Surg.* 2006;35:681–690.

2.1c

Philipsen HP, Reichart PA, Nikai H, et al. Peripheral ameloblastoma: biological profile based on 160 cases from the literature. *Oral Oncol.* 2001;37:17–27.

2.1d

Bello IO, Alanen K, Slootweg PJ, et al. Alpha-smooth muscle actin within epithelial islands is predictive of ameloblastic carcinoma. *Oral Oncol.* 2009;45:760–765.

Cox DP, Muller S, Carlson GW, et al. Ameloblastic carcinoma ex ameloblastoma of the mandible with malignancy-associated hypercalcemia. *Oral Surg Oral Med Oral Pathol Oral Radiol Endod.* 2000;90:716–722.

2.2

Luo HY, Li TJ. Odontogenic tumors: a study of 1309 cases in a Chinese population. *Oral Oncol.* 2009;45:706–711.

Pathology and genetics of head and neck tumours. In: *World Health Organization Classification of Tumours.* Edited by Leon Barnes, MD, et al. IARC (International Agency for Research on Cancer) Press, Lyon; 2005.

2.3

Angadi PV, Rekha K. Calcifying epithelial odontogenic tumor (Pindborg tumor). *Head Neck Pathol.* 2011; 5(2):137–9.

Regezi JA. Odontogenic cysts, odontogenic tumors, fibro-osseous, and giant cell lesions of the jaws. *Mod Pathol.* 2002;15:331–341.

Solomon A, Murphy CL, Weaver K, et al. Calcifying epithelial odontogenic (Pindborg) tumor-associated amyloid consists of a novel human protein. *J Lab Clin Med.* 2003;142:348–355.

2.4

Buchner A. The central (intraosseous) calcifying odontogenic cyst: an analysis of 215 cases. *J Oral Maxillofac Surg.* 1991;49:330–339.

Hong SP, Ellis GL, Hartman KS. Calcifying odontogenic cyst. A review of ninety-two cases with reevaluation of their nature as cysts or neoplasms, the nature of ghost cells, and subclassification. *Oral Surg Oral Med Oral Pathol.* 1991;72:56–64.

Li TJ, Yu SF. Clinicopathologic spectrum of the so-called calcifying odontogenic cysts: a study of 21 intraosseous cases with reconsideration of the terminology and classification. *Am J Surg Pathol.* 2003;27:372–384.

2.5

Haghighat K, Kalmar JR, Mariotti AJ. Squamous odontogenic tumor: diagnosis and management. *J Periodontol.* 2002;73:653–656.

2.6

Chen Y, Wang J-M, Li T-J. Ameloblastic fibroma: a review of published studies with special reference to its nature and biological behavior. *Oral Oncol.* 2007;43:960–969.

2.7

Cohen DM, Bhattacharyya I. Ameloblastic fibroma, ameloblastic fibro-odontoma, and odontoma. *Oral Maxillofac Surg Clin North Am.* 2004;6:375–384.

2.8

DeLair D, Bejarano PA, Peleg M, et al. Ameloblastic carcinosarcoma of the mandible arising in ameloblastic fibroma: a case report and review of the literature. *Oral Surg Oral Med Oral Pathol Oral Radiol Endod.* 2007;103:516–520.

2.9

Hidalgo-Sánchez O, Leco-Berrocal MI, Martínez-González JM. Metaanalysis of the epidemiology and clinical manifestations of odontomas. *Med Oral Patol Oral Cir Bucal.* 2008;13(11):E730–4.

Soluk Tekkesin M, Pehlivan S, Olgac V, Aksakallı N, Alatlı C. Clinical and Histopathological Investigation of Odontomas: Review of the Literature and Presentation of 160 Cases. *J Oral Maxillofac Surg.* 2011 Epub ahead of print.

2.10

Simon EN, Merkx MA. Odontogenic myxoma: a clinicopathological study of 33 cases. *Int J Oral Maxillofac Surg.* 2004;33:333–337.

2.11

Handlers JP, Abrams AM, Melrose RJ, et al. Central odontogenic fibroma: clinicopathologic features of 19 cases and review of the literature. *J Oral Maxillofac Surg.* 1991;49:46–54.

2.12

Brannon RB, Fowler CB, Carpenter WM, et al. Cementoblastoma: an innocuous neoplasm? A clinicopathologic study of 44 cases and review of the literature with special emphasis on recurrence. *Oral Surg Oral Med Oral Pathol Oral Radiol Endod.* 2002;93:311–320.

Clear Cell Odontogenic Carcinoma

Bilodeau EA, Hoschar AP, Barnes EL, et al. Clear cell carcinoma and clear cell odontogenic carcinoma: a comparative clinicopathologic and immunohistochemical study. *Head Neck Pathol.* 2011;5:101–107.

CHAPTER

3

Salivary Gland Pathology

Mucocele
Necrotizing sialometaplasia
Pleomorphic adenoma
Myoepithelioma
Canalicular adenoma
Cystadenoma
Sialadenoma papilliferum
Mucoepidermoid carcinoma
Polymorphous low-grade adenocarcinoma
Adenoid cystic carcinoma
Acinic cell adenocarcinoma
Clear cell adenocarcinoma
Basal cell adenocarcinoma
Adenocarcinoma, NOS

Introduction

Situated under the oral mucosa are several hundred minor salivary glands. These 2- to 3-mm structures are located throughout the mouth, sparing, essentially, only the gingiva surrounding the teeth. Tumors arising in these glands are most common in the palate, upper lip, and buccal mucosa. Although the World Health Organization describes 40 histologic tumor types in its latest fascicle, only 12 will be highlighted here. The discussion also includes the common mucocele and necrotizing sialometaplasia, the latter a reactive process sometimes confused with malignancy.

Among these tumors, polymorphous low-grade adenocarcinoma (PLGA) deserves special mention. This tumor, which almost always occurs in minor salivary glands, can be confused with a cellular pleomorphic adenoma (one devoid of chondro-osseous tissue) or an adenoid cystic carcinoma. It is especially important to recognize that it is not adenoid cystic carcinoma, since PLGA calls for more conservative treatment and has a much better long-term prognosis.

Finally, a note on assessing malignancy in minor salivary gland tumors. Since, as a rule, cellular atypia, nuclear atypia, increased mitotic rate and necrosis are not usually encountered, invasion into adjacent normal tissues and/or the presence of tumor in a perineural or intravascular location must be used instead. Low and intermediate -power pattern recognition is especially helpful in differentiating mucoepidermoid, adenoid cystic, acinic cell and polymorphous low-grade carcinomas.

3.1 Mucocele

Definition

A cystic structure caused by the severance of minor intraoral salivary gland ducts, usually because of accidental biting of the lip or the cheek. The extravasated mucin accumulates and is walled off by granulation tissue, forming the cyst.

Presentation

A fluctuant, bluish, dome-shaped mucosal swelling. Usually on the lower lip or on the buccal mucosa, but it can also occur on the floor of the mouth or the tongue. Most common in children and young adults.

Microscopic Findings

- Mucin-filled cyst lined by compressed granulation tissue
- Abundant foamy histiocytes within fibrous wall and cyst lumen
- Variable inflammatory component

Treatment and Prognosis

Excision with removal of the involved minor salivary glands. Recurrence can occur if the ducts of the remaining glands are severed during the procedure.

Additional

- Rarely, a mucin-filled intraoral cyst will have a well-defined epithelial lining; the term for this is *salivary duct cyst.*
- A large mucocele in the floor of the mouth is known as a *ranula.*

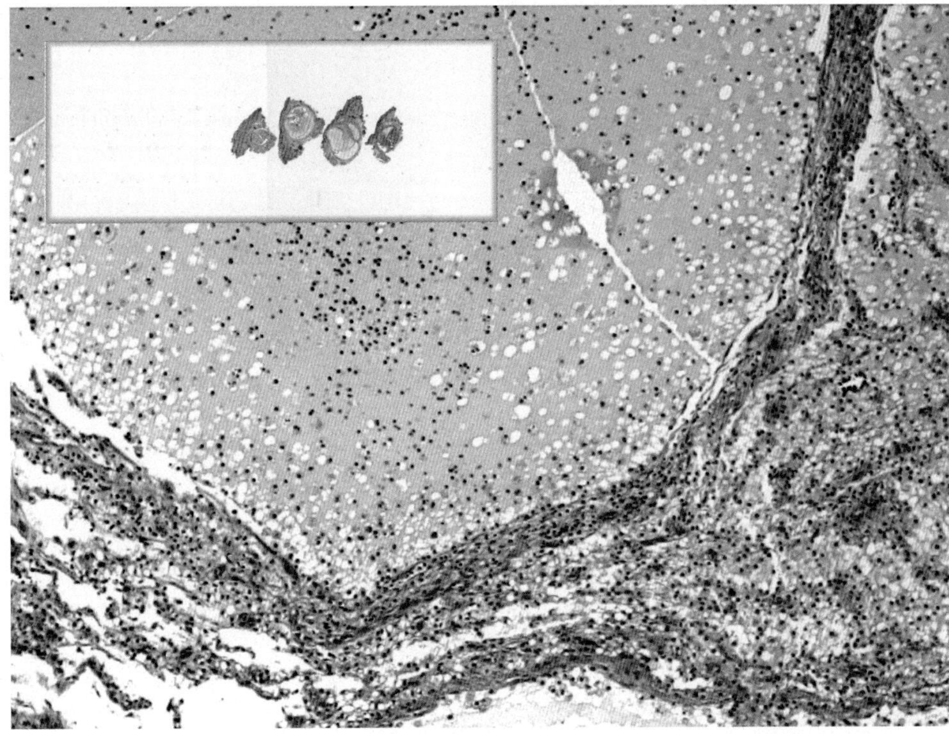

Figure 3.1.1.
Mucocele. A well-defined cystic structure filled with amphophilic mucinous material and inflammatory cells. The lining is compressed granulation tissue.

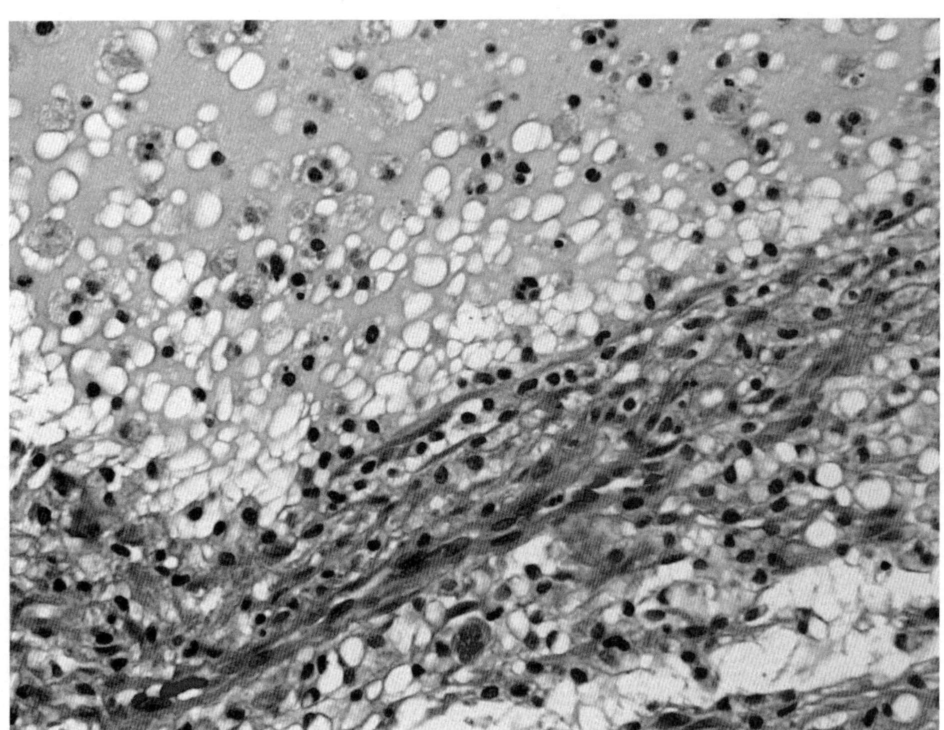

Figure 3.1.2.
Mucocele. The cyst lumen is filled with mucin, mucinophages, and other inflammatory cells.

3.2 Necrotizing Sialometaplasia

Definition

A reactive, self-healing condition of minor salivary glands that can be mistaken both clinically and histologically for a malignant tumor.

Presentation

Nodular swelling or crater-like ulcer of the palate, often of rapid onset. Usually asymptomatic but can present with pain or paresthesia. Often bilateral.

Microscopic Findings

- Necrotic salivary gland acini with thin fibrous strands preserving the lobular architecture
- Squamous metaplasia of ducts
- Pseudoepitheliomatous hyperplasia of the overlying mucosal epithelium
- Mild inflammatory and regenerative atypia of epithelial and myoepithelial cells
- Intense acute and chronic inflammatory cell infiltrate

Special Stains/Immunohistochemistry

- Myoepithelial cells amid the squamous nests will stain positive for S100 or other myoepithelial markers.

Histopathologic Differential

- *Mucoepidermoid carcinoma* does not have necrotic mucous acini, an intense inflammatory reaction, or S100-positive myoepithelial cells intermixed with the squamous cells of the metaplastic ducts.
- *Squamous cell carcinoma* has cellular pleomorphism and nuclear atypia and can also have individual cell keratinization and dysplastic changes of the overlying epithelium.

Treatment and Prognosis

No additional treatment after biopsy. Slow to heal but does not recur.

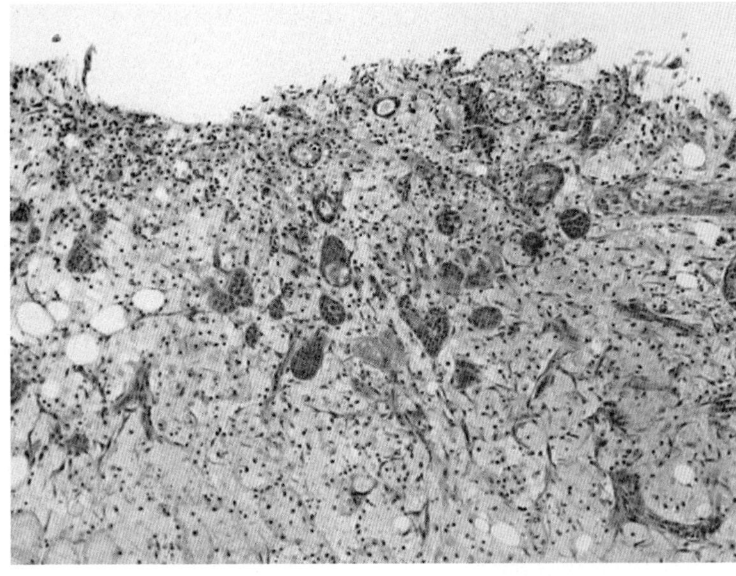

Figure 3.2.1.
Necrotizing sialometaplasia. Nests of squamous cells on the surface and, below, pools of mucin and outlines of acinar structures.

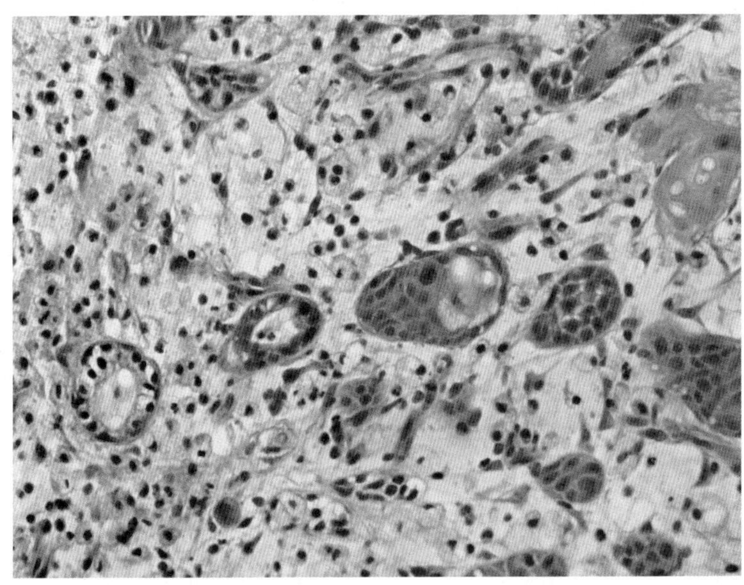

Figure 3.2.2.
Necrotizing sialometaplasia. Metaplastic ducts filled with squamous cells in a background of mucin and inflammatory cells. Note the two ductal structures on the left that have not yet undergone metaplasia.

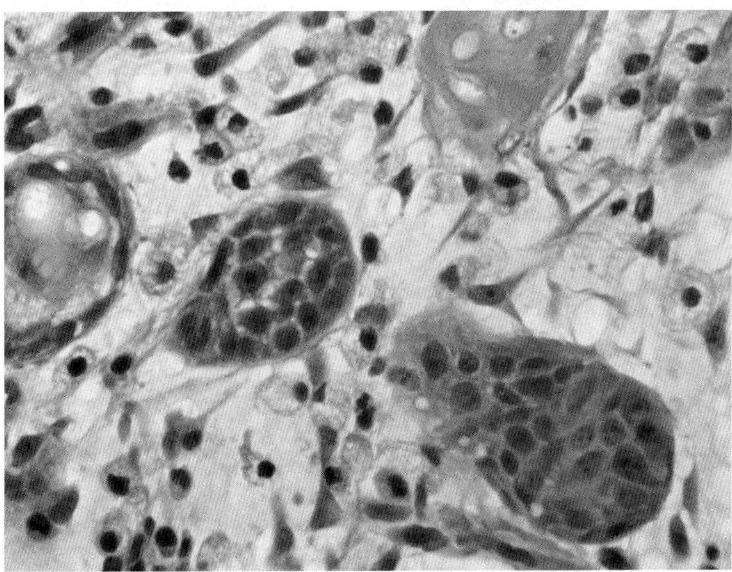

Figure 3.2.3.
Necrotizing sialometaplasia. The squamous cells filling these metaplastic ducts are atypical and form keratin pearls. Their growth pattern also suggests invasive tumor. Despite these worrisome features, the background is inflammatory: neutrophils, plasma cells, and tissue-culture fibroblasts.

3.3 Pleomorphic Adenoma

Presentation

Asymptomatic, slow-growing tumor. Most common intraoral sites are the palate, upper lip, and buccal mucosa.

Microscopic Findings

- Well-circumscribed, sometimes partially encapsulated.
- Nests of myoepithelial cells and ductal structures within a mesenchymal background.
- Myoepithelial cells form large nests or broad, interconnecting trabeculae containing small ducts or tubular structures. These ducts consist of an inner single layer of cuboidal-lining cells and an outer layer of clear myoepithelial cells.
- Myoepithelial cells can take on a variety of forms: spindle, hyaline (plasmacytoid), or clear cell.
- Mesenchyme-like stroma can be myxoid, chondroid, hyalinized, fibrous, or even osseous.
- Tumor nests sometimes extend into the capsule but do not infiltrate the surrounding tissues.

Special Stains/Immunohistochemistry

- Duct-lining cells are positive for cytokeratins.
- Myoepithelial cells are positive for smooth muscle actin, S100, GFAP, calponin, and p63.

Histopathologic Differential

- *Myoepithelioma* is more monomorphic, lacking mesenchymal areas and ductal structures.
- *Polymorphous low-grade adenocarcinoma* infiltrates the lamina propria and residual mucous glands; it also invades small nerves.

Treatment and Prognosis

Complete surgical excision

Additional

Pleomorphic adenoma is the most common minor salivary gland tumor and is well known for its diverse architecture and cytomorphology. The mesenchymal tissues are thought to be a metaplastic product of the myoepithelial cells.

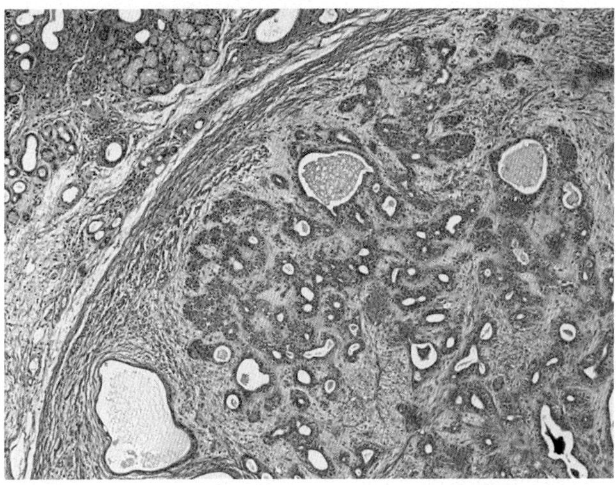

Figure 3.3.1.
Pleomorphic adenoma. Although usually well circumscribed, this particular pleomorphic adenoma is encapsulated.

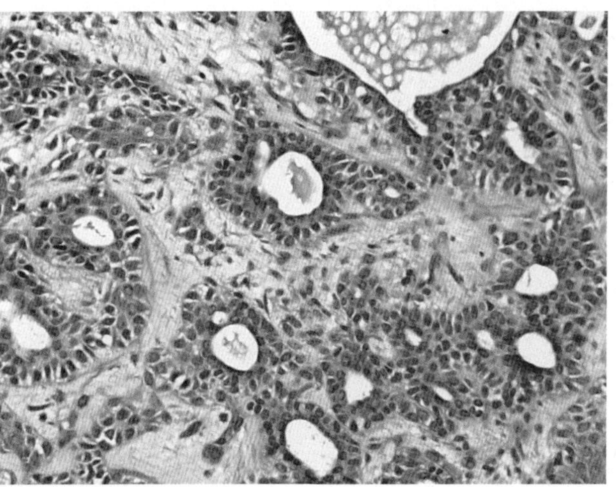

Figure 3.3.2.
Pleomorphic adenoma. Epithelial nests within the tumor recapitulate normal salivary ducts: luminal cuboidal ductal epithelium surrounded by myoepithelial cells with clear cytoplasm and angulated nuclei.

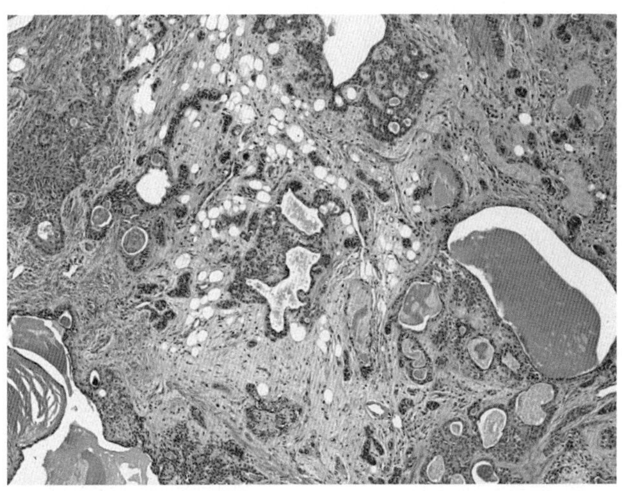

Figure 3.3.3.
Pleomorphic adenoma. The tumor is composed of large and small cystic spaces with ductal structures and solid epithelial nests. The stroma is myxoid and fibrous.

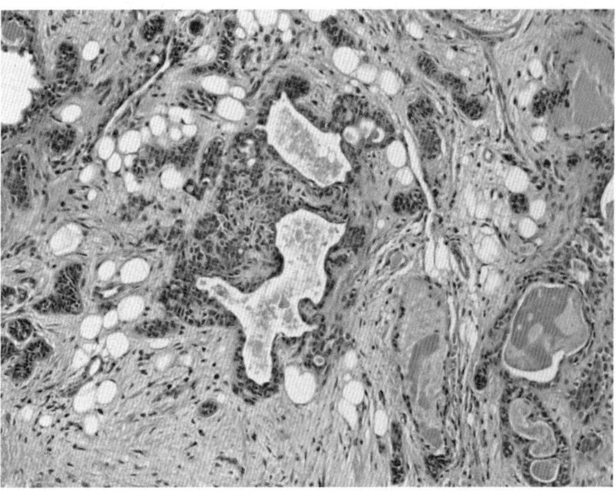

Figure 3.3.4.
Pleomorphic adenoma. The stroma consists of a mixture of myxoid and fibrous tissues. The adipocytes in this case are an unusual finding.

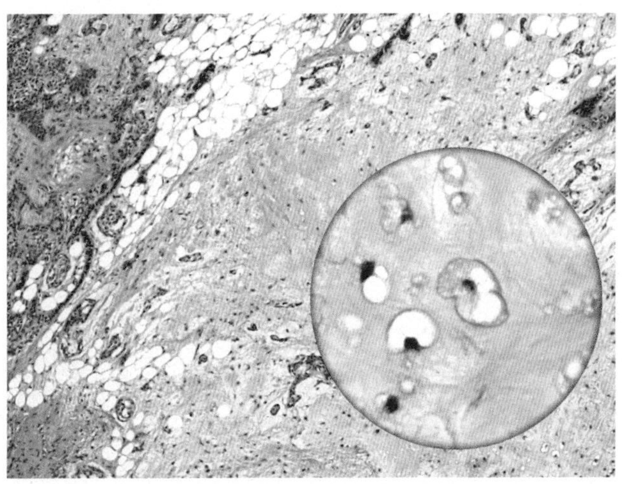

Figure 3.3.5.
Pleomorphic adenoma. An area of predominantly myxochondroid stroma. Chondrocytes can be seen in the inset.

3.4 Myoepithelioma

Definition

The myoepithelioma is composed of a proliferation of myoepithelial cells without the formation of ductal structures.

Presentation

Asymptomatic, slow-growing tumor. The most common intraoral site is the palate.

Microscopic Findings

- Well circumscribed, partially encapsulated.
- The myoepithelial proliferation can take on different forms. One is interdigitating fascicles of spindle cells in a myxoid stroma; another, sheets of plasmacytoid cells. A variety of growth patterns and myoepithelial cell types are seen in some tumors.
- Most palatal myoepitheliomas are plasmacytoid.

Special Stains/Immunohistochemistry

Positive for smooth muscle actin, S100, GFAP, calponin, and p63.

Histopathologic Differential

Pleomorphic adenoma has ductal structures and myxochondroid areas.

Treatment and Prognosis

Complete surgical excision

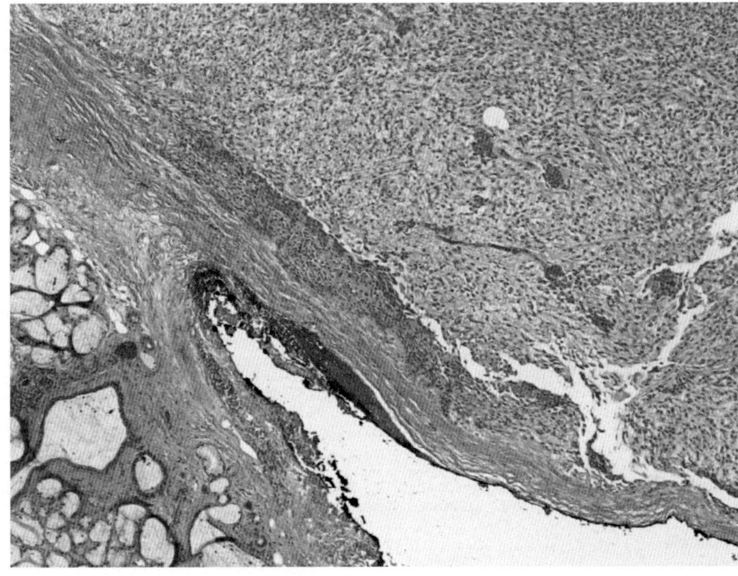

Figure 3.4.1.
Myoepithelioma. Cellular tumor composed of small, spindled epithelial cells. It is separated from the residual mucous glands (lower left) by a fibrous capsule.

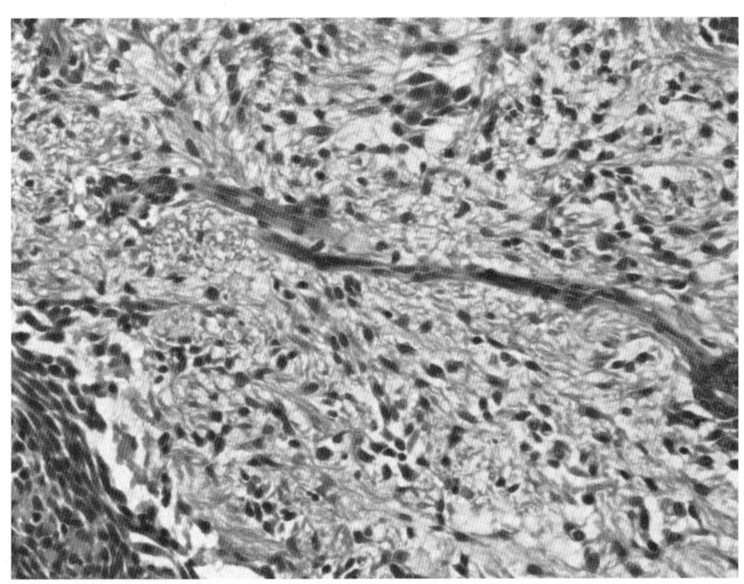

Figure 3.4.2.
Myoepithelioma. A mixture of two myoepithelial cell types: spindled and, at lower left, plasmacytoid.

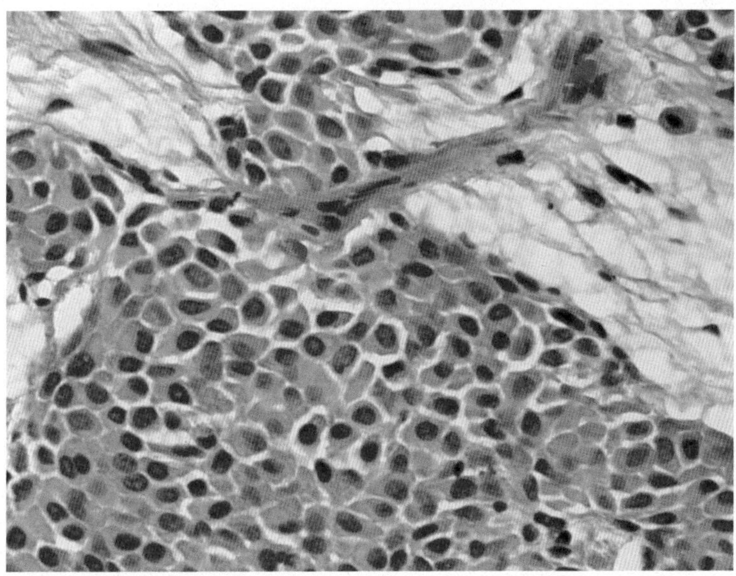

Figure 3.4.3.
Myoepithelioma. The myoepithelial cells in this tumor are plasmacytoid, with an amphophilic cytoplasm, well-defined cell borders, and an eccentrically placed nucleus.

3.5 Canalicular Adenoma

Presentation

Slowly enlarging, painless nodule. Most common in the upper lip, but it can also be seen in the buccal mucosa adjacent to the upper lip. Sometimes multifocal. Uncommon under the age of 50.

Microscopic Findings

- Well circumscribed, usually encapsulated.
- Thin, branching, interconnecting cords of columnar and cuboidal epithelial cells with uniform, deeply basophilic nuclei.
- Cords resemble a string of beads, widening in areas to form elongated, narrow canals.
- Background stroma consists of a well-vascularized, loose fibrous connective tissue.

Special Stains/Immunopathology

Positive for cytokeratins; negative for most myoepithelial markers (smooth muscle actin, GFAP, calponin, and p63).

Treatment and Prognosis

Surgical excision

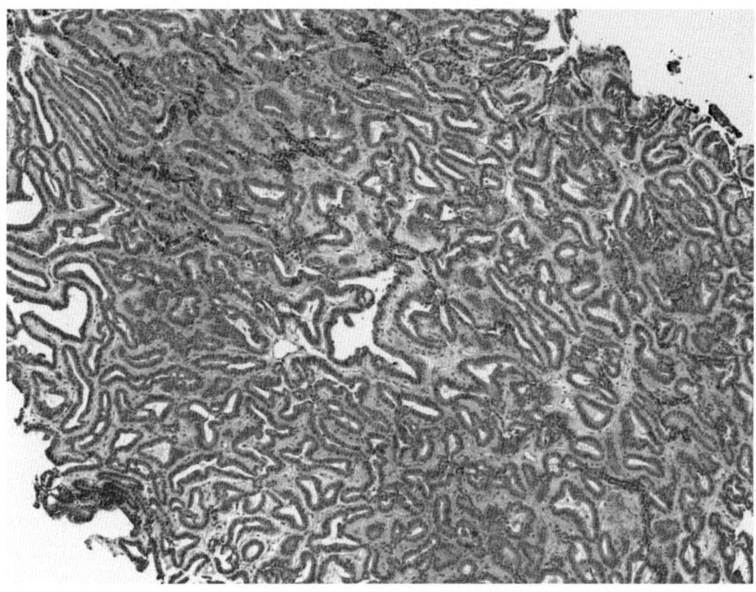

Figure 3.5.1.
Canalicular adenoma. Branching, interconnecting epithelial cords set in scant fibrous stroma.

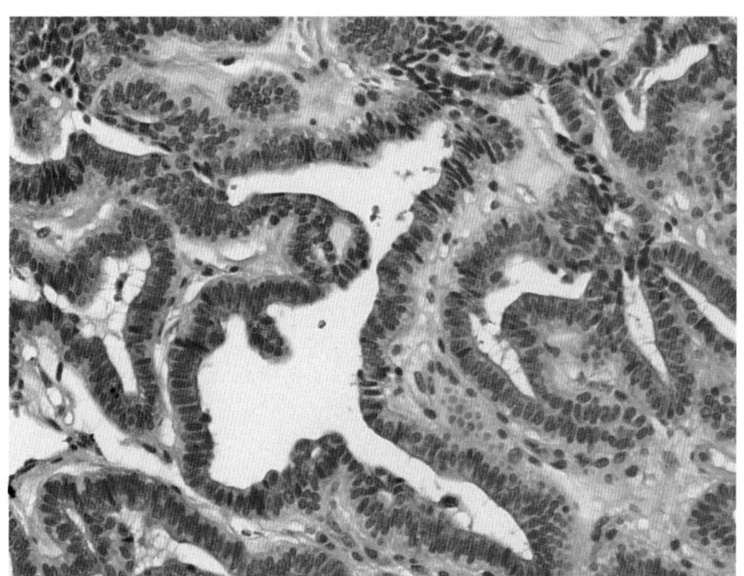

Figure 3.5.2.
Canalicular adenoma. The cords widen in areas to take on the form of canals. The stroma is a well-vascularized, loose fibrous connective tissue.

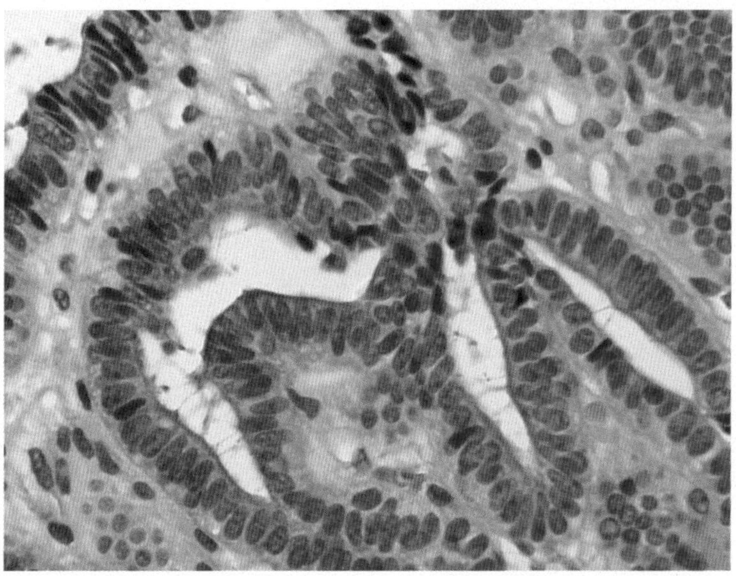

Figure 3.5.3.
Canalicular adenoma. The tubules are lined by cuboidal to columnar cells with an amphophilic cytoplasm and deeply basophilic nuclei. The nuclei are uniform in areas and resemble a string of beads.

3.6 Cystadenoma

Presentation

A fluctuant, submucosal nodule in the lips or the buccal mucosa. Small, under 1 cm. More common in older adults.

Microscopic Findings

- Well circumscribed, occasionally encapsulated.
- Cystic space with luminal, often papillary, epithelial proliferations; can be polycystic.
- Lining cells are columnar, cuboidal, mucous, or oncocytic.
- When a prominent lymphoid component is present, the cystadenoma can resemble a Warthin tumor.

Histopathologic Differential

Duct ectasia secondary to obstruction. In this case, dilated ductal structures are surrounded by inflamed fibrous tissue and generally lack luminal proliferation.

Treatment and Prognosis

Excision. Does not recur.

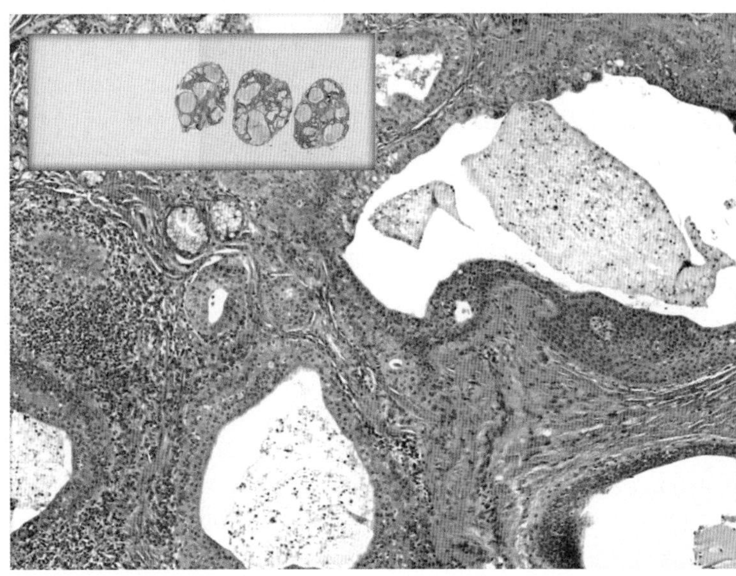

Figure 3.6.1.
Cystadenoma. A well-circumscribed nodule containing cystic spaces of variable size.

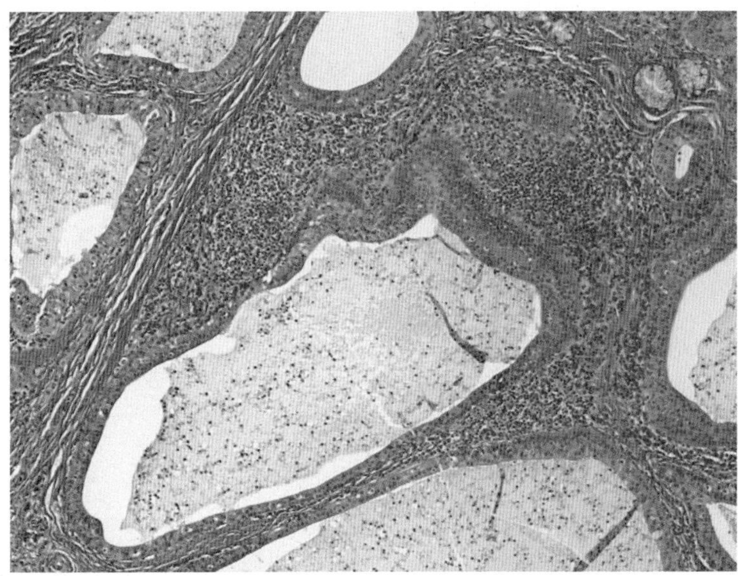

Figure 3.6.2.
Cystadenoma. The collections of lymphocytes seen in this tumor are not typical of most cystadenomas.

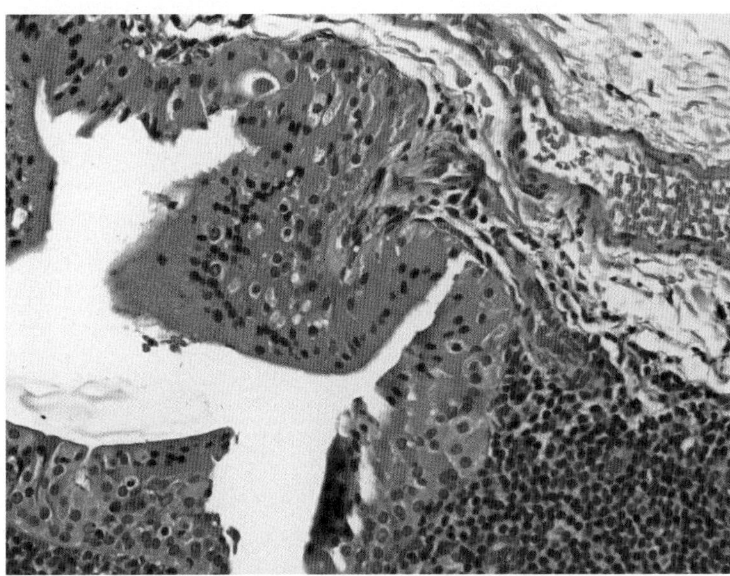

Figure 3.6.3.
Cystadenoma. The oncocytic, papillary lining and nodular lymphoid infiltrate recall the morphology of a Warthin tumor.

3.7 Sialadenoma Papilliferum

Presentation

Red, raised, papillomatous lesion on the palate. In older adults.

Microscopic Findings

- Circumscribed mass with papillary surface.
- Papillary projections covered by stratified squamous epithelium merge at their base with proliferating ductal structures.

Treatment and Prognosis

Excision. Recurrence rare.

Additional

- Sialadenoma papilliferum is the only salivary gland tumor to manifest itself clinically as a papillary excrescence; the clinical impression is usually squamous papilloma.
- The ductal structures at the base of the lesion are usually not circumscribed and can suggest invasive adenocarcinoma.

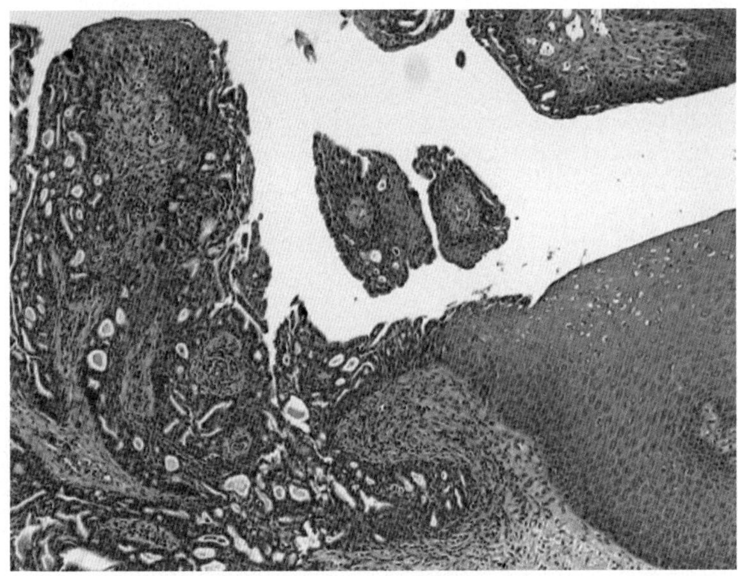

Figure 3.7.1.
Sialadenoma papilliferum. The tumor is largely exophytic and consists of papillary glandular structures covered by stratified squamous epithelium with an underlying proliferation of ducts.

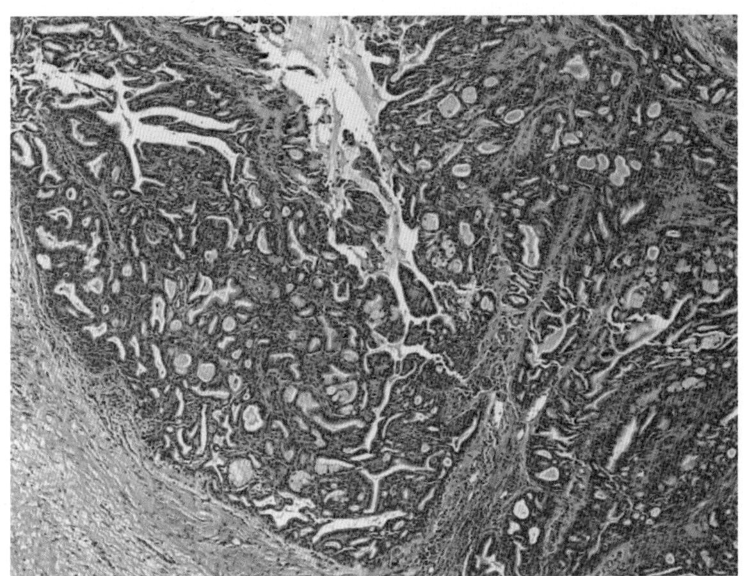

Figure 3.7.2.
Sialadenoma papilliferum. Ducts of variable size extend into the underlying submucosa. The deep margin of these tumors is not always as well circumscribed as in this example, and the glandular structures can be mistaken for a low-grade, invasive adenocarcinoma.

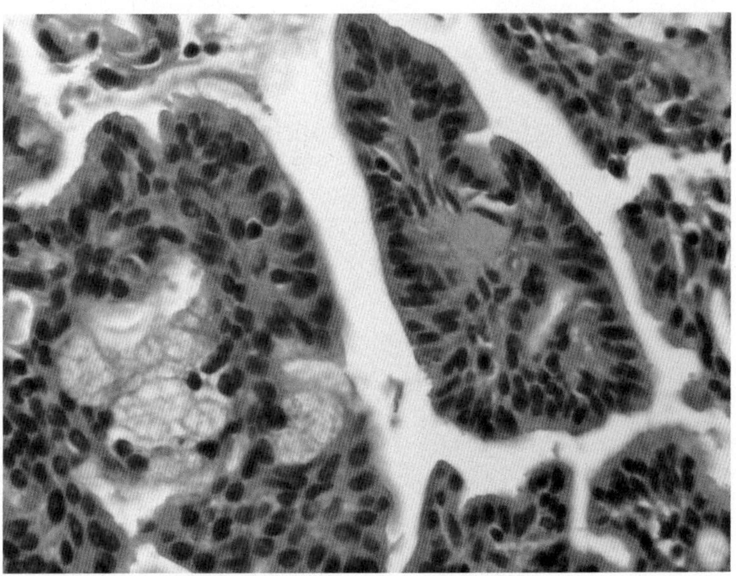

Figure 3.7.3.
Sialadenoma papilliferum. The papillary structures are composed of columnar eosinophilic cells with nests of embedded mucous cells.

3.8 Mucoepidermoid Carcinoma

Presentation

Low-grade tumors typically present as a fluctuant swelling that can resemble a mucocele; high-grade tumors are often accompanied by pain or paresthesia. The palate and the buccal mucosa are the most common intraoral sites.

Microscopic Findings

- Unencapsulated, infiltrative tumor
- Mixture of cystic spaces and solid growth
- Three main cell types: epidermoid, mucous, and intermediate (between basal and epidermoid in size, sometimes with a clear perinuclear space)

Special Stains/Immunopathology

Mucous cells stain positive for mucin.

Grading

The grading of mucoepidermoid carcinomas is essential for determining treatment and prognosis. Several systems are in use, but most agree that the following adverse parameters should be reported. Two or more of these findings will generally put the tumor in a higher grade.

- Solid (not cystic) growth
- Neural invasion
- Necrosis
- Anaplasia
- Mitotic rate of over 3 to 4 per 10 high-power fields

Histopathologic Differential

- *Squamous cell carcinoma* has cellular pleomorphism and nuclear atypia and can also have individual cell keratinization and dysplastic changes of the overlying epithelium.
- *Necrotizing sialometaplasia* has recognizable residual lobular architecture, necrosis of mucous gland acini, and an inflammatory background.

Treatment and Prognosis

Surgical excision. High-grade lesions frequently metastasize to cervical nodes. Prognosis depends on the grade and stage of tumor.

Additional

A small number of mucoepidermoid carcinomas occur centrally within the maxilla and the mandible. Over half are associated with odontogenic cysts or impacted teeth.

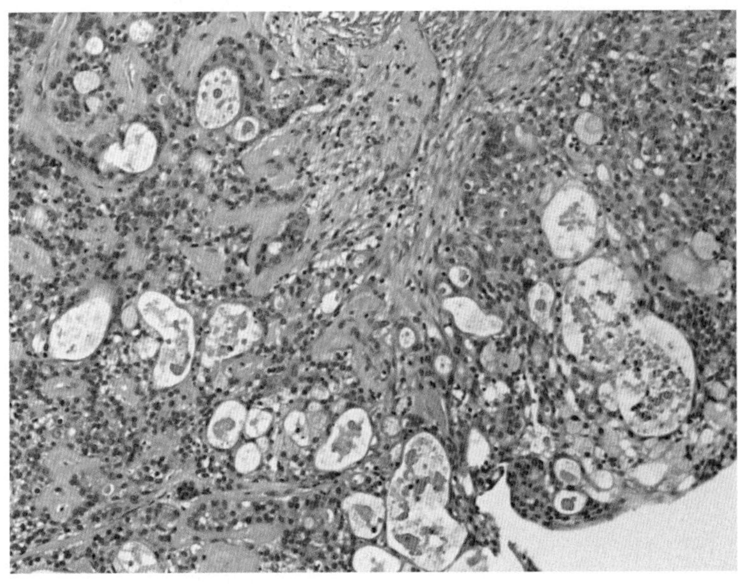

Figure 3.8.1.
Mucoepidermoid carcinoma, low grade. Infiltrating epithelial islands with prominent mucin-filled cystic spaces. The stroma is loose and fibrous.

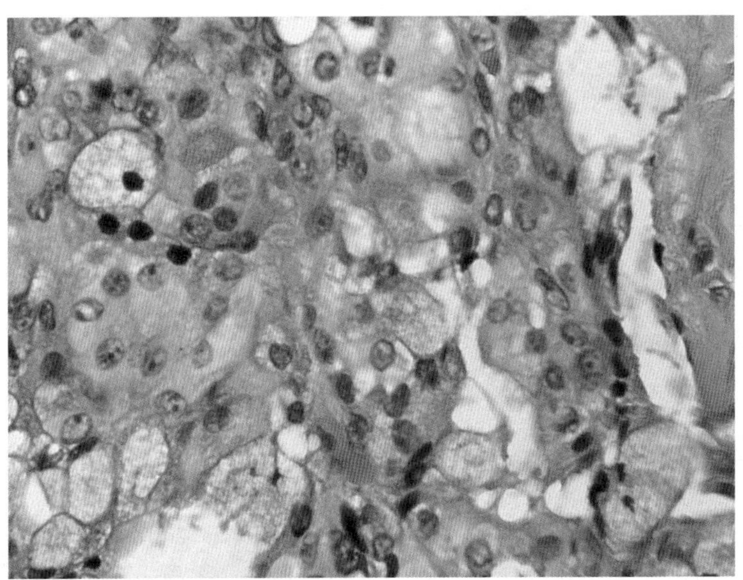

Figure 3.8.2.
Mucoepidermoid carcinoma, low grade. All three cell types of mucoepidermoid carcinoma are present in this field: epidermoid, intermediate, and mucous.

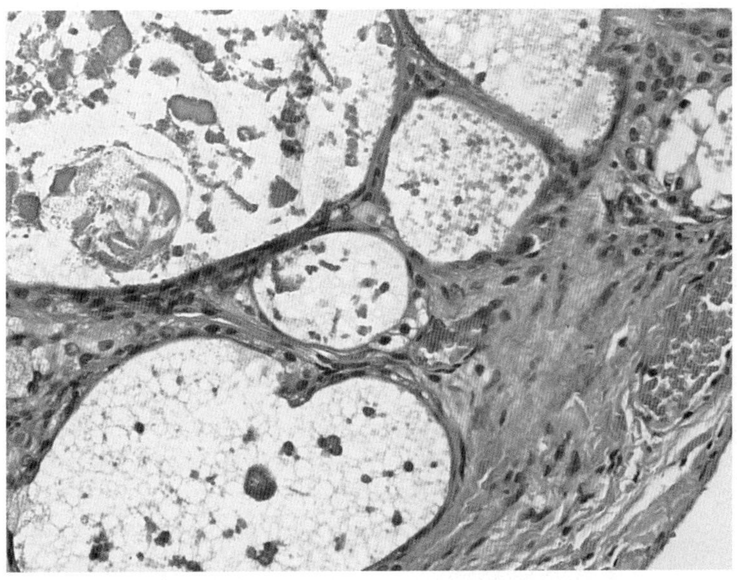

Figure 3.8.3.
Mucoepidermoid carcinoma, low grade. Large cystic spaces are filled with mucin and lined by low cuboidal epithelium. This histology can be misinterpreted as a mucocele.

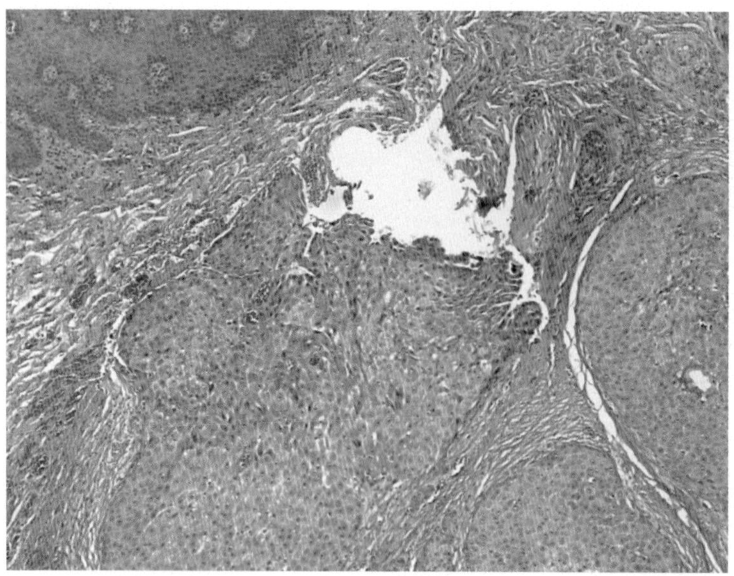

Figure 3.8.4.
Mucoepidermoid carcinoma, intermediate grade. The growth is solid and the tumor is infiltrative.

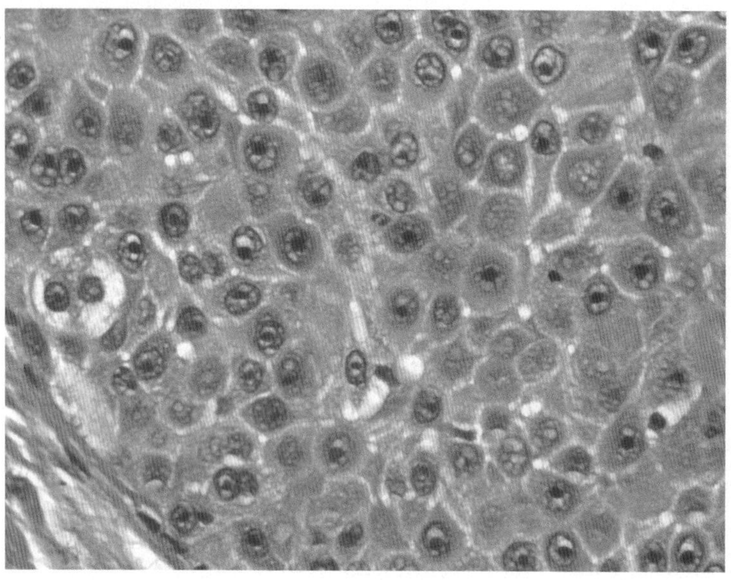

Figure 3.8.5.
Mucoepidermoid carcinoma, intermediate grade. Epidermoid cells have squamous features, including intercellular bridges. The nuclei are pleomorphic and have prominent nucleoli.

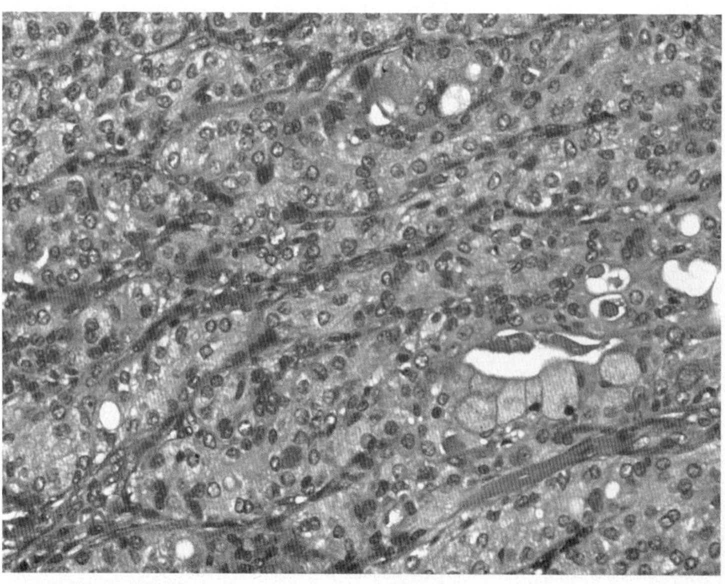

Figure 3.8.6.
Mucoepidermoid carcinoma, intermediate grade. This example consists of intermediate cells with scattered mucin-containing goblet cells.

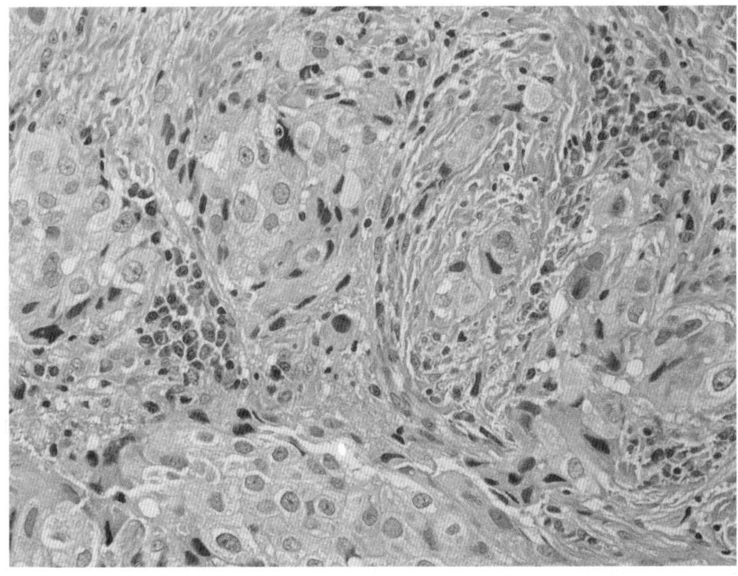

Figure 3.8.7.
Mucoepidermoid carcinoma, high grade. The tumor consists of solid, infiltrating nests of epidermoid and clear cells. Some cells have atypical nuclear forms.

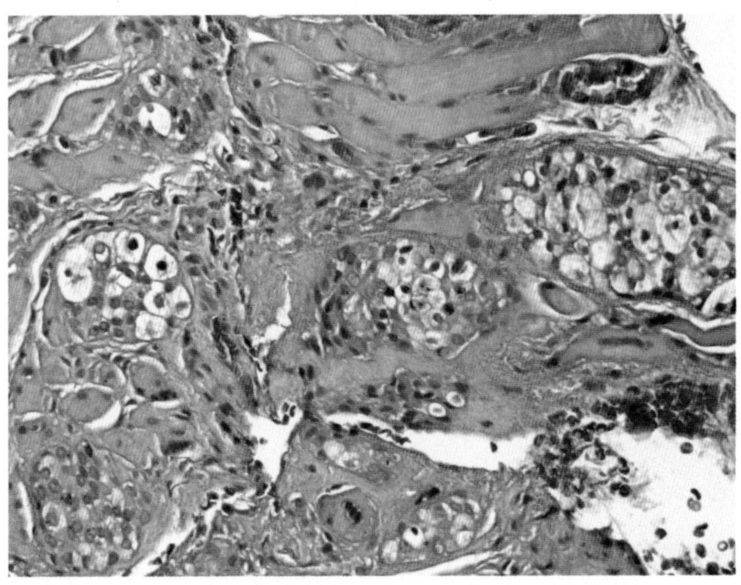

Figure 3.8.8.
Mucoepidermoid carcinoma, high grade, mucicarmine stain. Nests of epidermoid cells with clear cell features invade the regional striated muscle and the fibrous connective tissue. Mucin is present in some of the cells.

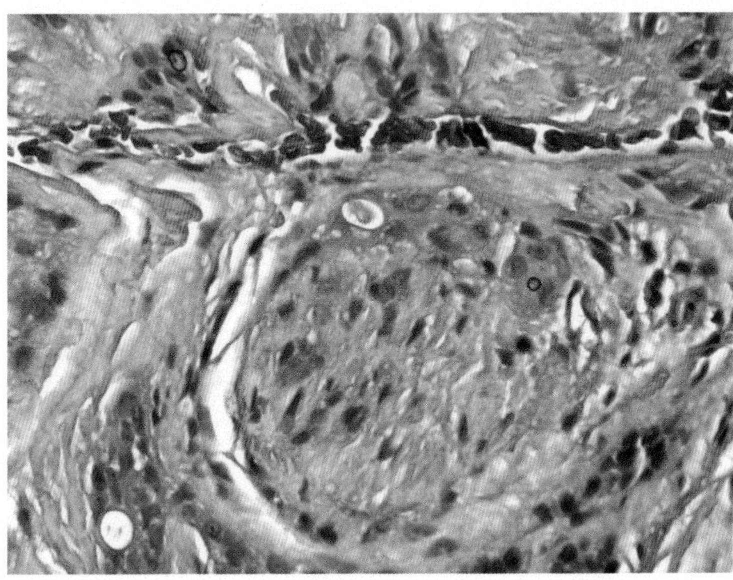

Figure 3.8.9.
Mucoepidermoid carcinoma, high grade, mucicarmine stain. Perineural invasion by tumor cells, some of which stain for mucin.

3.9 Polymorphous Low-grade Adenocarcinoma

Definition

A multipatterned, salivary gland adenocarcinoma composed of small, uniform epithelial cells exhibiting neurotropism and single-file growth

Presentation

Asymptomatic submucosal swelling of the palate or the buccal mucosa. Most tumors are less than 2 cm in diameter.

Microscopic Findings

- Infiltrative tumor; nonencapsulated
- Nests of isomorphic cells with uniform, ovoid nuclei and scant eosinophilic cytoplasm
- Parallel rows of cells streaming in single file, especially at the periphery of the tumor
- Prominent perineural infiltration
- Targetoid, onion-skin growth around cell nests or small nerves
- Small tubules lined by a single layer of cuboidal cells
- Myxoid and hyalinized stroma

Histopathologic Differential

The greatest challenge is distinguishing PLGA from adenoid cystic carcinoma. The criteria given in Table 3.1 are important to consider.

Table 3.1 • PLGA Versus Adenoid Cystic Carcinoma

	PLGA	Adenoid Cystic Carcinoma
Small epithelial cells with large round nuclei	Yes	No
Clear cells with angular, hyperchromatic nuclei	No	Yes
Cells with eosinophilic cytoplasm	Yes	No
Prominent pseudocystic spaces filled with hyaline material	No	Yes
Solid tumor nests with nuclear pleomorphism, necrosis, and mitoses	No	Yes (Solid type)

- A *cellular pleomorphic adenoma* may exhibit extracapsular extension of cell nests but no actual invasion of surrounding tissues. Perineural invasion is also absent.

Treatment and Prognosis

Wide local excision. About 10% of patients will develop metastases to cervical lymph nodes. Recurrence, often late, has been reported in up to 20% of cases.

PLGA is found almost exclusively in the minor salivary glands.

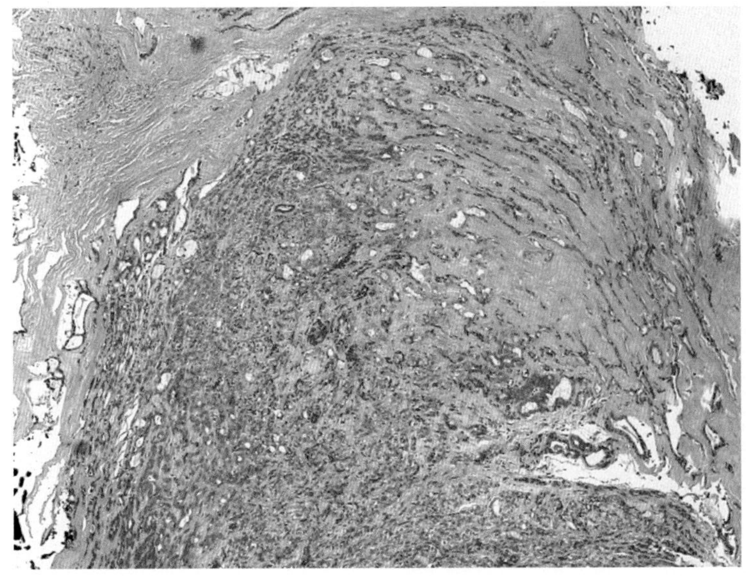

Figure 3.9.1.
Polymorphous low-grade adenocarcinoma. A central cellular area is surrounded by single-file ribbons of epithelial cells infiltrating the surrounding fibrous stroma.

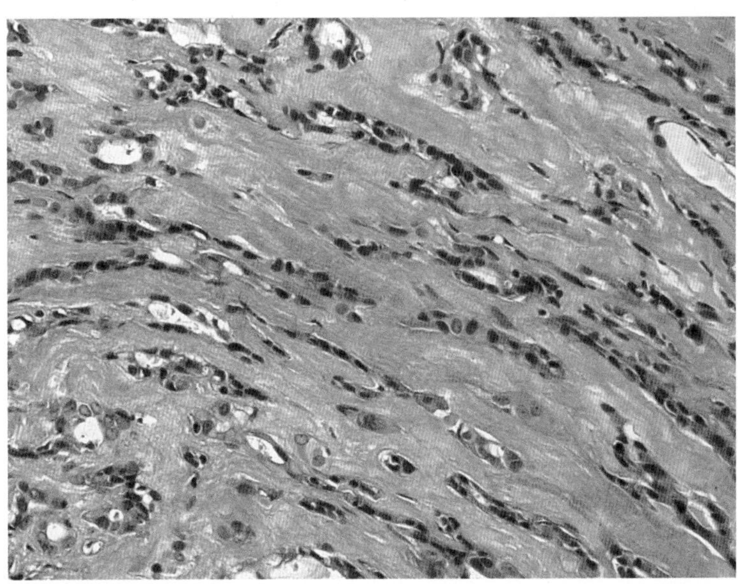

Figure 3.9.2.
Polymorphous low-grade adenocarcinoma. Small ducts lined by a single layer of cuboidal epithelial cells are seen at the left side of the image. Single-file growth is noted at the right. Some nuclei appear hyperchromatic, a compression artifact.

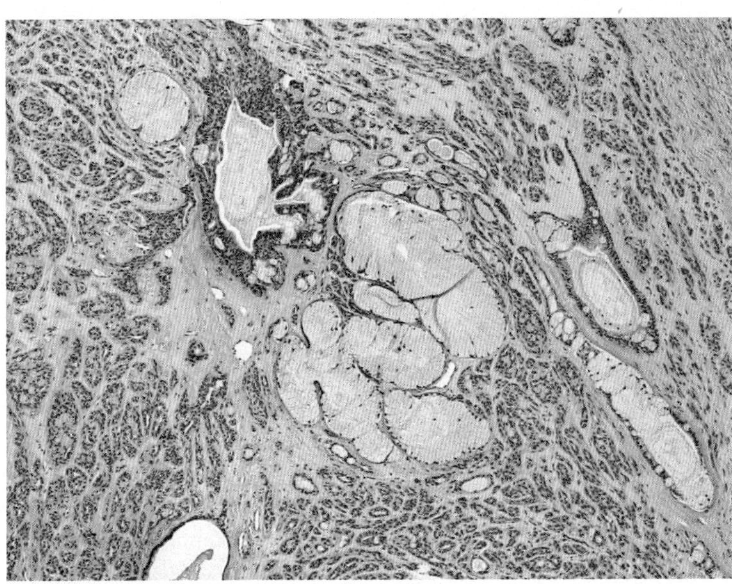

Figure 3.9.3.
Polymorphous low-grade adenocarcinoma. Tumor nests infiltrate residual mucous glands.

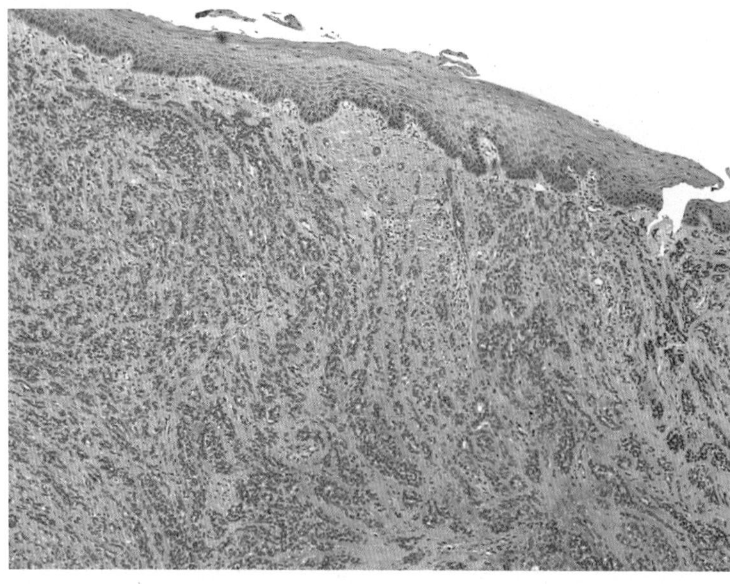

Figure 3.9.4.
Polymorphous low-grade adenocarcinoma. Infiltrating nests of small epithelial cells forming ductal structures infiltrate the lamina propria of the mucosa.

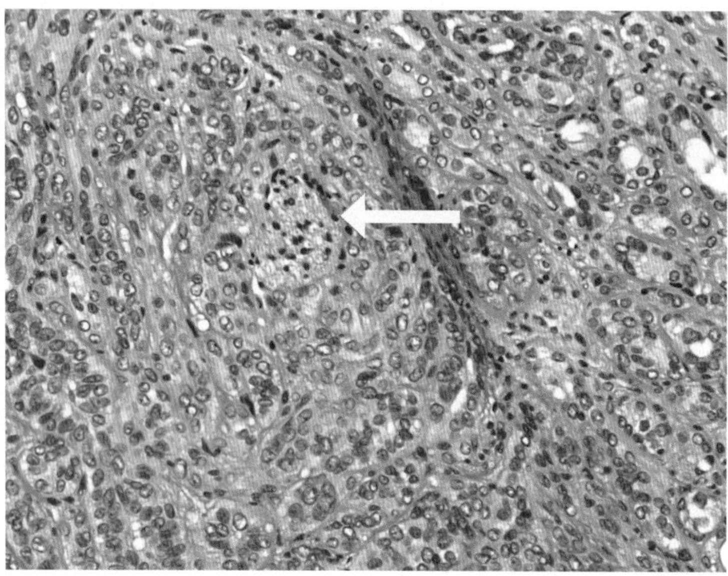

Figure 3.9.5.
Polymorphous low-grade adenocarcinoma. Nests of tumor cells encircle a tiny nerve trunk (arrow).

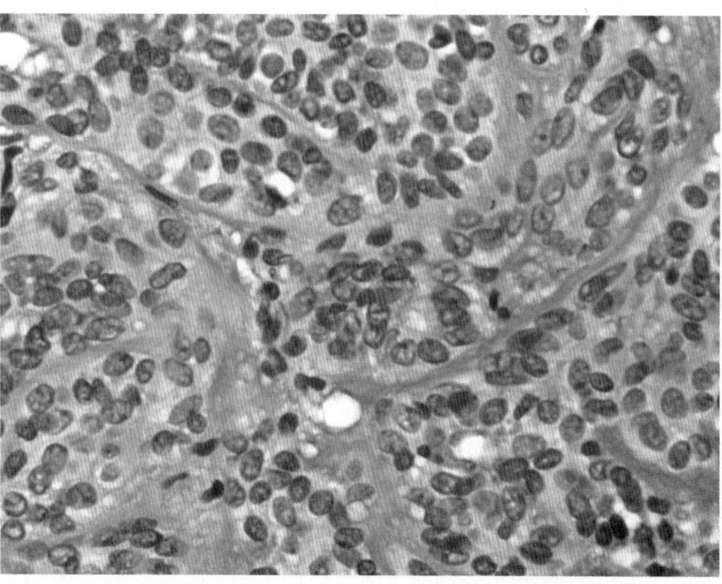

Figure 3.9.6.
Polymorphous low-grade adenocarcinoma. The tumor cells are monomorphic; the nuclei are uniform and ovoid and some are vesicular.

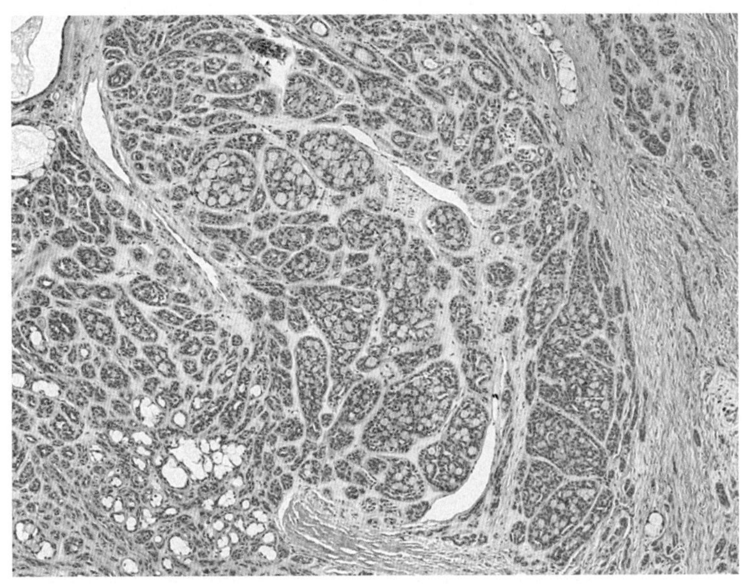

Figure 3.9.7.
Polymorphous low-grade adenocarcinoma. This part of the tumor has a cribriform pattern. Note the cells infiltrating single file at far right.

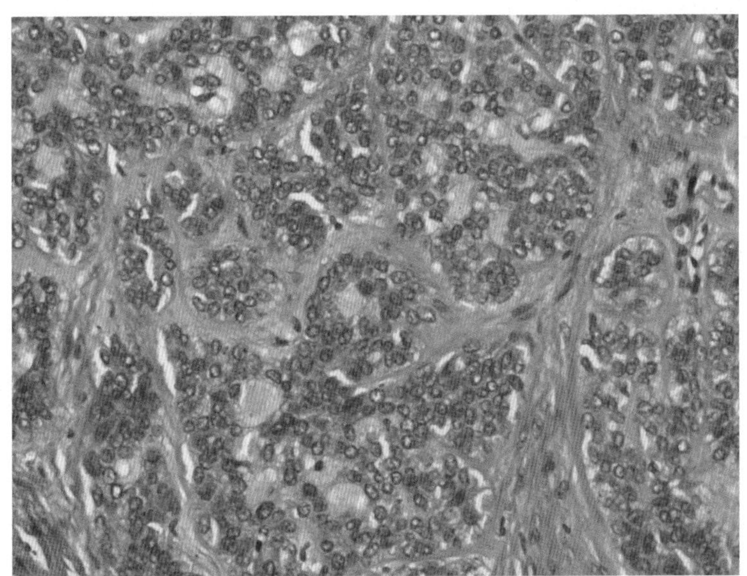

Figure 3.9.8.
Polymorphous low-grade adenocarcinoma. Small ductal structures lined by cuboidal cells with uniform ovoid nuclei.

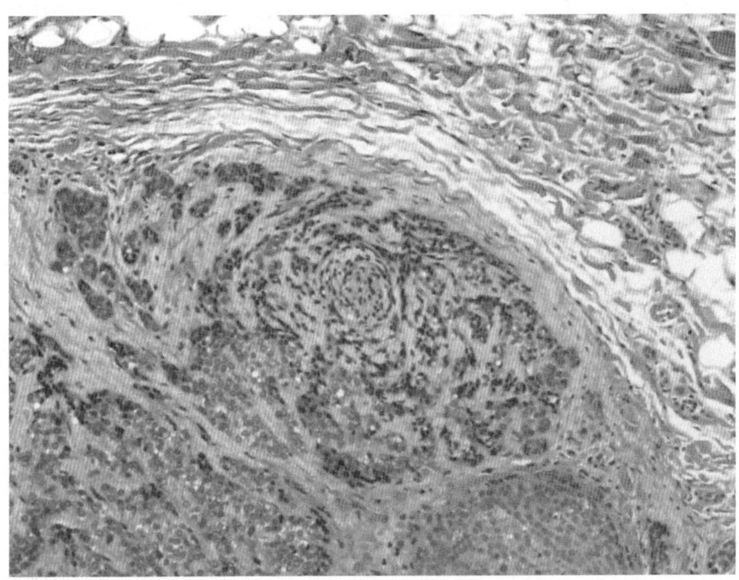

Figure 3.9.9.
Polymorphous low-grade adenocarcinoma. Infiltrating lobules of small epithelial cells with concentric, perineural growth.

3.10 Adenoid Cystic Carcinoma

Presentation

Submucosal swelling of the palate or the buccal mucosa. Can be ulcerated and/or painful.

Microscopic Findings

The main histologic patterns are cribriform, tubular, and solid. A mixture of patterns is common. Perineural invasion of small and large nerve trunks.

CRIBRIFORM

- Sheets of epithelial cells with hyperchromatic, angular nuclei surrounding pseudoluminal spaces filled with hyalinized or amorphous, frothy basophilic material producing a Swiss cheese appearance
- Inconspicuous, small ducts of cuboidal epithelial cells within the mass of tumor cells
- Fibrous or myxoid stroma

TUBULAR

- Histopathology as in cribriform, but small ducts are plentiful and form tubular structures.

SOLID

- Sheets or large islands of cells
- Increased mitotic rate and comedonecrosis

Special Stains/Immunopathology

Immunohistochemistry can be useful in attempting to identify the dual ductal and myoepithelial nature of the tumor. Ductal cells are positive for epithelial markers; the surrounding myoepithelial cells are positive for myoepithelial markers.

Histopathologic Differential

See Table 3.1: PLGA versus adenoid cystic carcinoma (page 76).

Treatment and Prognosis

Radical surgery with or without radiation. Growth is slow and relentless; difficult to eradicate. The presence of a solid component imparts a worse prognosis.

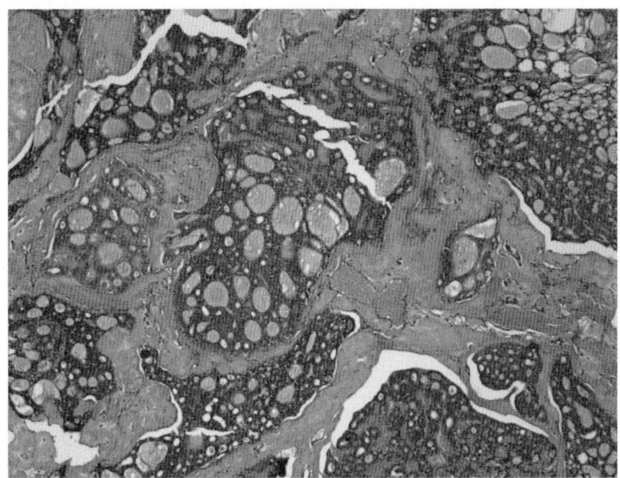

Figure 3.10.1.
Adenoid cystic carcinoma, cribriform variant. Tumor nests have a prominent Swiss cheese pattern. Dense fibrous stroma. Pseudocystic spaces are filled with lightly basophilic, frothy material.

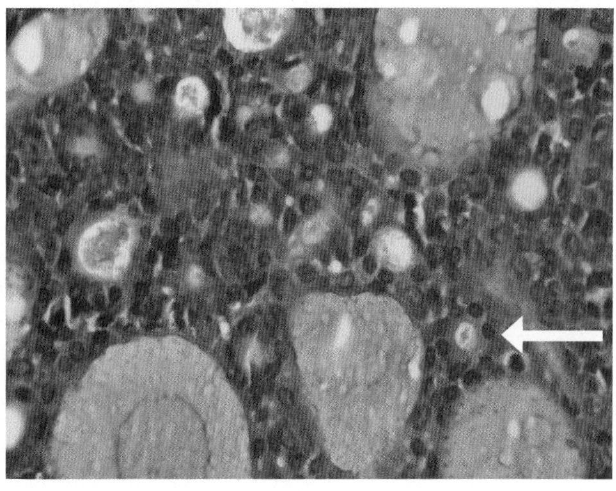

Figure 3.10.2.
Adenoid cystic carcinoma. Note the area of true ductal differentiation. The other cells in this field are predominantly myoepithelial, some with angular, hyperchromatic nuclei and indistinct cell borders.

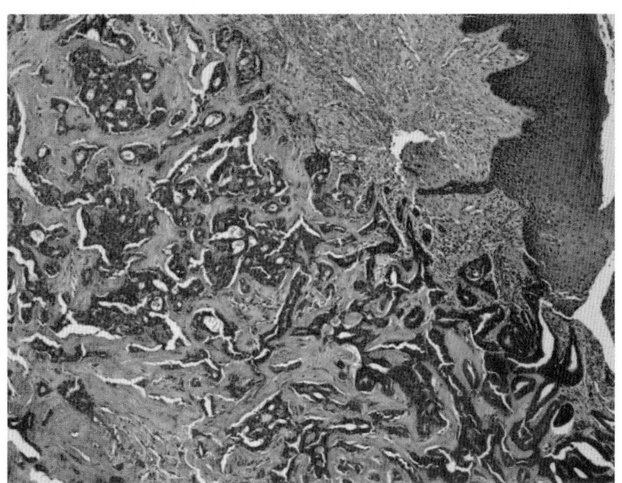

Figure 3.10.3.
Adenoid cystic carcinoma. Submucosal glandular nests of small tumor cells infiltrate the submucosa and ulcerate the mucosal epithelium.

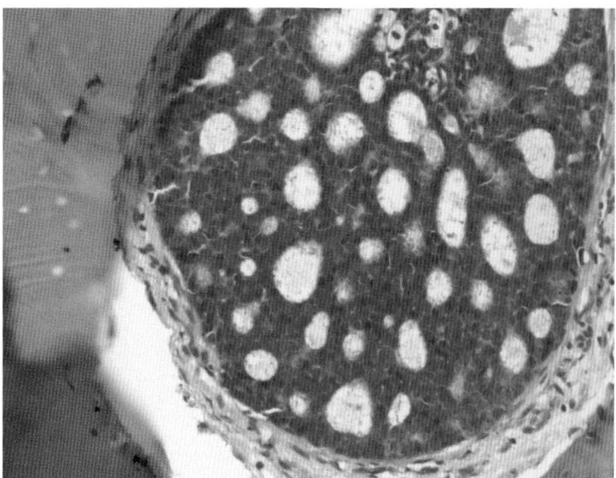

Figure 3.10.4.
Adenoid cystic carcinoma. A nest of tumor cells with a cribriform pattern infiltrates the bone of the maxilla.

3.11 Acinic Cell Adenocarcinoma

Presentation

Submucosal mass of buccal mucosa, upper lip, or palate

Microscopic Findings

- Multiple architectural patterns. Solid and microcystic with papillary epithelial proliferations is the most common; tumors with larger cystic spaces can resemble thyroid tissue. Lymphocytic infiltrate is frequent.
- Multiple cell types: Intercalated duct (small, with basophilic to amphophilic cytoplasm and centrally placed nucleus), vacuolated, acinar, or clear cell.
- Scant fibrous stroma

Special Stains/Immunopathology

Acinar and vacuolated cells contain PAS-positive, diastase-resistant zymogen-like granules and are negative for glycogen.

Histopathologic Differential

When clear cells are prominent, the following tumors enter into the differential:

- The cells of a *clear cell adenocarcinoma* usually contain glycogen and are thus PAS-positive, diastase-labile.
- The cells of a clear cell *myoepithelioma* are positive for myoepithelial markers (S100, calponin, p63, SMA, and GFAP).

Treatment and Prognosis

Complete surgical excision. Tumors of the intraoral minor glands are less aggressive than parotid acinic cell carcinomas.

Additional

At low power, most minor gland acinic cell carcinomas have a basophilic or amphophilic quality.

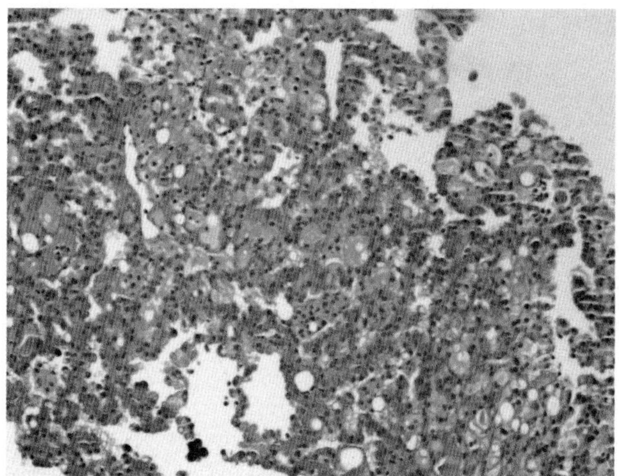

Figure 3.11.1.
Acinic cell adenocarcinoma. Acinic cell tumors often have a distinctive pale basophilic to amphophilic staining quality.

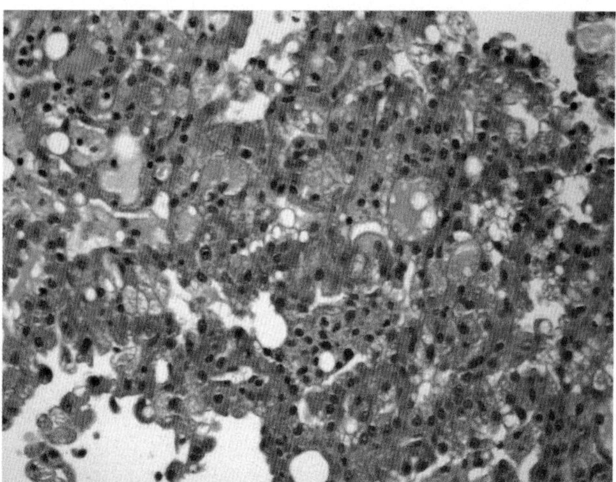

Figure 3.11.2.
Acinic cell adenocarcinoma. Most tumors of the minor glands have a papillary-microcystic growth pattern similar to the one seen here.

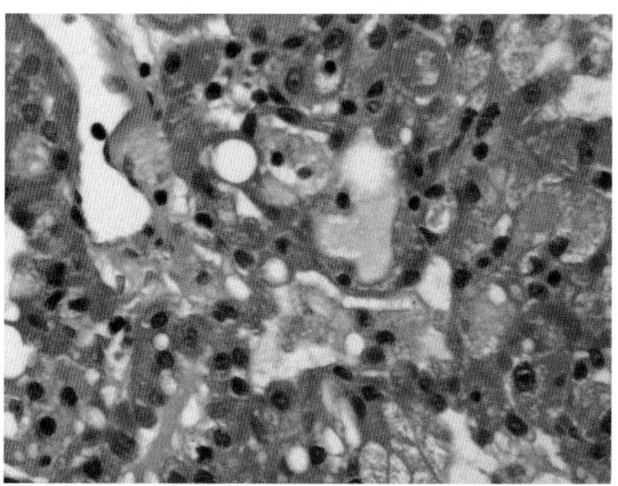

Figure 3.11.3.
Acinic cell adenocarcinoma. Most of the cells in this field are of the intercalated duct type. They are large, basaloid, with amphophilic granular cytoplasm and small, round nuclei. Interspersed are vacuolated cells and microcystic spaces.

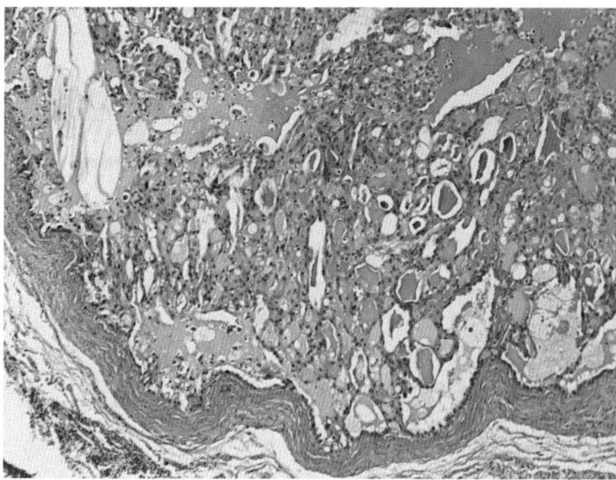

Figure 3.11.4.
Acinic cell adenocarcinoma. This tumor is largely microcystic, but some areas have fluid-filled cysts resembling thyroid follicles. The prominent capsule here is an unusual finding.

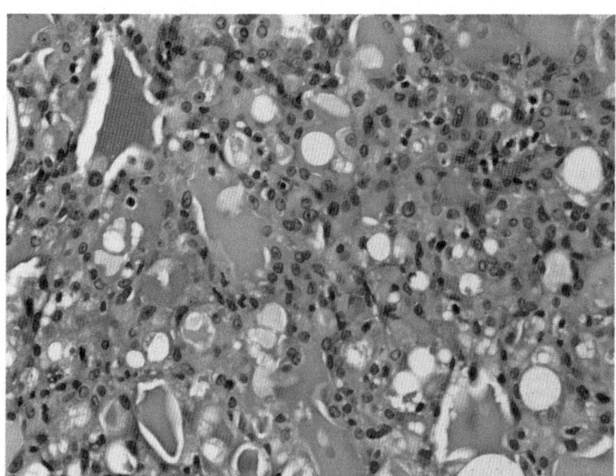

Figure 3.11.5.
Acinic cell adenocarcinoma. Small basaloid epithelial cells with amphophilic granular cytoplasm and round nuclei form solid nests and thyroid-like follicles.

3.12 Clear Cell Adenocarcinoma

Presentation

A swelling of the palate, buccal mucosa, or tongue. A hyalinizing variant is common in the base of the tongue. Older adults.

Microscopic Findings

- Poorly circumscribed; infiltrative.
- Medium-size, round-to-polygonal cells with a clear or eosinophilic cytoplasm.
- The hyalinizing variant has prominent intervening stroma ranging from feathery wisps to thick, hyalinized bands.

Special Stains/Immunopathology

The clear cells are usually positive for glycogen (PAS-positive, diastase-labile).

Histopathologic Differential

Several other salivary gland neoplasms have a clear cell component.

- The clear cells of a *mucoepidermoid carcinoma* will be positive for mucin.
- The vacuolated cells of *acinic cell carcinoma* can contain PAS-positive, diastase-resistant zymogen-like granules.
- The clear cells of *epithelial–myoepithelial carcinoma,* which is rare in the minor glands, are positive for myoepithelial markers.
- *Metastatic renal cell carcinoma* has CD10-positive clear cells accompanied by a prominent vascularity.

Treatment and Prognosis

Surgical excision. A low-grade malignancy.

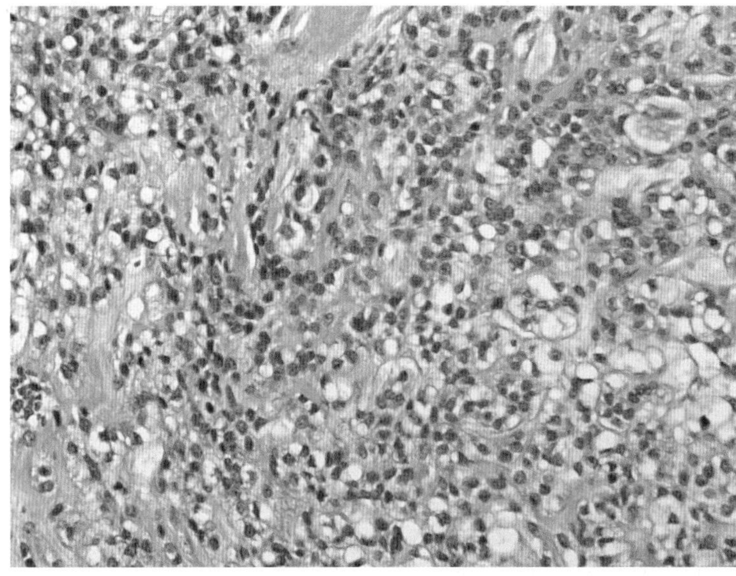

Figure 3.12.1.
Clear cell adenocarcinoma. Infiltrating nests of small epithelial cells admixed with foci of clear cells. Stroma is scant and fibrous.

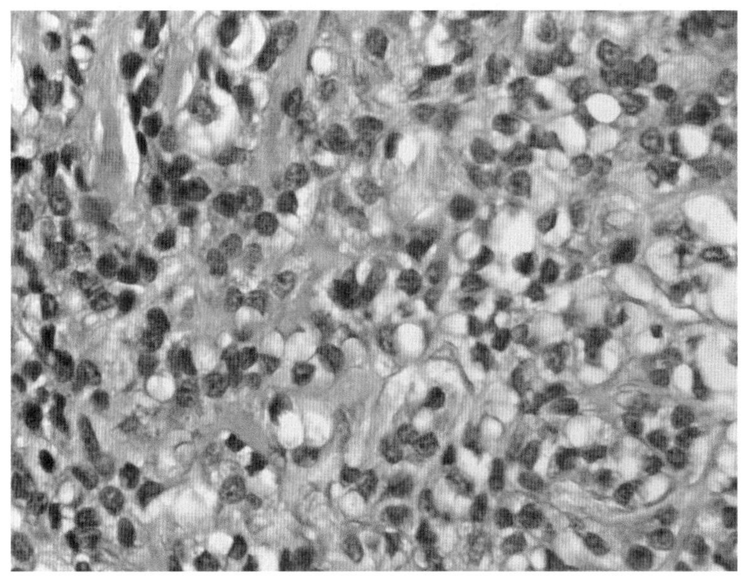

Figure 3.12.2.
Clear cell adenocarcinoma. The tumor cells are polyhedral, with a clear cytoplasm and hyperchromatic nuclei. The cytoplasm is usually positive for glycogen.

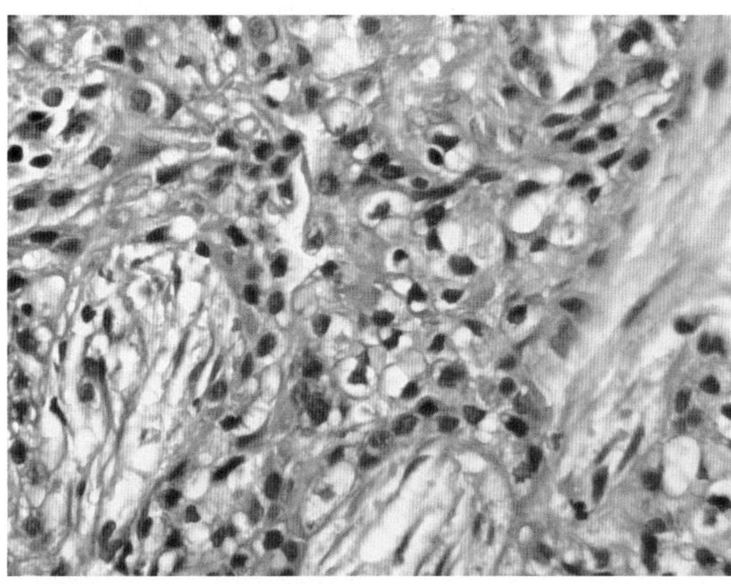

Figure 3.12.3.
Clear cell adenocarcinoma. Not all cells are clear; some have a granular, eosinophilic cytoplasm.

3.13 Basal Cell Adenocarcinoma

Presentation

Slow-growing mass of the buccal mucosa, palate, lip, or tongue. In older adults.

Microscopic Findings

- Sheets and large nests of basaloid cells with peripheral palisading of nuclei
- Invasive growth pattern: infiltration into adjacent tissue, perineural invasion
- Mitotic figures and cellular pleomorphism sometimes seen
- Prominent eosinophilic, hyaline bands in the membranous variant
- Fibrous stroma

Histopathologic Differential

- The *basal cell adenoma* does invade local structures and/or nerves or vessels.
- The solid variant of *adenoid cystic carcinoma* has dark, angulated nuclei in contrast to the paler-staining, round, vesicular nuclei of basal cell adenocarcinoma. In addition, the cells' nests of adenoid cystic carcinoma will lack peripheral palisading and almost always have at least a few cribriform areas.

Treatment and Prognosis

Wide local excision. The diagnosis of malignancy is based on demonstrating invasion; cellular pleomorphism is not a constant feature.

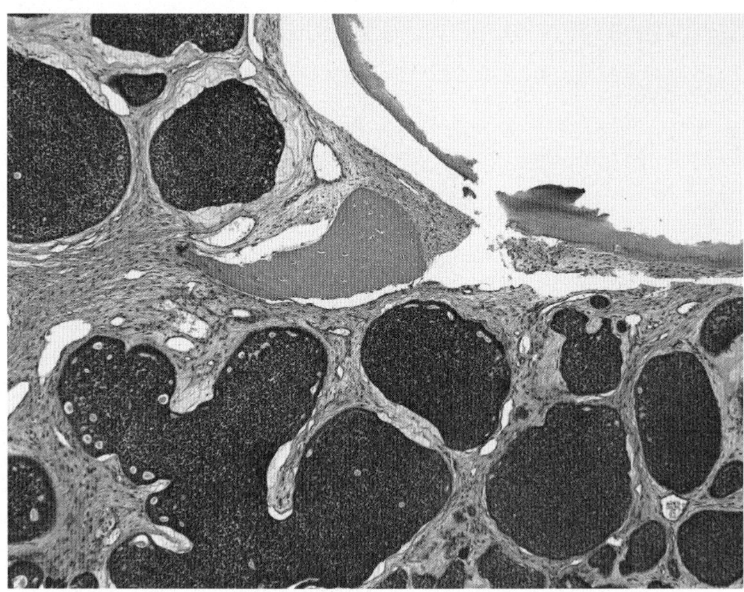

Figure 3.13.1.
Basal cell adenocarcinoma. Islands of densely packed, deeply basophilic epithelial cells infiltrate the fibrous tissue and bone.

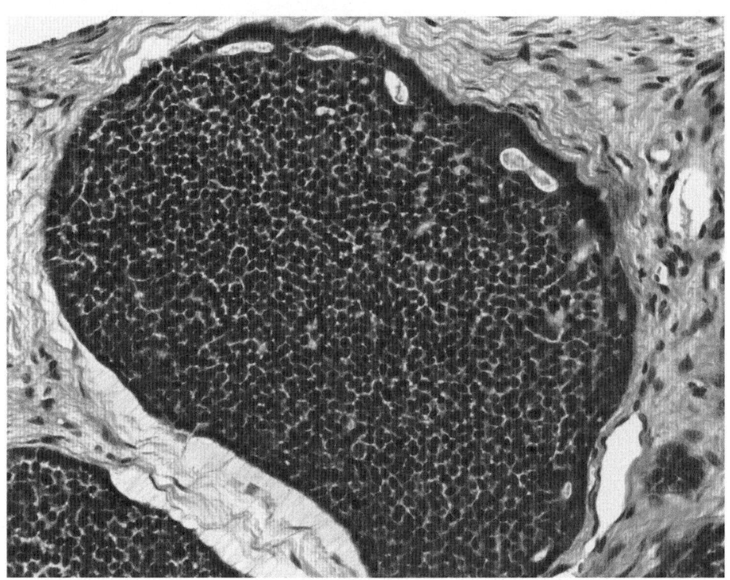

Figure 3.13.2.
Basal cell adenocarcinoma. Irregularly shaped nodules of basaloid tumor cells contain scattered ductal structures at the periphery.

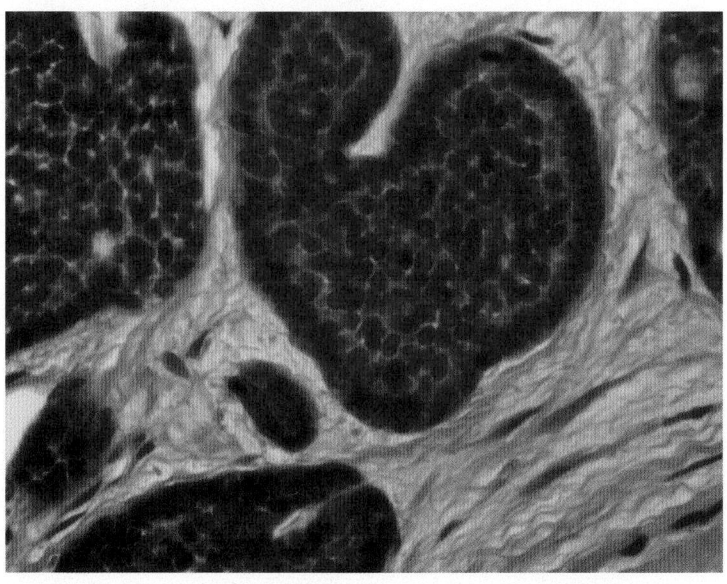

Figure 3.13.3.
Basal cell adenocarcinoma. Palisading of nuclei along the periphery of the tumor nests. Cytologic atypia is minimal; cellular density and nuclear hyperchromaticity are prominent.

3.14 Adenocarcinoma, Not otherwise specified (NOS)

Definition

A salivary gland carcinoma that cannot be easily placed histologically into any of the other, better-defined adenocarcinoma categories

Presentation

Slow-growing mass, often of the palate. In older adults.

Microscopic Findings

- A wide variety of growth patterns: all demonstrate glandular or duct-like structures and infiltrative growth.
- Cytomorphology and mitotic rate are used to divide these tumors into low, intermediate, and high grades.

Histopathologic Differential

- Adenocarcinoma, NOS is by definition a diagnosis of exclusion. Before arriving at the diagnosis, the pathologist has to rule out the other established salivary gland malignancies.

Treatment and Prognosis

Surgical excision. Prognosis depends on the grade and stage of tumor.

Additional

Many cases of adenocarcinoma, NOS from older series would probably now be classified as PLGAs.

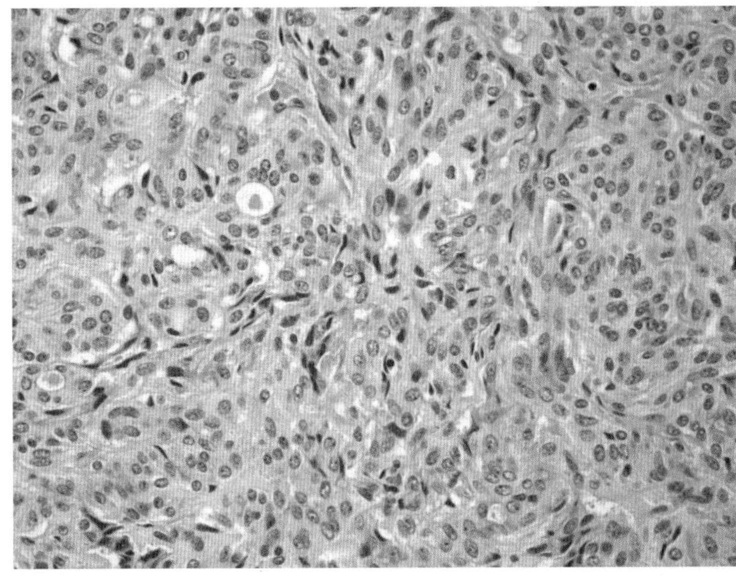

Figure 3.14.1.
Adenocarcinoma, NOS, low grade. Closely packed epithelial islands contain occasional ducts. The intervening fibrovascular tissue is scant.

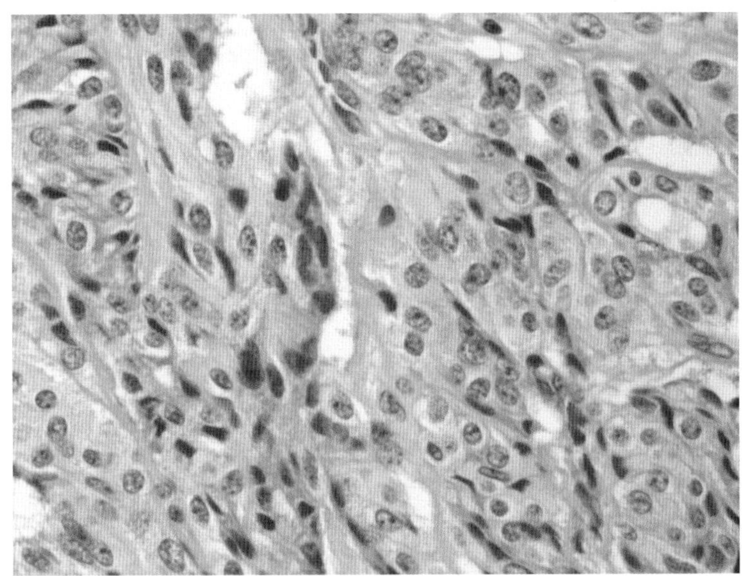

Figure 3.14.2.
Adenocarcinoma, NOS, low grade. The tumor is cytologically bland. Nuclear pleomorphism is minimal, and cells have abundant cytoplasm.

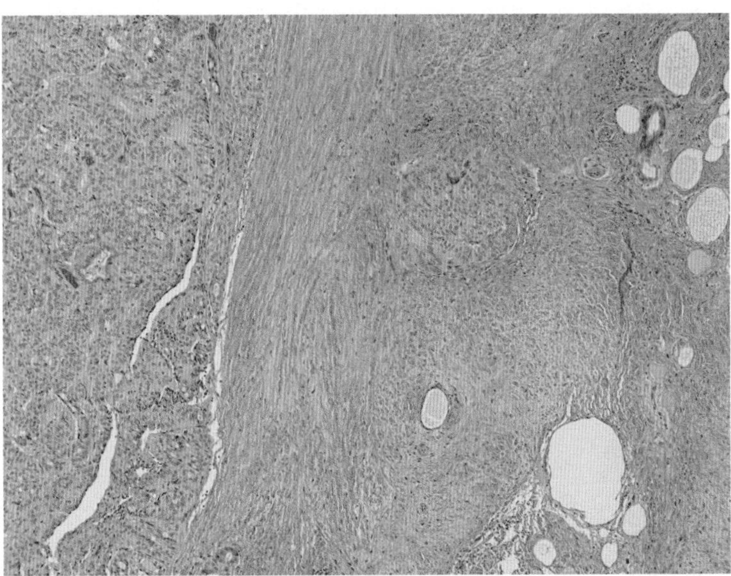

Figure 3.14.3.
Adenocarcinoma, NOS, low grade. Nests of tumor (one large, several smaller) infiltrate the adjacent fibrous stroma.

Bibliography and Suggested Reading

3.2

Carlson DL. Necrotizing sialometaplasia: a practical approach to the diagnosis. *Arch Pathol Lab Med.* 2009;133:692–698.

3.4

Zormpa MT, Sarigelou AS, Eleftheriou AN, et al. Plasmacytoid myoepithelioma of the palate: case report. *Head Neck Pathol.* 2011;5:154–158.

3.5

Smullin SE, Fielding AF, Susarla SM, Pringle G, Eichstaedt R. Canalicular adenoma of the palate: case report and literature review. *Oral Surg Oral Med Oral Pathol Oral Radiol Endod.* 2004;98(1):32–36.

3.6

Lim CS, Ngu I, Collins AP, et al. Papillary cystadenoma of a minor salivary gland: report of a case involving cytological analysis and review of the literature. *Oral Surg Oral Med Oral Pathol Oral Radiol Endod.* 2008;105:e28–e33.

3.7

Argyres MI, Golitz LE. Sialadenoma papilliferum of the palate: case report and literature review. *J Cutan Pathol.* 1999;26(5):259–262.

3.8

Brandwein MS, Ivanov K, Wallace DI, et al. Mucoepidermoid carcinoma: a clinicopathologic study of 80 patients with special reference to histological grading. *Am J Surg Pathol.* 2001;25:835–845.

Chenevert J, Barnes LE, Chiosea SI. Mucoepidermoid carcinoma: a five-decade journey. *Virchows Arch.* 2011;458:133–140.

3.9

Freedman PD, Lumerman H. Lobular carcinoma of intraoral minor salivary gland origin. Report of twelve cases. *Oral Surg Oral Med Oral Pathol.* 1983;56:157–166.

Seethala RR, Johnson JT, Barnes EL, et al. Polymorphous low-grade adenocarcinoma: the University of Pittsburgh experience. *Arch Otolaryngol Head Neck Surg.* 2010;136:385–392.

3.10

Woo VL, Bhuiya T, Kelsch R. Assessment of CD43 expression in adenoid cystic carcinomas, polymorphous low-grade adenocarcinomas, and monomorphic adenomas. *Oral Surg Oral Med Oral Pathol Oral Radiol Endod.* 2006;102:495–500.

3.11

Omlie JE, Koutlas IG. Acinic cell carcinoma of minor salivary glands: a clinicopathologic study of 21 cases. *J Oral Maxillofac Surg.* 2010;68:2053–2057.

Triantafillidou K, Iordanidis F, Psomaderis K, et al. Acinic cell carcinoma of minor salivary glands: a clinical and immunohistochemical study. *J Oral Maxillofac Surg.* 2010;68:2489–2496.

3.12

Casani AP, Marchetti M, Seccia V, et al. Clear cell adenocarcinoma of the base of the tongue: a case report and review of the literature. *Ear Nose Throat J.* 2011;90:E9–E16.

3.13

Ward BK, Seethala RR, Barnes EL, et al. Basal cell adenocarcinoma of a hard palate minor salivary gland: case report and review of the literature. *Head Neck Oncol.* 2009;1:41.

CHAPTER

4

Epithelial Pathology and Selected Mucosal Diseases

Epithelial hyperplasia and hyperkeratosis
Epithelial dysplasia
Tobacco pouch keratosis
Verrucous hyperplasia/verrucous carcinoma
Squamous cell carcinoma
Basaloid squamous cell carcinoma
Spindle cell carcinoma
Leukoedema
Migratory glossitis (geographic tongue)
Cheek/tongue chewing lesion
Oral hairy leukoplakia
Verruciform xanthoma
Condyloma acuminatum
Aphthous ulcer
CMV ulcer
Oral lichen planus
Lichenoid mucositis
Mucous membrane pemphigoid
Pemphigus vulgaris
Amalgam tattoo
Oral melanotic macule
Intramucosal nevus
Oral mucosal melanoma
Sjögren syndrome
Sarcoidosis

Introduction

Leukoplakias and erythroplakias (white and red patches) are the most common oral mucosal lesions submitted to the pathology laboratory. In about 80% of the cases, leukoplakias result from hyperplasia of the lesional epithelium or hyperplasia and hyperkeratosis. In 20%, the histologic diagnosis is epithelial dysplasia, Carcinoma in situ (CIS), or invasive squamous carcinoma. At initial histologic examination, 90% of the erythroplakias show severe epithelial dysplasia, CIS, or superficial invasive carcinoma. Overall, the leukoplakias have a 4% transformation rate to squamous carcinoma, and the dysplastic lesions show about a 20% transformation rate. The degree of dysplasia directly correlates with the transformation to invasive carcinoma.

In most instances, oral squamous carcinoma is easily diagnosed, but for two aggressive variants, basaloid squamous and spindle cell, diagnosis may require immunohistochemical stains and attentive study of the overlying epithelium. At the other end of the dysplasia spectrum are two lesions with minimal cytologic atypia—verrucous hyperplasia and verrucous carcinoma. Since their histology is similar, accurate orientation of the specimen, the presence of *en masse* invasion, and knowledge of the clinical history become necessary to render the correct diagnosis. These features are further discussed in the outline of these lesions.

4.1 Epithelial Hyperplasia and Hyperkeratosis

Presentation

A white patch (leukoplakia) on the tongue, gingiva, or buccal mucosa

Microscopic Findings

- Increased thickness of stratified squamous epithelium and the overlying keratin
- Mild chronic inflammatory cell infiltrate in the lamina propria

Histopathologic Differential

Epithelial dysplasia has a loss of the normal organization of the epithelial strata, tear drop-shaped rete ridges, and atypical cells and nuclei.

Treatment and Prognosis

Follow-up or excision

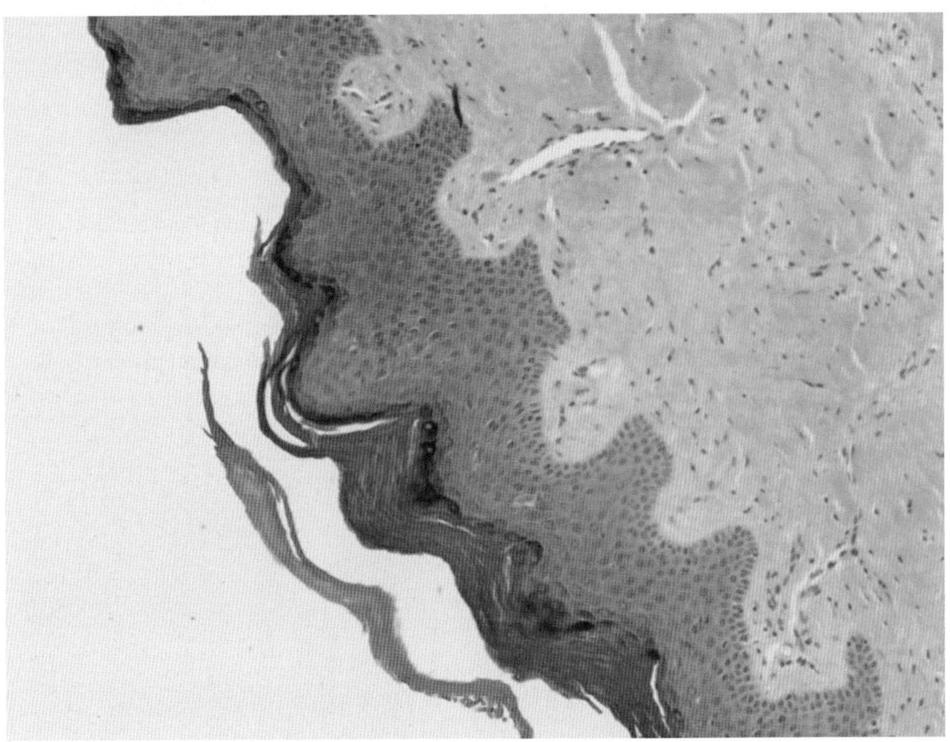

Figure 4.1.1.
Hyperkeratosis. This mucosal leukoplakia consists of marked hyperkeratosis.

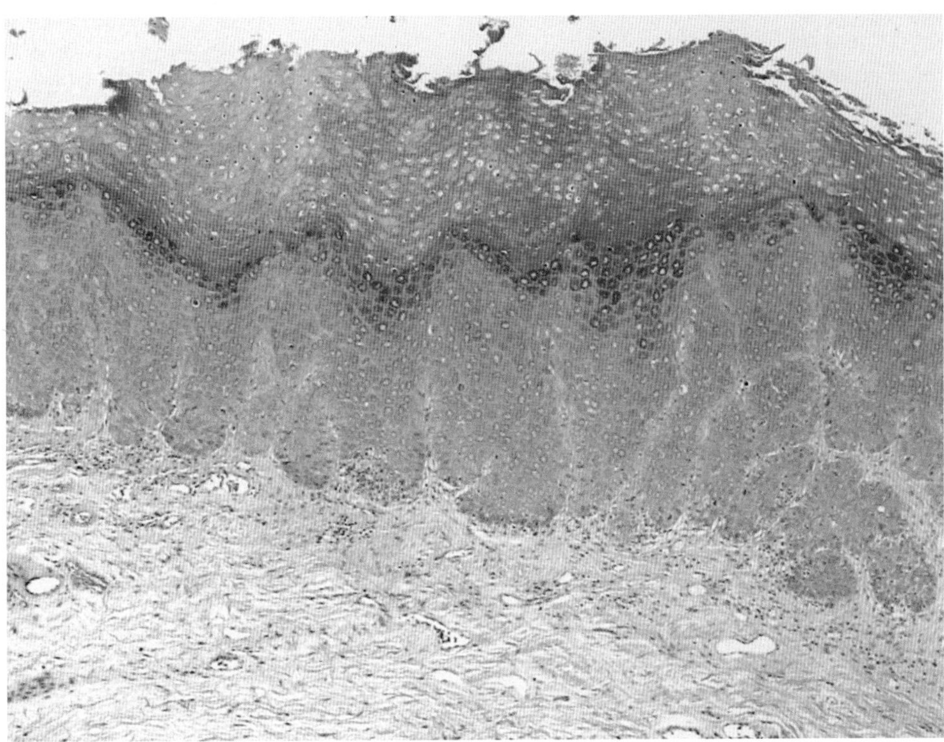

Figure 4.1.2.
Hyperkeratosis and epithelial hyperplasia. In this example, the epithelium shows hyperparakeratosis and marked epithelial hyperplasia. Epithelial islands in the lamina propria are results of the trangential cut.

4.2 Epithelial Dysplasia

Presentation

A white patch (leukoplakia) or velvety red area (erythroplakia) of the oral mucosa

Microscopic Findings

The accepted criteria for the evaluation of dysplasia are architectural changes and cellular atypia.

Architectural changes:

- Disturbances in normal stratification of the mucosal stratified squamous epithelium
- Dyskeratosis (keratinization of parabasal cells and improper keratinization pattern)
- Loss of cell cohesion
- Teardrop-shaped rete ridges
- Mitotic figures above the basal cell layer

Cellular atypia:

- Nuclear enlargement
- Nuclear pleomorphism
- Nuclear hyperchromasia
- Atypical mitotic figures
- Increased nuclear to cytoplasmic ratio

Based upon the above architectural and cellular features, the dysplasia is graded as follows:

- Mild, when changes are confined to the lower one-third of the epithelium
- Moderate, when changes involve less than two-thirds of the epithelium
- Severe, when changes involve more than two-thirds of the epithelium
- Carcinoma in situ, when the entire lesional epithelium shows undifferentiated basaloid or other atypical squamous cells with cytologic atypia and often no keratinization

Treatment and Prognosis

Excision and discontinuation of the use of tobacco products and alcohol. Close follow-up.

Additional

In cases of moderate to severe dysplasia, it is important to examine the specimen at multiple levels to rule out foci of microinvasion.

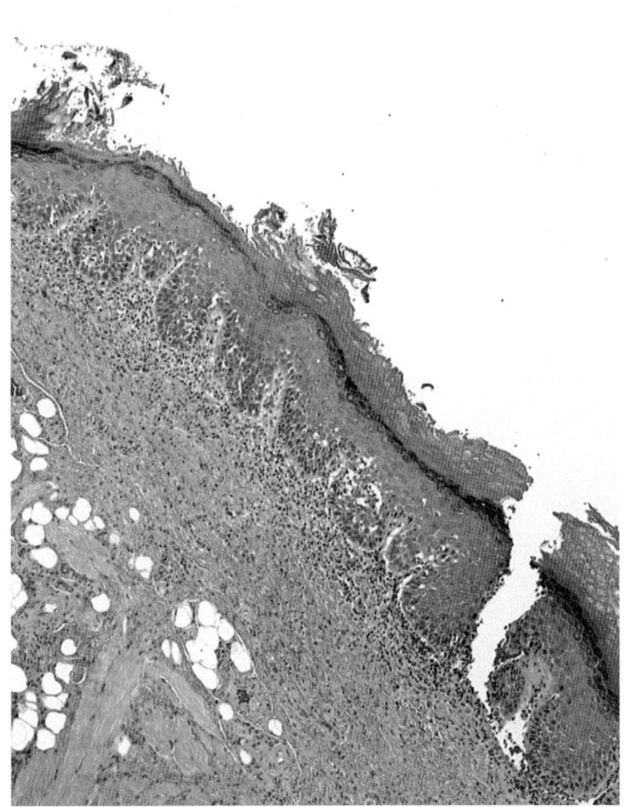

Figure 4.2.1.
Epithelial dysplasia, mild. Hyperkeratosis and teardrop-shaped rete ridges. The lamina propria contains a mild inflammatory cell infiltrate.

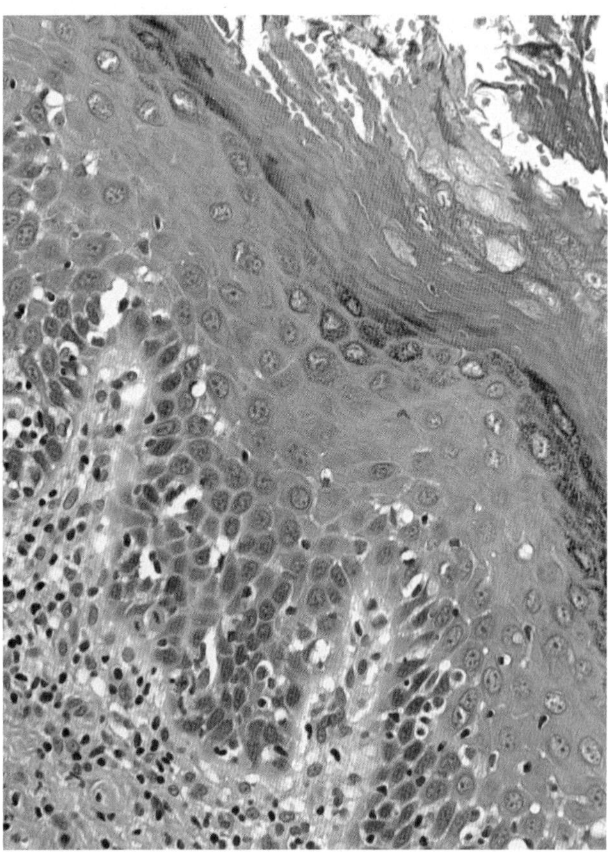

Figure 4.2.2.
Epithelial dysplasia, mild. Loss of cell cohesion in the basilar layer, basilar hyperplasia, spindling, and hyperchromasia of basal cell nuclei. Changes are confined to the lower one-third of the epithelium.

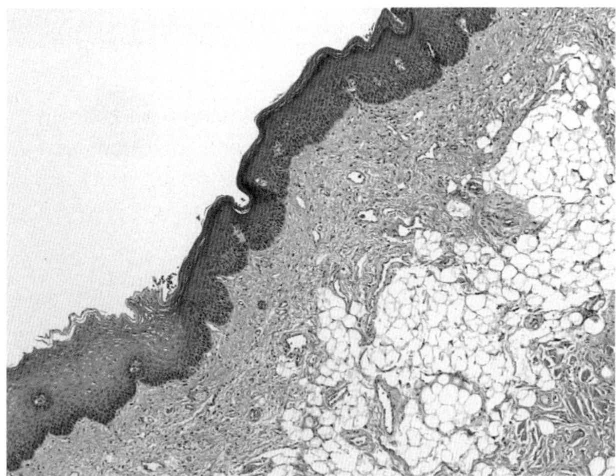

Figure 4.2.3.
Epithelial dysplasia, moderate. Hyperkeratosis with mild epithelial hyperplasia and variation in the shape of rete ridges. Note the abrupt change from normal squamous epithelium on the left.

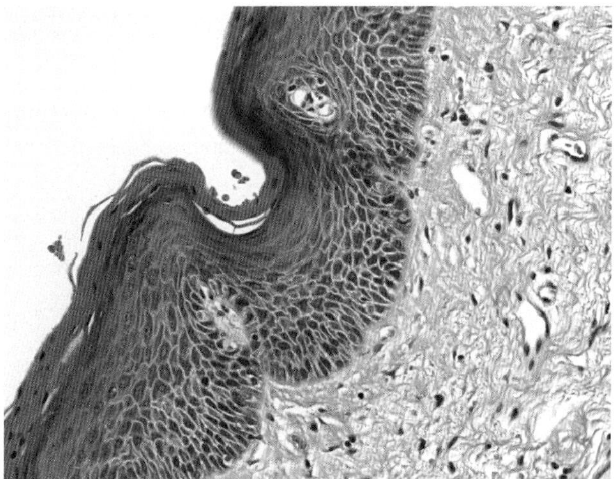

Figure 4.2.4.
Epithelial dysplasia, moderate. Tear drop-shaped rete ridges, loss of normal stratification, and nuclear hyperchromasia limited to the lower half of the epithelium.

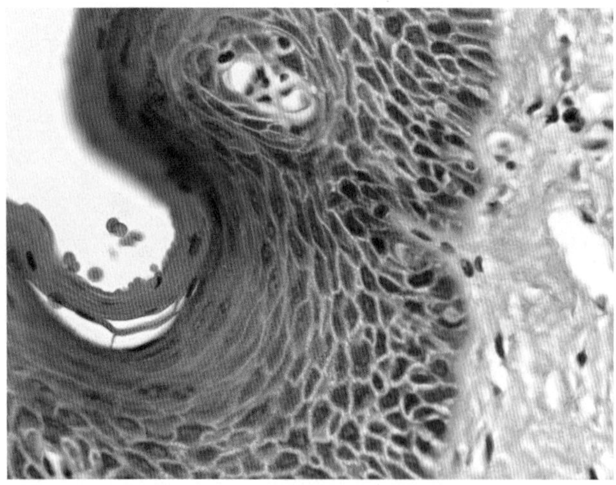

Figure 4.2.5.
Epithelial dysplasia, moderate. Basal cell hyperplasia and loss of normal orientation.

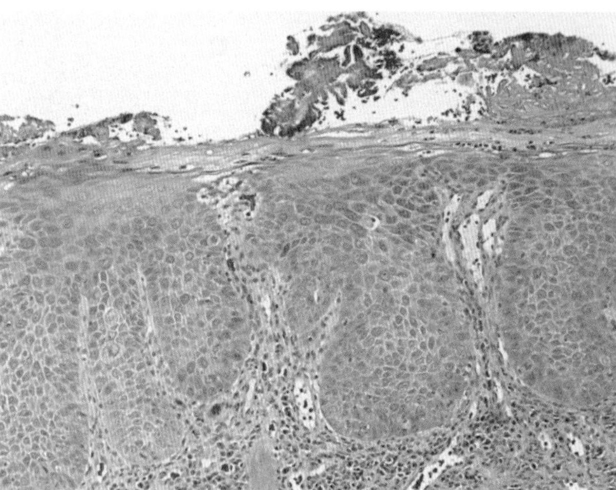

Figure 4.2.6.
Epithelial dysplasia, severe. Loss of epithelial stratification with intense inflammatory response and teardrop-shaped rete ridges.

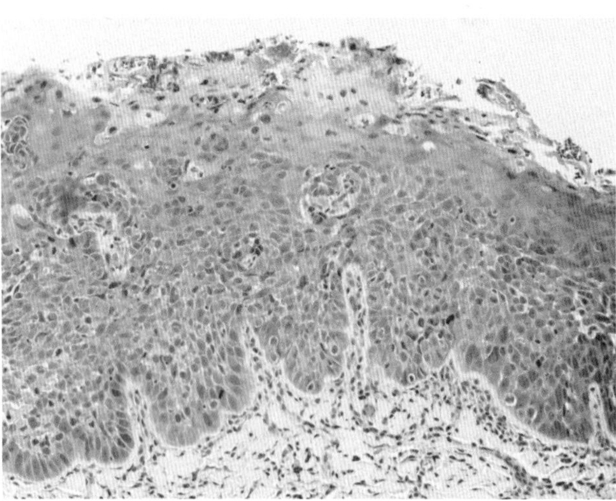

Figure 4.2.7.
Epithelial dysplasia, severe. Dysplasia involves almost the entire lesional thickness of the stratified squamous epithelium.

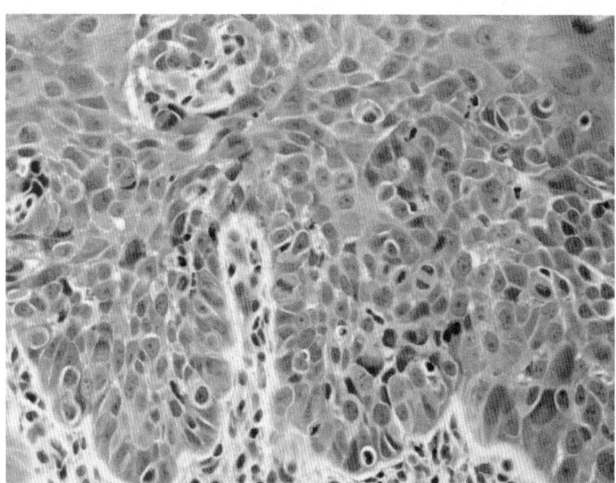

Figure 4.2.8.
Epithelial dysplasia, severe. Normal epithelial stratification is lost. Cells are pleomorphic, with enlarged, hyperchromatic nuclei. Cells are dyskeratotic, and mitoses are numerous and not limited to the basal layer.

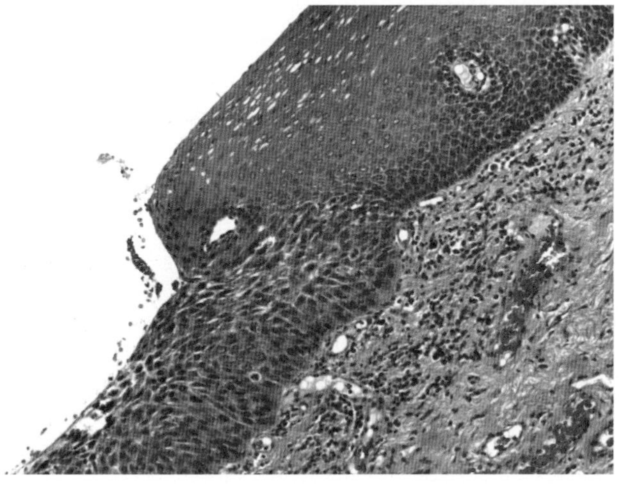

Figure 4.2.9.
Carcinoma in situ. Dysplastic epithelial cells are seen throughout the entire thickness of the epithelium. Note the area of abrupt transition from the relatively normal epithelium on the upper right.

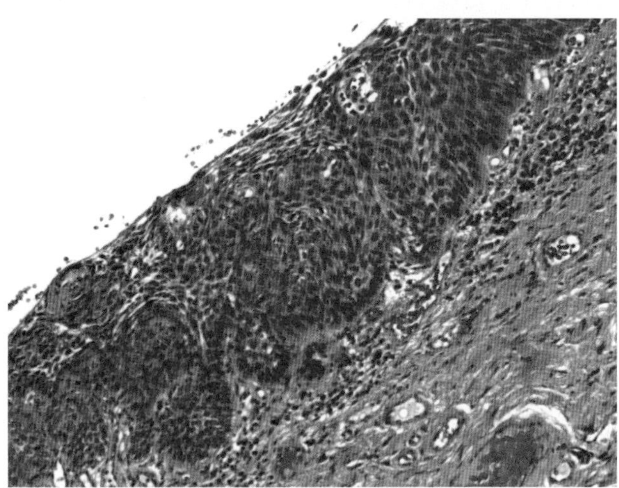

Figure 4.2.10.
Carcinoma in situ. Loss of normal cell orientation, hyperchromasia of nuclei, tear drop-shaped rete ridges. The entire epithelial thickness is involved.

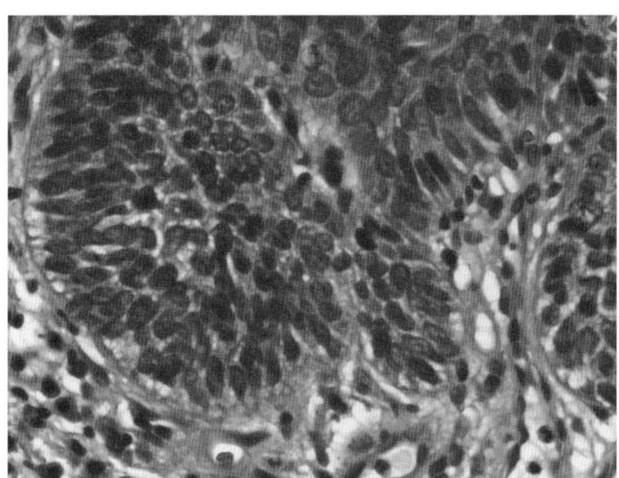

Figure 4.2.11.
Carcinoma in situ. Densely packed, poorly differentiated basaloid dysplastic cells.

4.3 Tobacco Pouch Keratosis

Definition

A translucent white lesion produced by the chronic use of chewing tobacco and snuff, both moist and dry

Presentation

- Painless leukoplakia ranging from thin, translucent, and fissured to thick, white, and corrugated
- Retraction of gingival tissue from teeth where tobacco is held

Microscopic Findings

- Epithelial hyperplasia
- Hyperkeratosis with chevron tips (church spires)
- Superficial epithelial edema
- Eosinophilic, hyalinized material in the lamina propria and around mucous glands

Treatment and Prognosis

- After discontinuation of tobacco product, lesions generally disappear within 2 to 3 weeks.
- The risk of transformation to squamous carcinoma is greatest with dry snuff used over a period of many years.

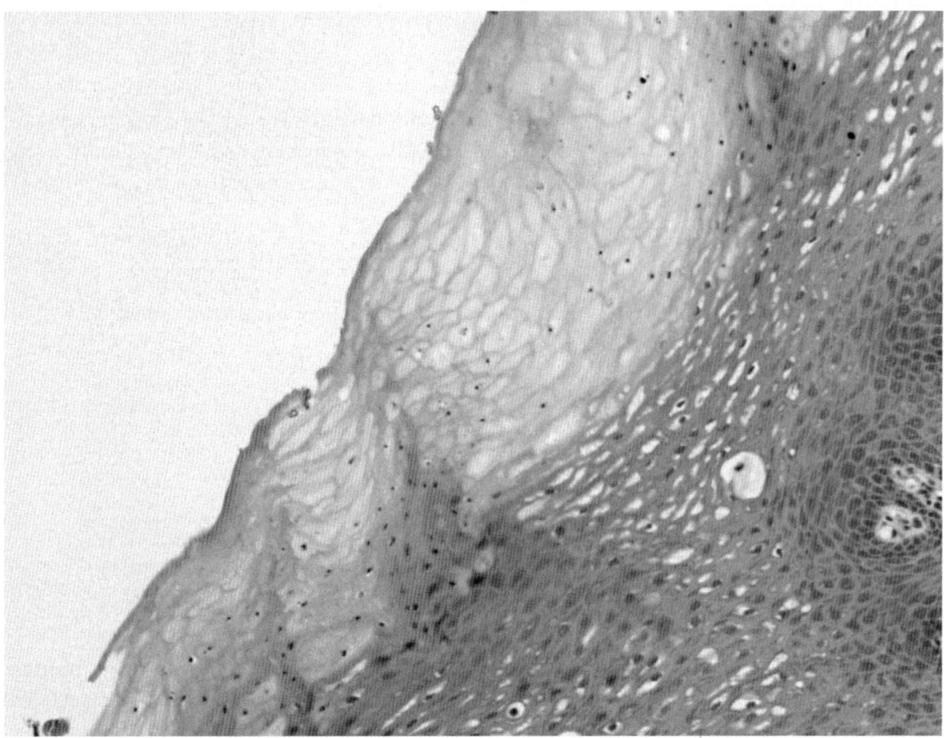

Figure 4.3.1.
Tobacco pouch keratosis. Marked hyperkeratosis and epithelial edema. The pyknotic nuclei of the parakeratin layer condense in spots to form chevron tips (church spires).

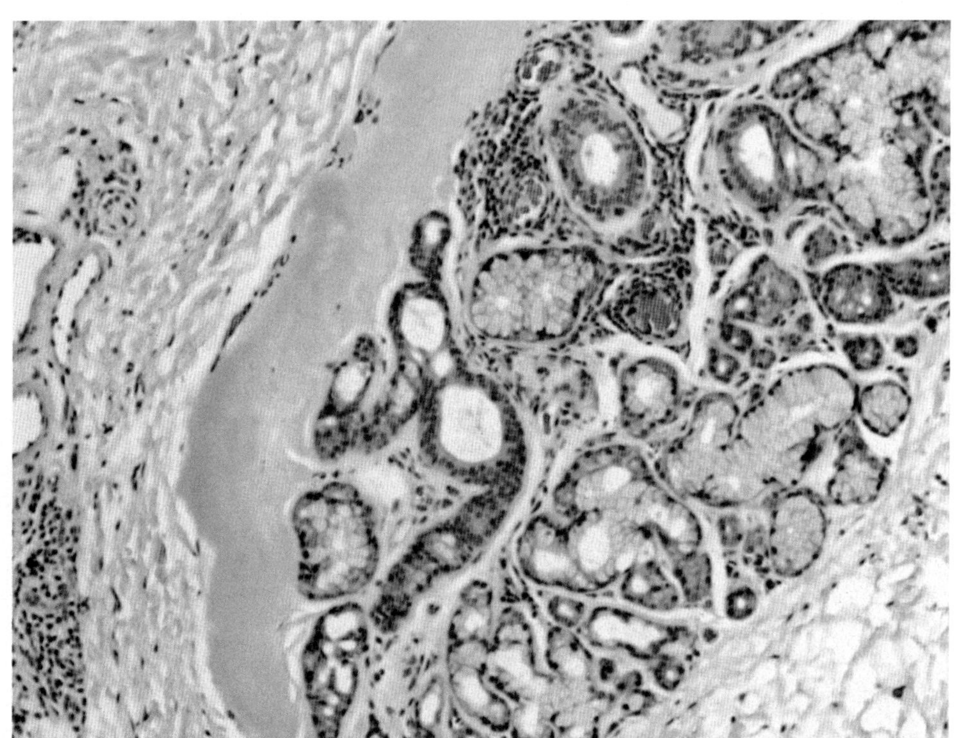

Figure 4.3.2.
Tobacco pouch keratosis. Eosinophilic, hyalinized material around submucosal mucous glands.

4.4 Verrucous Hyperplasia/Verrucous Carcinoma

Definition

Verrucous carcinoma is a highly differentiated, locally destructive squamous *en masse* carcinoma that does not metastasize. Verrucous hyperplasia, a clinically and histologically similar—but purely exophytic—epithelial lesion, is benign but associated with an increased risk of transformation to invasive carcinoma.

Presentation

Large, white, exophytic, papillary tumor. Mandibular mucobuccal fold, gingiva, buccal mucosa, or tongue. In older adults, mostly males.

Microscopic Findings

COMMON TO BOTH LESIONS

- Exophytic mass of hyperplastic epithelium
- Broad, bulbous, pushing rete pegs
- Hyperkeratotic, warty surface
- Infiltrate of lymphocytes and plasma cells at the epithelial-stromal interface

HISTOLOGICAL DIFFERENCES

- In verrucous hyperplasia, the base of the lesion is at the same level as the adjacent normal mucosal epithelium, which can show various degrees of epithelial dysplasia.
- In verrucous carcinoma, the base of the lesion extends below the level of the adjacent normal mucosal epithelium.

Treatment and Prognosis

Excision with close follow-up. Increased risk of transformation to invasive squamous cell carcinoma.

Careful physical examination of the entire oral cavity and follow-up of the patient should be done to rule out *proliferative verrucous leukoplakia*, a clinicopathologic entity characterized by a progressive leukoplakia that spreads and eventually, in almost all cases, evolves into squamous cell carcinoma. Verrucous hyperplasia and verrucous carcinoma are stages that the proliferative verrucous leukoplakia goes through before invasive squamous cell carcinoma develops.

Additional

Verrucous carcinoma's *en masse* pushing front and lack of frank dysplasia make the diagnosis of carcinoma difficult. The final diagnosis is best reserved for the examination of the entire tumor.

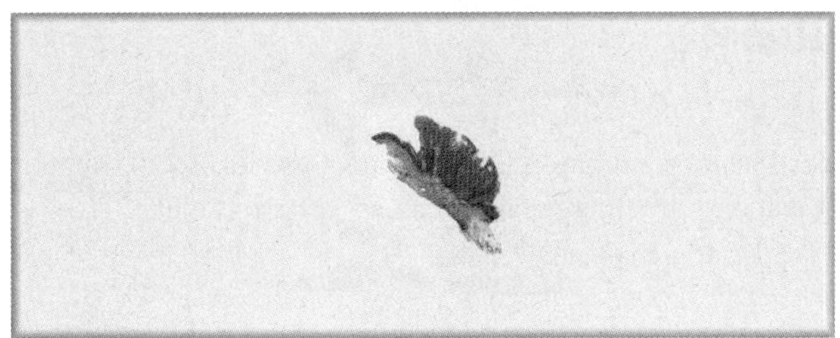

Figure 4.4.1.
Verrucous hyperplasia. Broad nests of epithelium extend up and outward but not below the level of the surrounding mucosal epithelium. The surface is hyperkeratotic and verrucous.

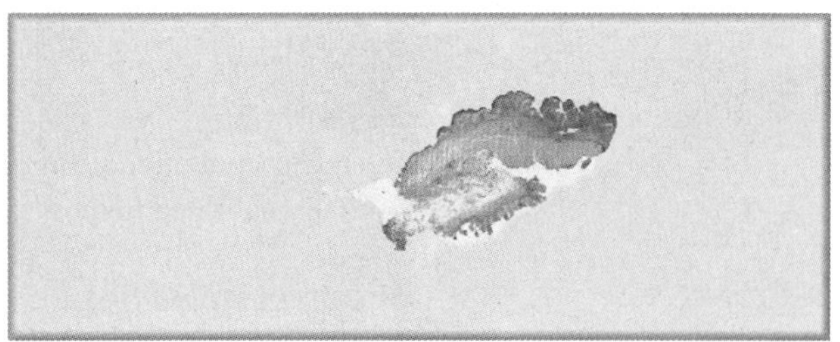

Figure 4.4.2.
Verrucous carcinoma. Broad nests of epithelium extend below the level of the surrounding mucosal epithelium.

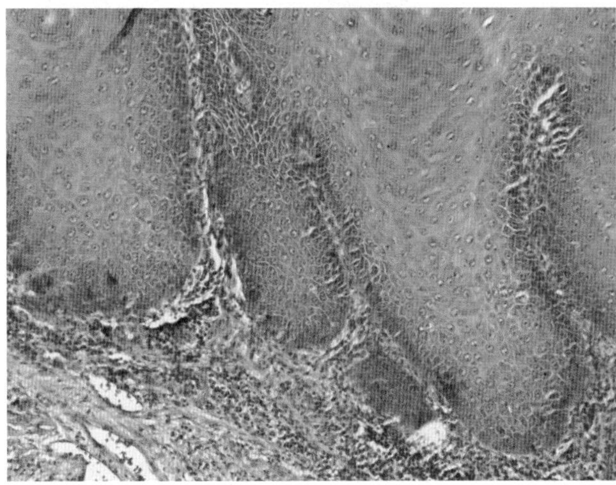

Figure 4.4.3.
Verrucous hyperplasia/ verrucous carcinoma. Broad-based rete ridges with minimal epithelial atypia are seen in both verrucous hyperplasia and verrucous carcinoma.

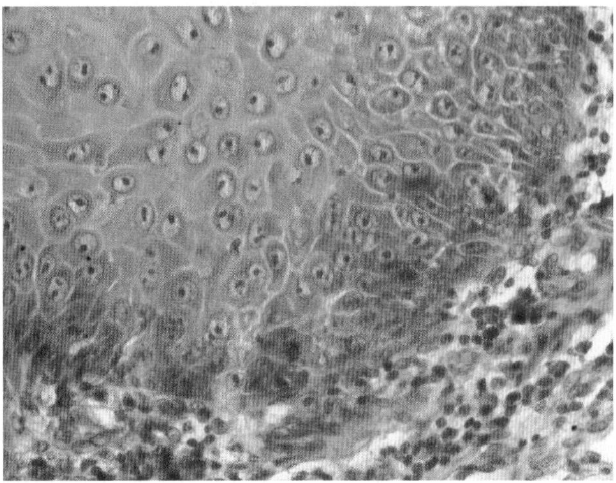

Figure 4.4.4.
Verrucous hyperplasia/verrucous carcinoma. Epithelial cells of basal layer have slight loss of cohesion and orientation and minimal atypia. Verrucous hyperplasia often shows considerable dysplasia, whereas verrucous carcinoma has minimal atypia confined to the basal layers.

4.5 Squamous Cell Carcinoma

Presentation

Indurated ulcer or endophytic mass. The most common locations are posterior lateral tongue, ventral tongue and floor of mouth. Patients are usually older than 60 years and male.

Microscopic Findings

- Well-differentiated squamous cell carcinoma
- Moderately differentiated
- Poorly differentiated

Treatment and Prognosis

Surgical excision and/or radiation and chemotherapy

Additional

When squamous cell carcinomas occur on the gingiva adjacent to teeth, they are often misdiagnosed as periodontal disease, resulting in delay in diagnosis and treatment. Oral squamous cell carcinomas represent 3% to 4% of all cancers.

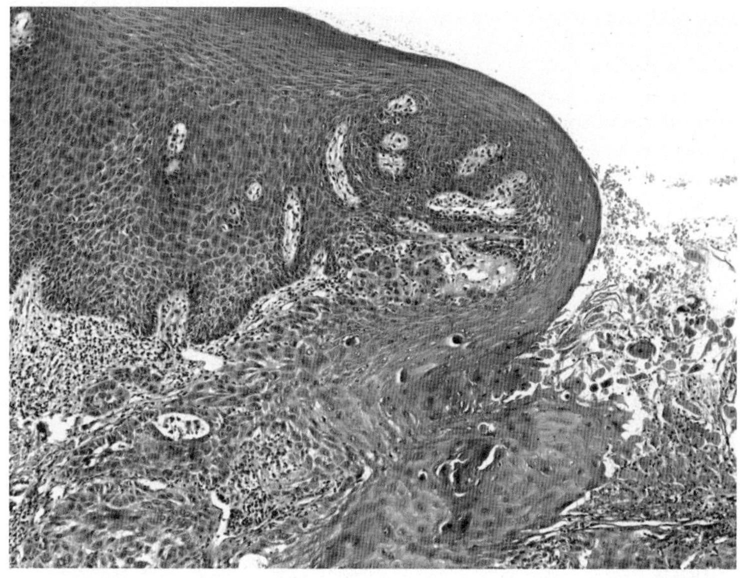

Figure 4.5.1.
Squamous cell carcinoma, well differentiated. Normal stratified squamous epithelium exhibits abrupt change to infiltrating squamous cell carcinoma.

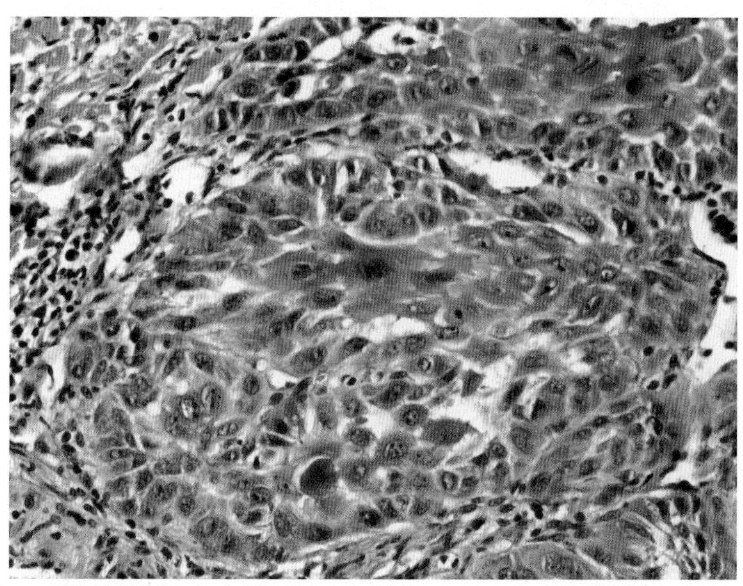

Figure 4.5.2.
Squamous cell carcinoma, well differentiated. Dyskeratosis (individual cell keratinization), loss of cellular cohesion, and nuclear hyperchromasia.

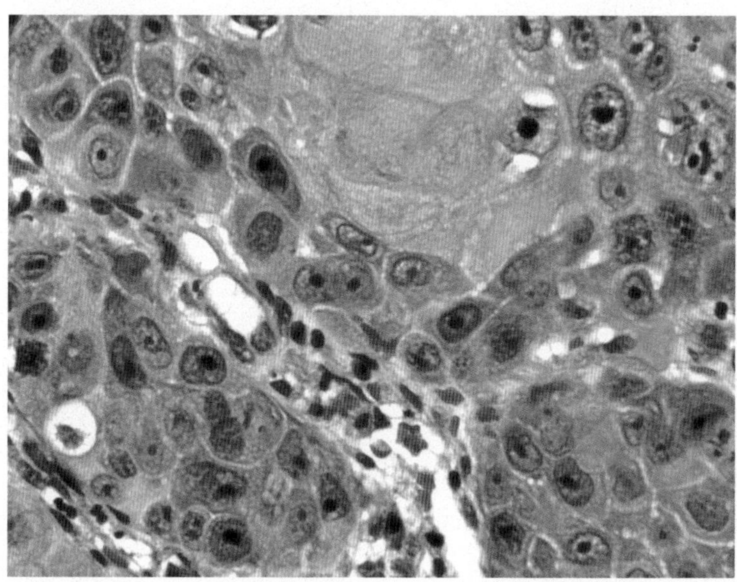

Figure 4.5.3.
Squamous cell carcinoma, well differentiated. Cells have large nuclei and prominent nucleoli. Note intercellular bridges at lower left.

4.6 Basaloid Squamous Cell Carcinoma

Definition

A high-grade, aggressive variant of squamous cell carcinoma

Presentation

Painful mass in the posterior base of the tongue. Most patients are older than 60 years and predominantly male.

Microscopic Findings

- Molding nests of basophilic tumor cells separated by eosinophilic bands and fibrous connective tissue
- Nuclear palisading at the periphery of the tumor nests
- Comedo necrosis; numerous mitoses
- Evidence of surface dysplasia or foci of invasive squamous carcinoma in the overlying epithelium

Treatment and Prognosis

Surgery with postoperative radiation. Local and distant metastases common.

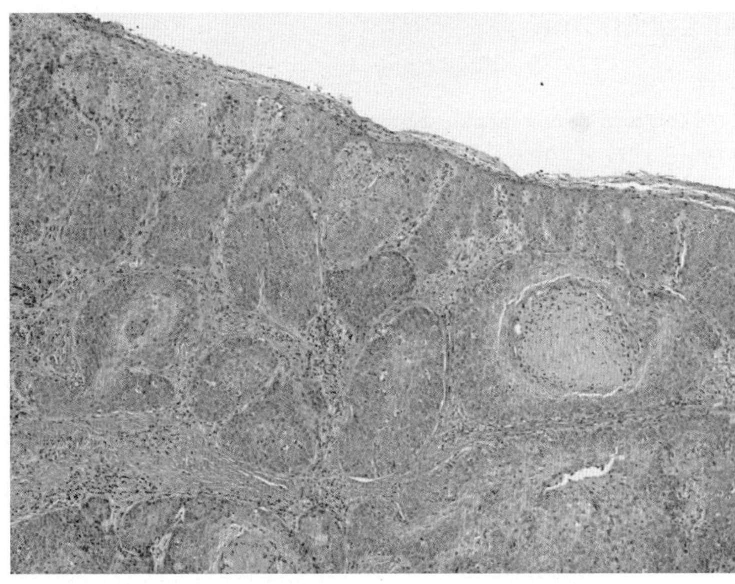

Figure 4.6.1.
Basaloid squamous cell carcinoma. Nests of basaloid squamous cells invade the fibrous submucosal stroma. The mucosal epithelium shows carcinoma in situ.

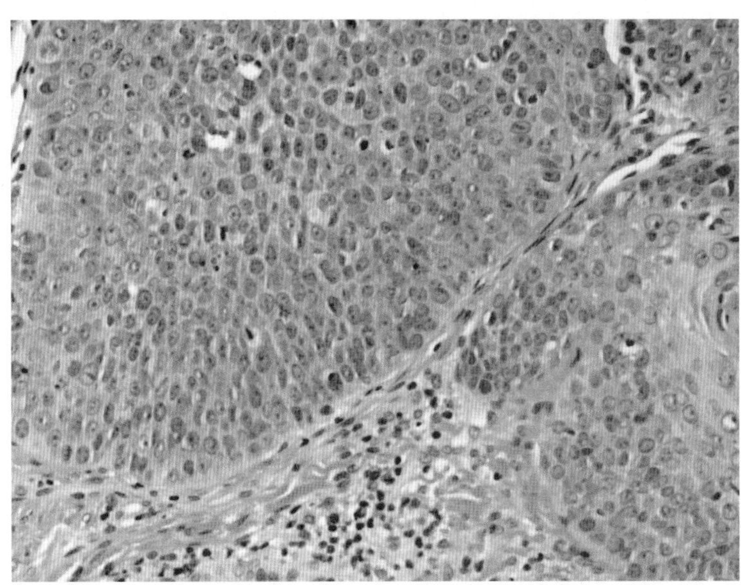

Figure 4.6.2.
Basaloid squamous cell carcinoma. Nests of malignant squamous cells with basaloid features and a suggestion of peripheral palisading.

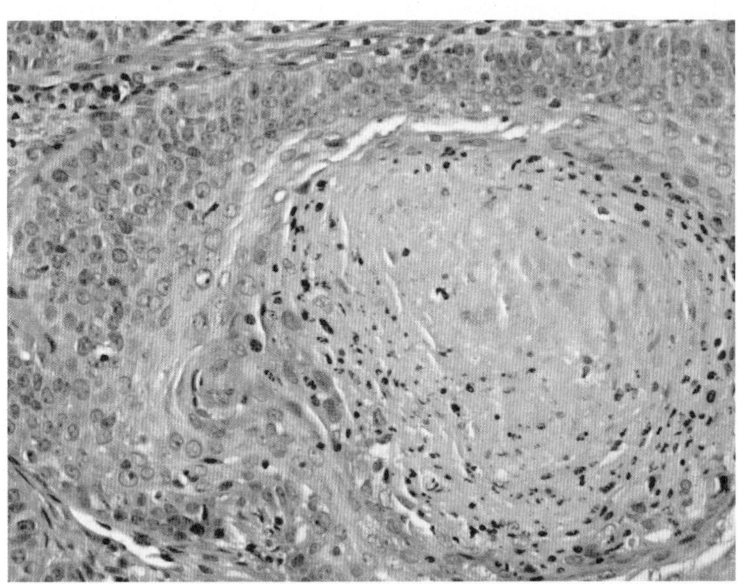

Figure 4.6.3.
Basaloid squamous cell carcinoma. Basaloid tumor nest with central comedo necrosis.

4.7 Spindle Cell Carcinoma

Definition

A high-grade carcinoma characterized by variable degrees of dysplasia in the overlying epithelium in addition to invasive nests of poorly differentiated spindled epithelial cells.

Presentation

Rapidly growing, exophytic, polypoid tumor accompanied by pain and paresthesia. Tongue, lower lip, and gingiva are the most common oral sites. The average age of the patient (mainly males) is about 60 years.

Microscopic Findings

- Proliferation of polymorphic, spindled cells
- Numerous mitotic figures
- Scattered malignant squamous cells
- Evidence of overlying epithelial dysplasia or carcinoma in situ
- Dense, intercellular collagen in some cases

Special Stains/Immunopathology

- Positive for cytokeratins and p63
- Negative for smooth muscle actin

Treatment and Prognosis

Radical surgery with neck dissection in the presence of clinically positive node. The 5-year survival rate is reported as 30%.

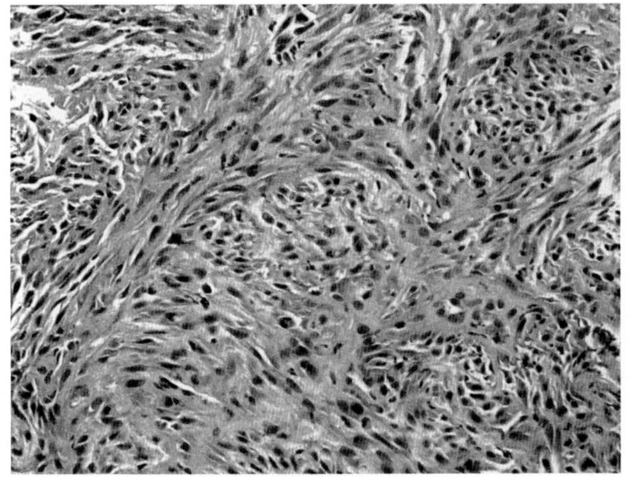

Figure 4.7.1.
Spindle cell carcinoma. Nests of atypical spindle cells in a storiform pattern seen in a biopsy of a large tumor of the buccal mucosa.

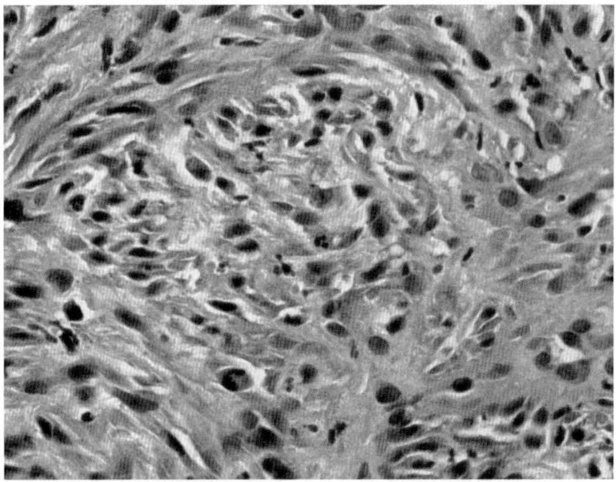

Figure 4.7.2.
Spindle cell carcinoma. Pleomorphic, spindled tumor cells.

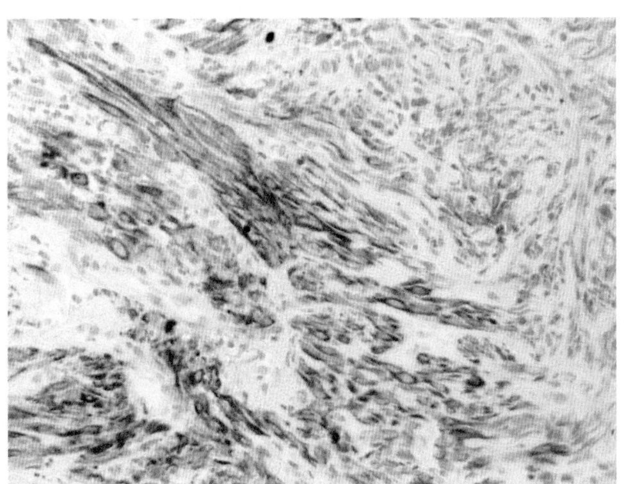

Figure 4.7.3.
Spindle cell carcinoma. Tumor cells are positive for CK5/6 and other epithelial markers.

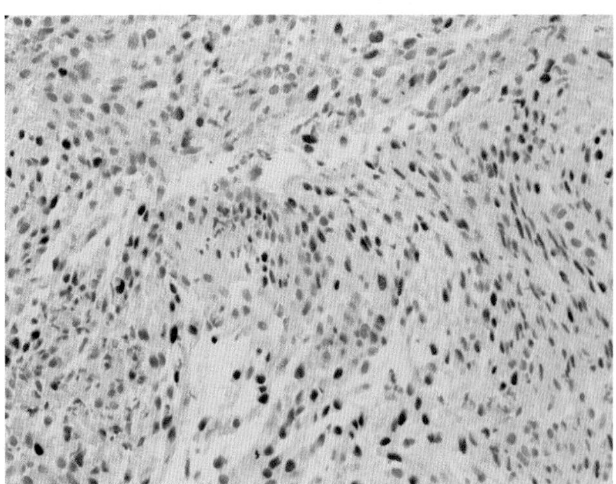

Figure 4.7.4.
Spindle cell carcinoma. The P67 stain reveals a high proliferative index.

4.8 Leukoedema

Definition

A diffuse white change to the buccal mucosa. Relatively common.

Presentation

Buccal mucosa is gray-white and wrinkled, with striae. The whiteness disappears when the mucosa is stretched.

Microscopic Findings

- Epithelial hyperplasia.
- Spinous epithelial cells are edematous and vacuolated and have pyknotic nuclei.
- Rete ridges elongated.

Treatment and Prognosis

None

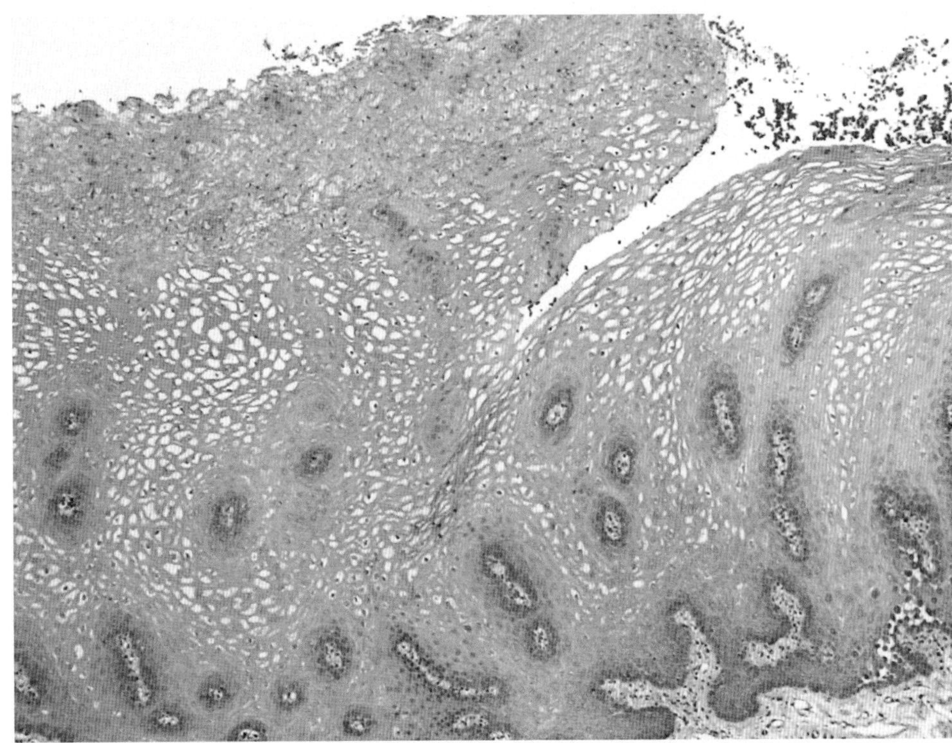

Figure 4.8.1.
Leukoedema. Epithelial hyperplasia and edema of the upper layers.

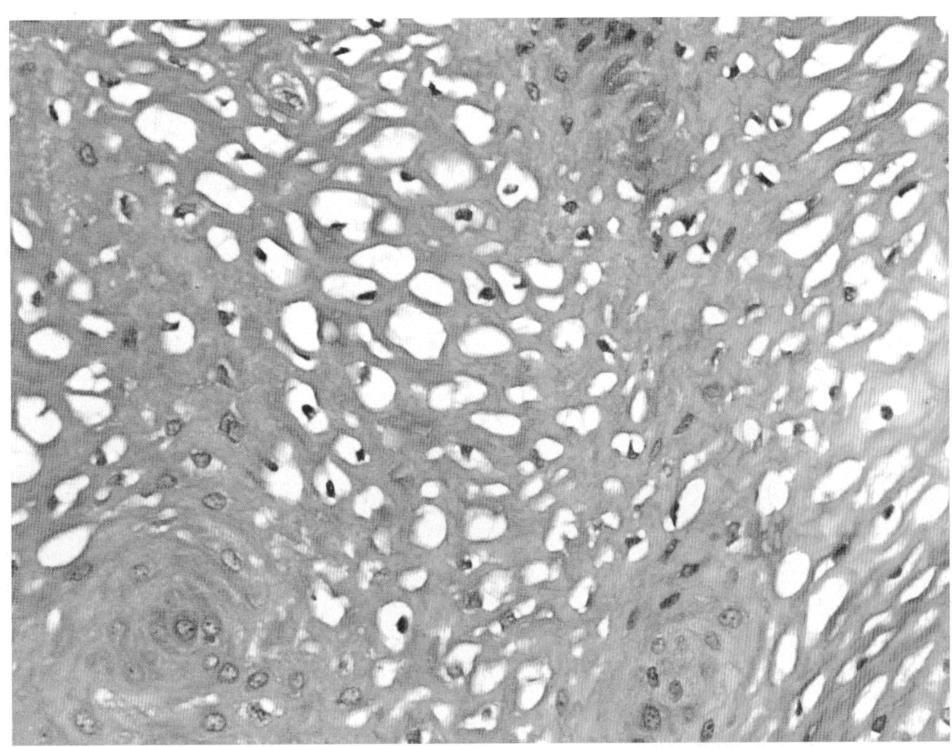

Figure 4.8.2.
Leukoedema. Marked epithelial edema with pyknosis of nuclei.

4.9 Migratory Glossitis (Geographic Tongue)

Presentation

Multiple, painless erythematous areas surrounded by a yellowish-white, slightly raised border. Recurs in different sites of the tongue.

Microscopic Findings

- Psoriasiform changes: elongated, interconnecting epithelial rete ridges and neutrophilic microabscesses within the superficial epithelium

Histopathologic Differential

A negative PAS or methenamine silver stain will rule out *candidiasis.*

Treatment and Prognosis

Generally, none. Topical steroids in symptomatic patients.

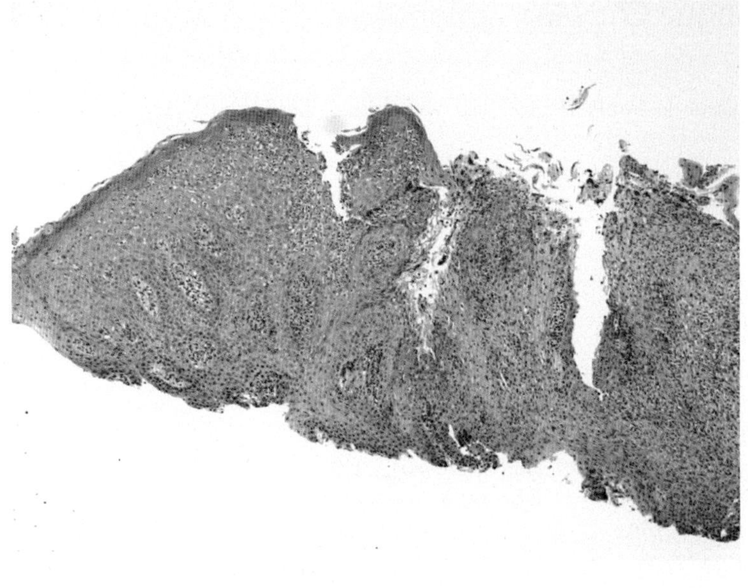

Figure 4.9.1.
Migratory glossitis. Epithelial hyperplasia with interconnected, elongated rete ridges.

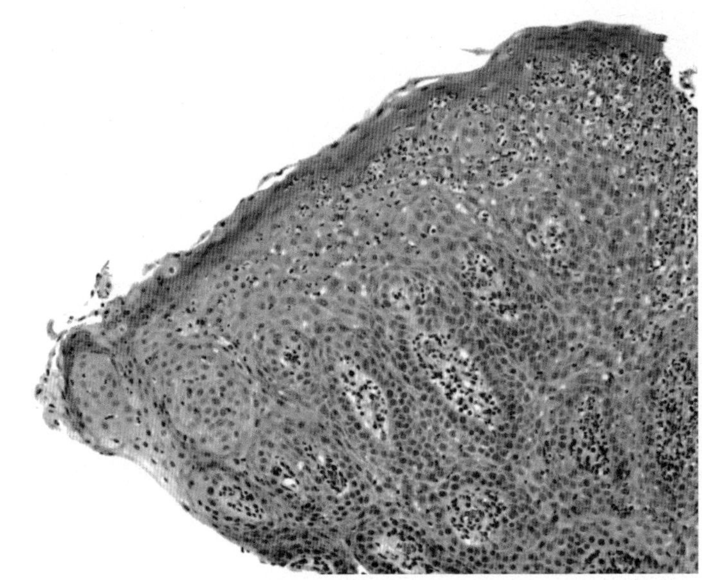

Figure 4.9.2.
Migratory glossitis. The epithelium is hyperplastic with interconnecting rete ridges and infiltrated by neutrophils simulating psoriasiform mucositis.

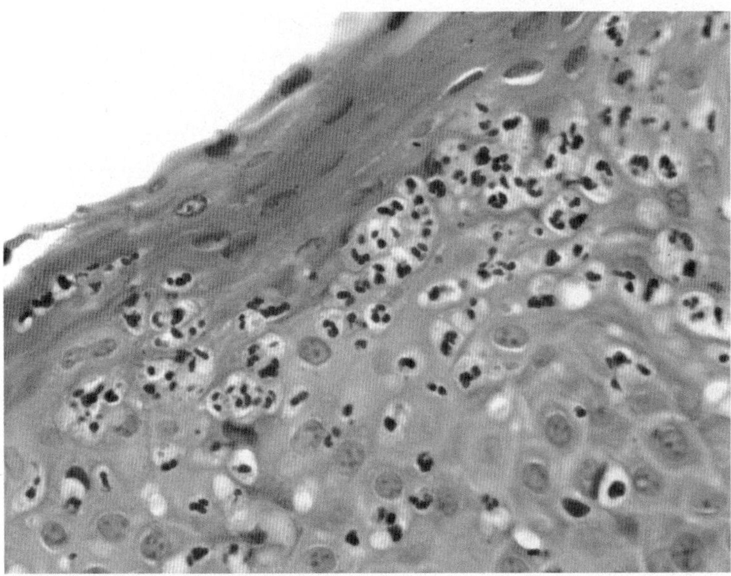

Figure 4.9.3.
Migratory glossitis. Neutrophilic microabscesses in the superficial portion of the epithelium. This histology is similar to that of candidal leukoplakia, in which fungal pseudohyphae are found within the hyperkeratotic layer. A negative PAS stain will rule out fungal infection.

4.10 Cheek/Tongue Chewing Lesion

Definition

A roughened, hyperplastic leukoplakia produced by habitual chewing or biting of cheek or tongue

Presentation

Buccal mucosa, tongue

Microscopic Findings

Irregular epithelial hyperplasia with elongated, ragged, and heaped-up parakeratotic surface covered with basophilic bacterial colonies

Special Stains/Immunopathology

EBER (EBV)-negative (see Histopathologic Differential)

Histopathologic Differential

The epithelial cells of *oral hairy leukoplakia* will have a koilocytic appearance with beading of the chromatin around the periphery of the nuclei. The nuclei of the keratinocytes will stain for the Epstein-Barr virus antigen (positive EBER stain).

Treatment and Prognosis

Discontinuation of habit or fabrication of protective dental appliance (night guard). The lesion generally resolves upon cessation of habit.

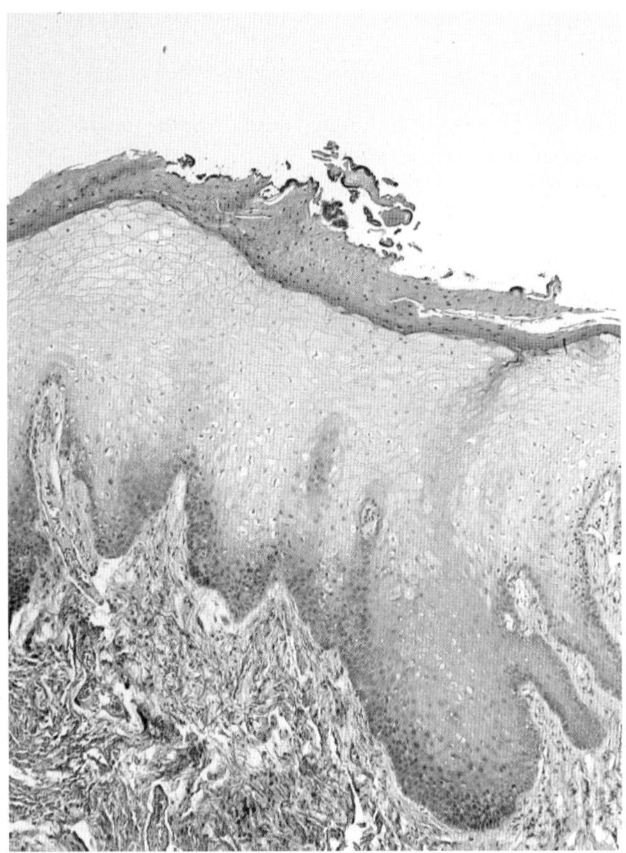

Figure 4.10.1.
Cheek/tongue chewing lesion. Irregular epithelial hyperplasia with hyperkeratosis. Basophilic bacterial colonies cover the ragged, heaped-up parakeratotic surface.

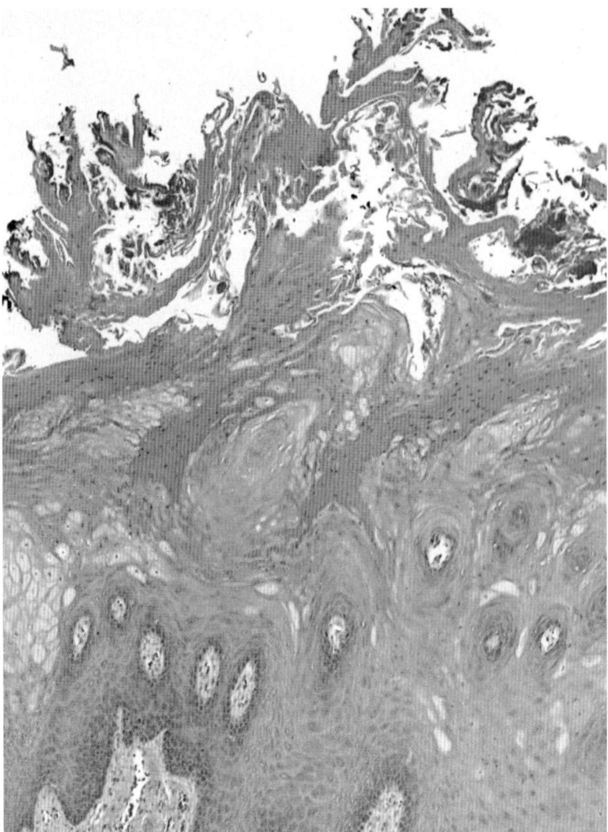

Figure 4.10.2.
Cheek/tongue chewing lesion. Basophilic bacterial colonies cover the ragged, heaped-up parakeratotic surface.

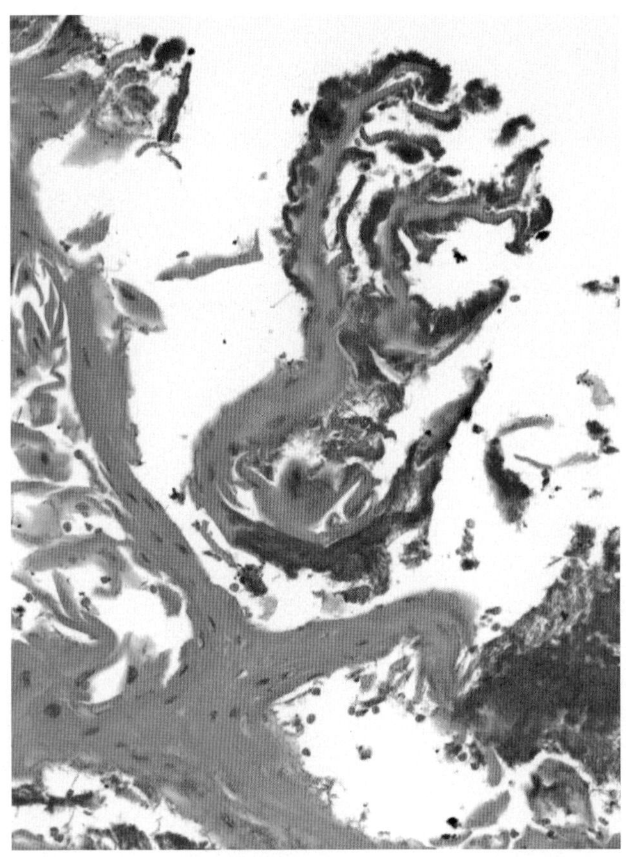

Figure 4.10.3.
Cheek/tongue chewing lesion. Fragments of bacteria-covered epithelium appear to float above the ragged parakeratotic surface.

4.11 Oral Hairy Leukoplakia

Presentation

Roughened leukoplakic lesion mostly seen bilaterally on the lateral surface of the tongue. Seen in HIV-positive and other immunocompromised patients.

Microscopic Findings

- Irregular epithelial hyperplasia with ragged and heaped-up parakeratotic surface covered with bacterial colonies.
- Epithelial cells have a koilocytic appearance, with beading of the chromatin around the periphery of the nuclei.

Special Stains/Immunopathology

With EBER in situ hybridization, nuclei are positive for Epstein-Barr virus–encoded RNA.

Histopathologic Differential

The epithelium of *cheek/tongue biting lesion* lacks koilocytosis and beaded chromatin around keratinocyte nuclei.

Treatment and Prognosis

This lesion was commonly seen in the early days of the AIDS epidemic, before the introduction of highly active antiretroviral therapy.

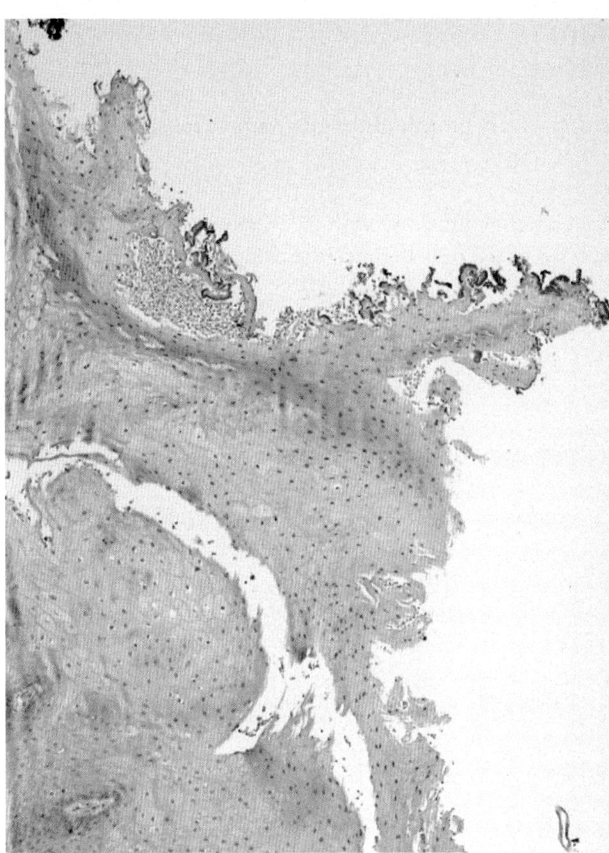

Figure 4.11.1.
Oral hairy leukoplakia. The surface of the leukoplakic lesion shows epithelial hyperplasia with hyperkeratosis and edema. Thick projections of the parakeratotic surface are covered with bacterial colonies.

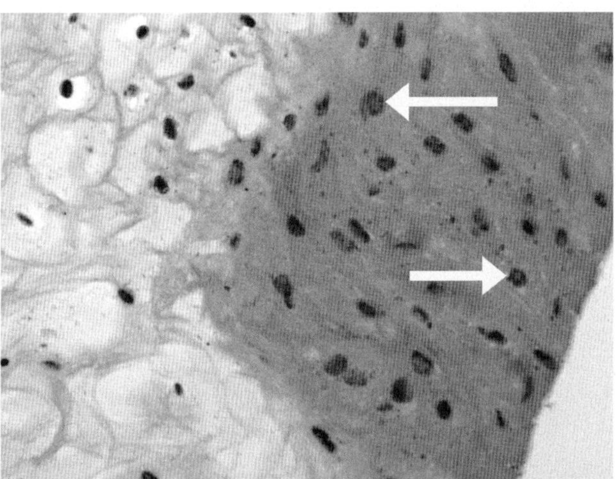

Figure 4.11.2.
Oral hairy leukoplakia. Edema of prickle cells along with beading of chromatin around the periphery of keratinocyte nuclei.

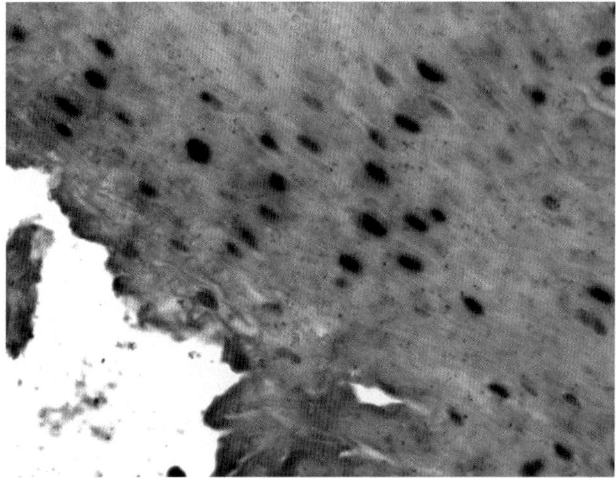

Figure 4.11.3.
Oral hairy leukoplakia, EBER in situ hybridization. Nuclei are positive for Epstein-Barr virus–encoded RNA.

4.12 Verruciform Xanthoma

Presentation

White to yellowish soft, broad-based, papillary growth of the gingiva. In adults.

Microscopic Findings

- Papillary, hyperplastic stratified squamous epithelium with parakeratotic surface
- Foamy macrophages (xanthoma cells) found only between the elongated rete ridges

Special Stains/Immunopathology

- Xanthoma cells are CD68-positive and PAS-positive, diastase-resistant.

Histopathologic Differential

- The epithelial proliferation of a *squamous papilloma* is more finger-like, and xanthoma cells are absent.
- The epithelial proliferation of a *condyloma acuminatum* has koilocytic change and lacks xanthoma cells.

Treatment and Prognosis

Excision. Does not recur.

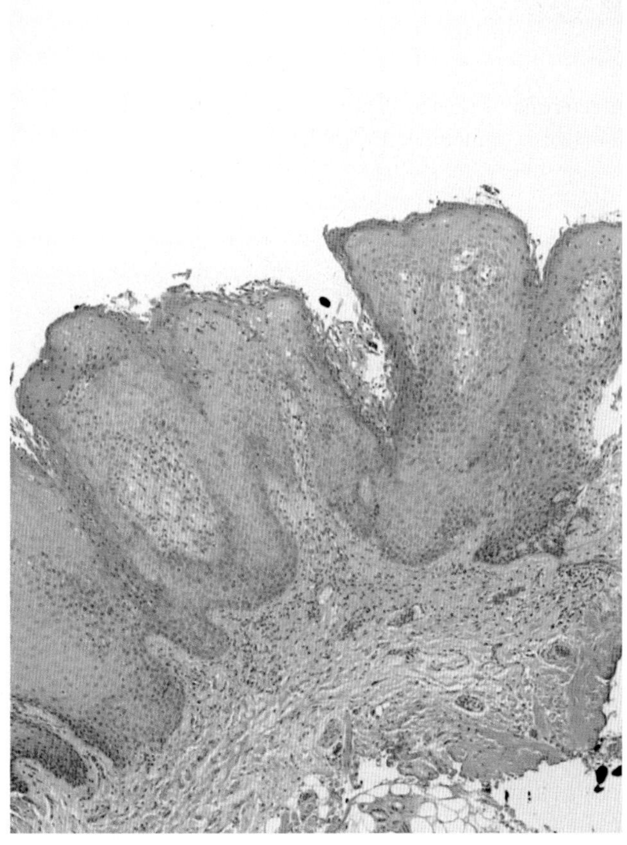

Figure 4.12.1.
Verruciform xanthoma. Papillary, parakeratotic, and acanthotic stratified squamous epithelium with elongated, interconnecting rete ridges.

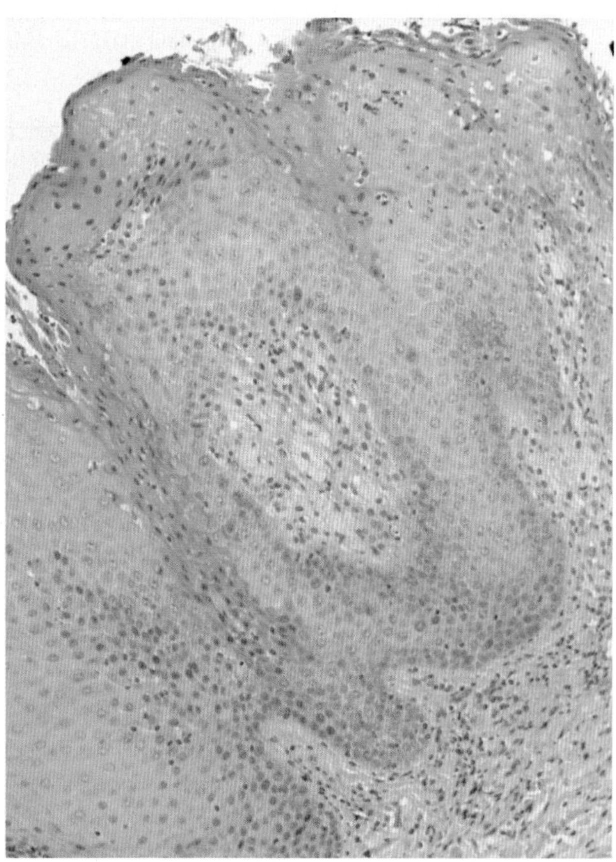

Figure 4.12.2.
Verruciform xanthoma. The fibrous stroma between the epithelial ridges is filled with a mixture of inflammatory and foamy cells.

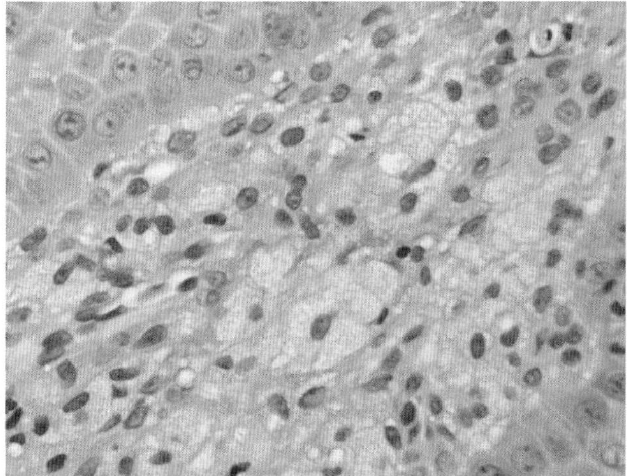

Figure 4.12.3.
Verruciform xanthoma. Foamy histiocytes are seen admixed with mononuclear inflammatory cells.

4.13 Condyloma Acuminatum

Definition

An exophytic, papillary lesion characterized by the proliferation of stratified squamous epithelium caused by the human papilloma virus, sometimes high-risk types 16 and 18.

Presentation

Pink, papillary lesions, usually multiple, with flattened, smooth surface projections. A sexually transmitted disease. In young adults.

Microscopic Findings

- Mildly keratotic papillary surface projections of the mucosa
- Blunted and broad surfaces with keratin-filled crypts
- Koilocytes often seen in the lesional upper epithelium

Special Stains/Immunopathology

Immunohistochemistry and polymerase chain reaction tests to demonstrate human papilloma virus viral antigens

Treatment and Prognosis

Excision. Can recur.

Additional

Children presenting with condyloma acuminatum should be evaluated for sexual abuse. A squamous papilloma is similar in histology, usually smaller and single, and can have either pointed or blunt projections.

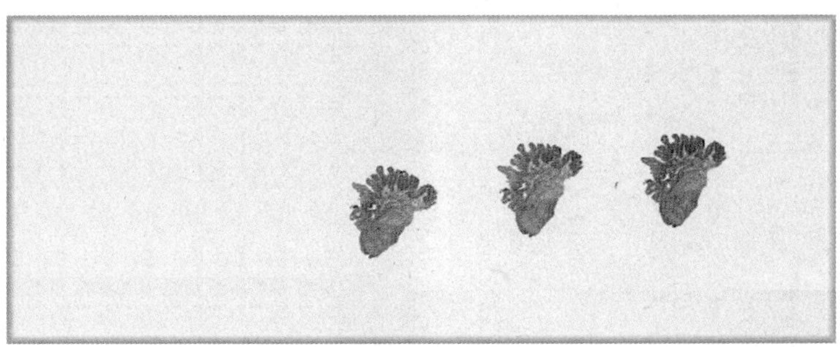

Figure 4.13.1.
Condyloma acuminatum. Blunted papillary epithelial proliferation.

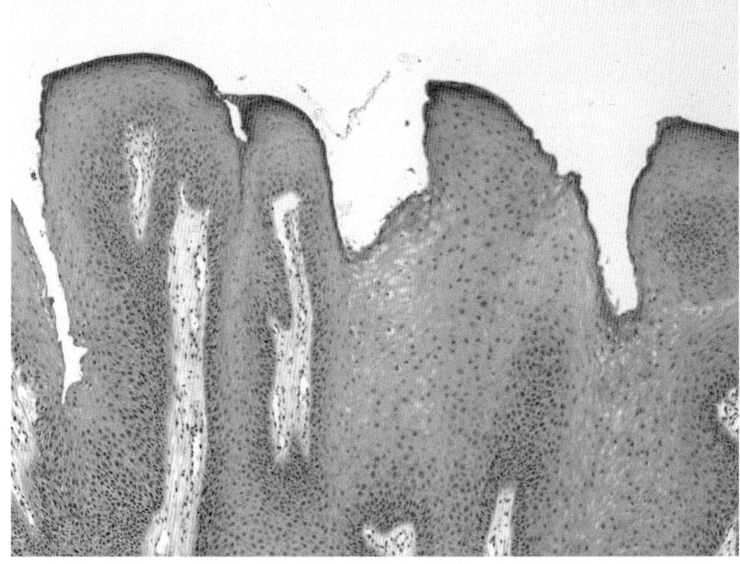

Figure 4.13.2.
Condyloma acuminatum. Hyperplastic, hyperkeratotic squamous epithelium forming blunted papillary projections. Clusters of koilocytes are present in the upper stratum spinosum.

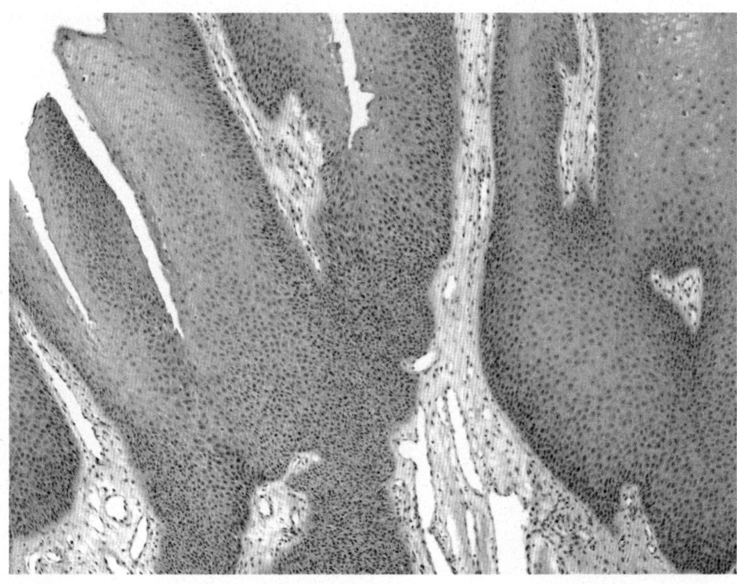

Figure 4.13.3.
Condyloma acuminatum. The supporting fibrous stroma shows prominent vascularity, and there is basilar hyperplasia. Scattered lymphocytes are seen in the lamina propria.

4.14 Aphthous Ulcer

Presentation
Multiple, recurrent ulcers of the movable oral mucosa (excluding palate and gingiva). In children and young adults.

Microscopic Findings
The features are that of a nonspecific ulcer:

- Ulcerated mucosa covered by a thin, fibrinous membrane
- Submucosal granulation tissue with acute and chronic inflammatory cell infiltrate

Treatment and Prognosis
Topical steroids

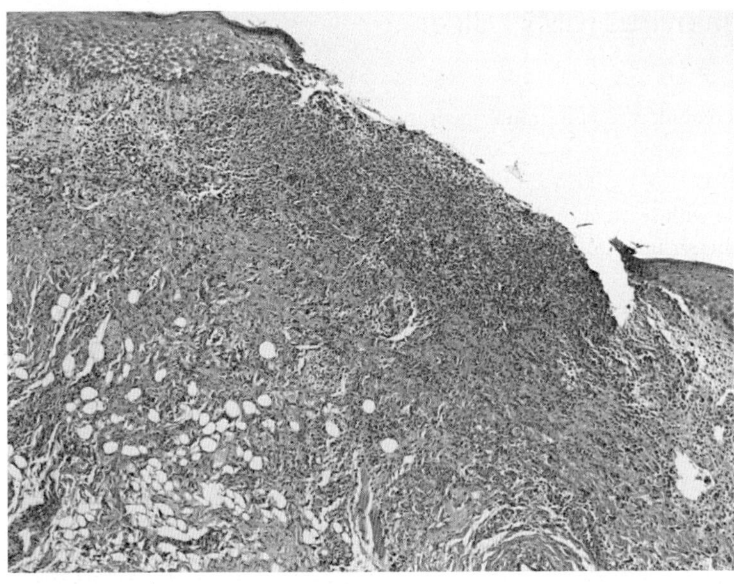

Figure 4.14.1.
Aphthous ulcer. Portion of mucosa exhibiting surface ulceration. There is a diffuse acute and chronic inflammatory cell infiltrate in the ulcer bed. The remaining mucosal epithelium is edematous.

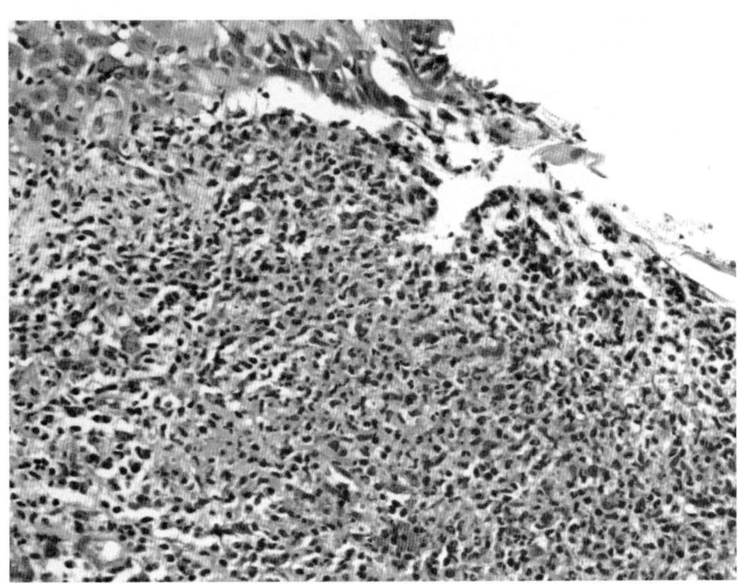

Figure 4.14.2.
Aphthous ulcer. Ulcerated surface with acute and chronic inflammatory cells.

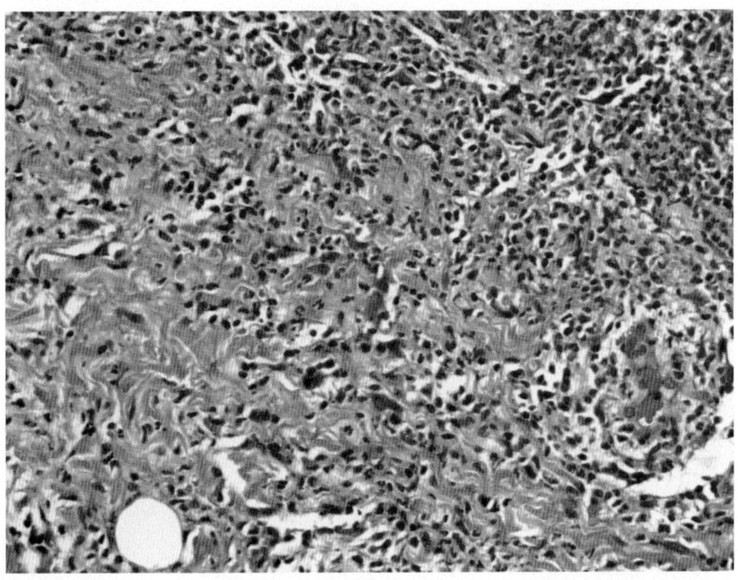

Figure 4.14.3.
Aphthous ulcer. Inflammatory cells, mostly mononuclear, are present in the fibrous connective tissue base.

4.15 Cytomegalovirus (CMV) Ulcer

Presentation

A chronic, deep mucosal ulcer seen in immunocompromised patients

Microscopic Findings

- Granulation tissue with scattered swollen endothelial cells
- "Owl eye" intranuclear inclusions

Special Stains/Immunopathology

Polymerase chain reaction tests for viral antigens

Treatment and Prognosis

Antivirals such as ganciclovir

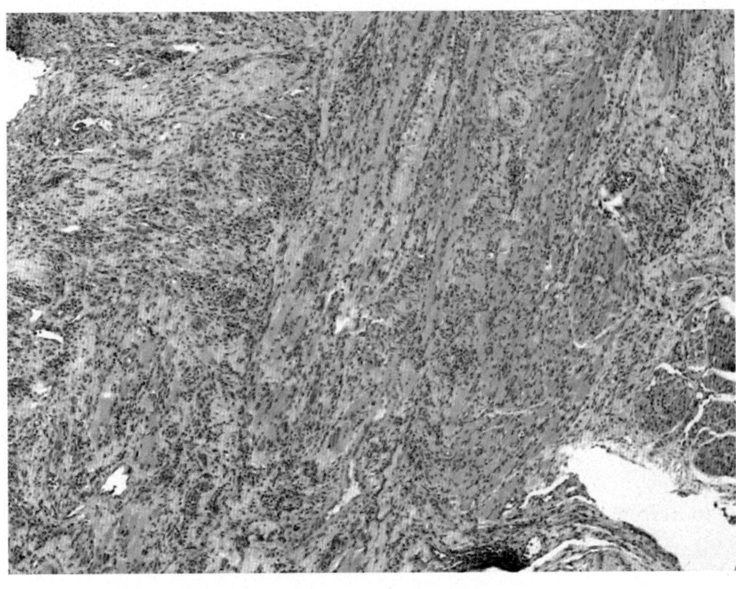

Figure 4.15.1.
CMV ulcer. Dense collections of inflammatory cells adjacent to an ulcer base.

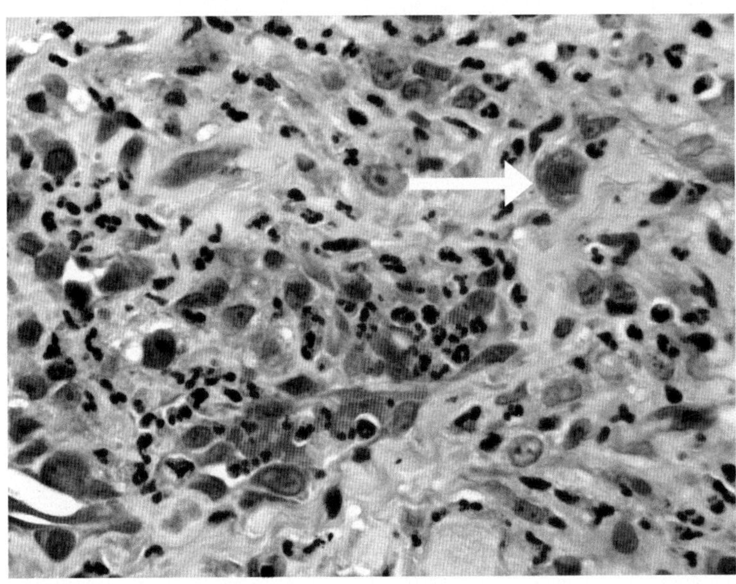

Figure 4.15.2.
CMV ulcer. Atypical, enlarged endothelial cells line capillaries. Some contain intracytoplasmic and intranuclear inclusions.

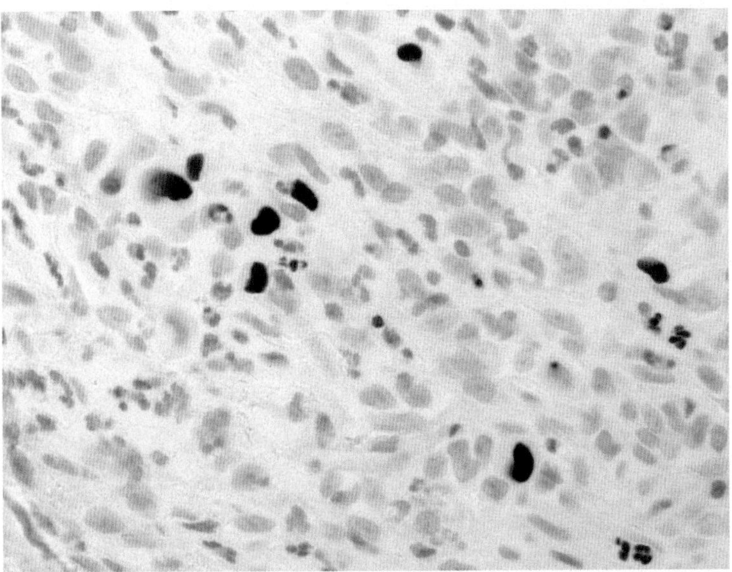

Figure 4.15.3.
CMV ulcer, CMV immuno stain. Several CMV-positive cells are noted.

4.16 Oral Lichen Planus

Presentation

Interconnecting white striae and papules on an erythematous background; can also present as a white patch or as a desquamative gingivitis. Buccal mucosa, tongue, and gingiva. In adults, more often females.

Microscopic Findings

- Parakeratosis, orthokeratosis, epithelial hyperplasia, or atrophy
- Pointed rete ridges (Saw-tooth-like)
- Band-like lymphocytic infiltrate of the lamina propria hugging the epithelium
- Loss of basal cells in the involved lesional epithelium
- Civatte bodies (apoptotic keratinocytes with pyknotic or anucleate forms)

Special Stains/Immunopathology

With direct immunofluorescence, an irregular band of fibrinogen is seen at the basement membrane.

Histopathologic Differential

Lichenoid mucositis has a deeper perivascular and nodular lymphocytic and plasmacytic infiltrate.

Treatment and Prognosis

Topical or systemic steroids

Additional

Oral lichen planus is a common disease and present in about 2% of the adult population.

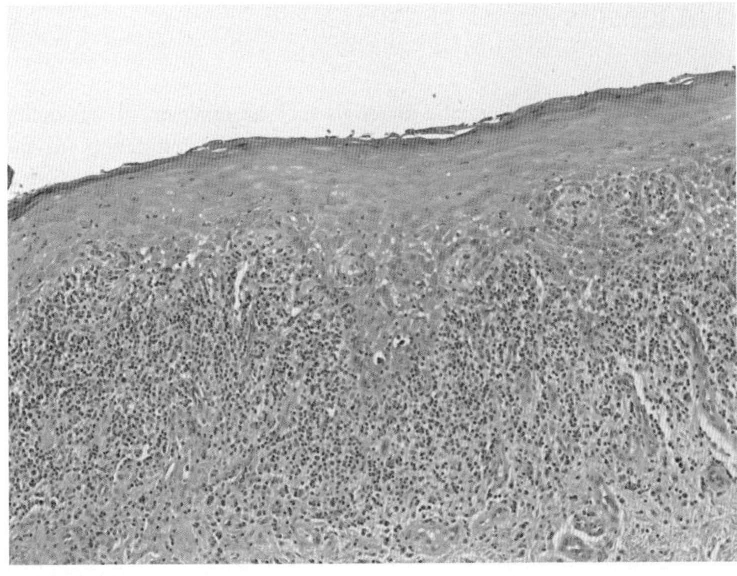

Figure 4.16.1.
Oral lichen planus. Parakeratotic stratified squamous epithelium closely hugged by a band-like infiltrate of inflammatory cells. The epithelial ridges are saw-toothed in areas.

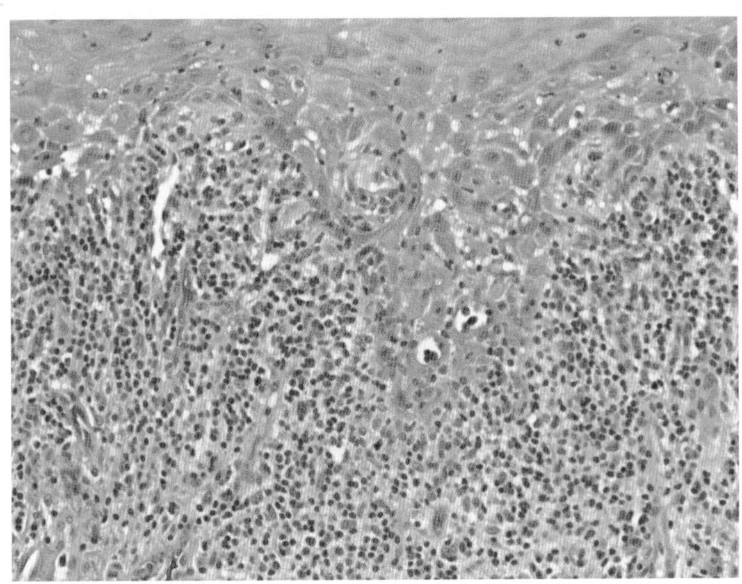

Figure 4.16.2.
Oral lichen planus. Lymphocytes are seen in a dense, band-like infiltrate as well as within the lesional epithelium.

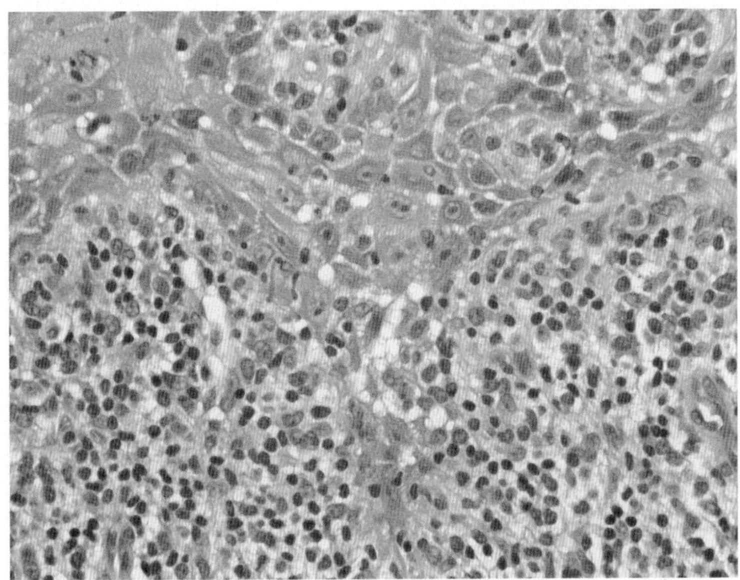

Figure 4.16.3.
Oral lichen planus. The rete ridges are edematous, and the basal cells are absent. Lymphocytes hug the saw-toothed epithelial ridge.

4.17 Lichenoid Mucositis

Definition

Reactive lesions caused by contact with allergenic materials such as amalgam fillings or ingestion of drugs such as nonsteroidal anti-inflammatories or angiotensin-converting enzyme inhibitors

Presentation

Interconnecting white striae and papules on an erythematous background; can also present as a white patch or as a desquamative gingivitis. Buccal mucosa, tongue, and gingiva. In adults, more often females. Usually related to drug intake.

Microscopic Findings

Same as oral lichen planus but with deep, perivascular inflammatory infiltrates, predominantly lymphocytes but also plasma cells.

Histopathologic Differential

Oral lichen planus has an identical histology but lacks the deeper perivascular and nodular lymphocytic infiltrate.

Treatment and Prognosis

Removal of the offending material or discontinuation of medication. Topical steroids.

Additional

Lichenoid mucositis resembles oral lichen planus both clinically and histologically. The diagnosis is established when the lesions resolve upon removal of the offending substance or drug.

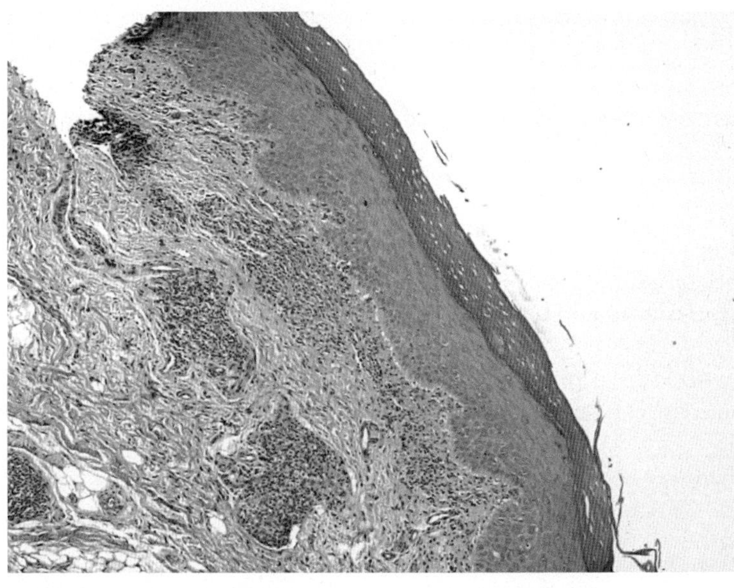

Figure 4.17.1.
Lichenoid mucositis. Hyperkeratotic stratified squamous epithelium covers a fibrous stroma containing nodules of mononuclear cells, mostly lymphocytes.

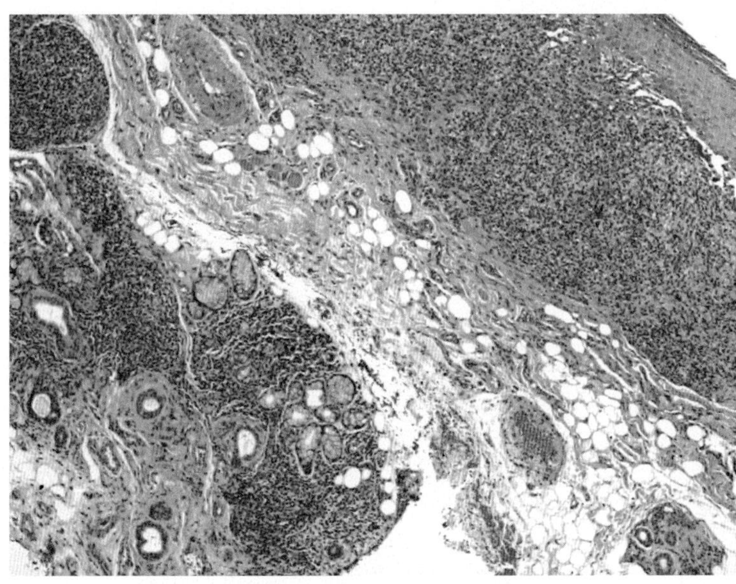

Figure 4.17.2.
Lichenoid mucositis. Dense foci of lymphocytes are seen hugging the basal cells as well as in the stroma surrounding regional mucous glands.

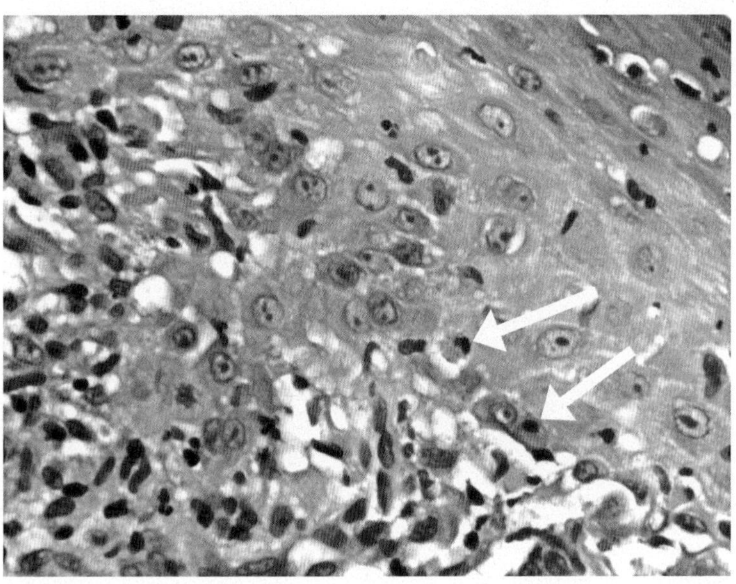

Figure 4.17.3.
Lichenoid mucositis. Apoptotic keratinocytes (Civatte bodies).

4.18 Mucous Membrane Pemphigoid

Presentation

Chronic, painful blisters and ulcers on the gingiva and buccal mucosa. In older adults, mainly females

Microscopic Findings

- Subepithelial clefting
- Fragments of epithelium with an intact basal layer
- Epithelium detaches cleanly from lamina propria, accentuating the clefting

Special Stains/Immunopathology

- Direct immunofluorescence: positive for basement membrane immunoreactants in almost all patients
- Indirect immunofluorescence: positive in only about 25% of the lesions

Treatment and Prognosis

Steroids, immunomodulators

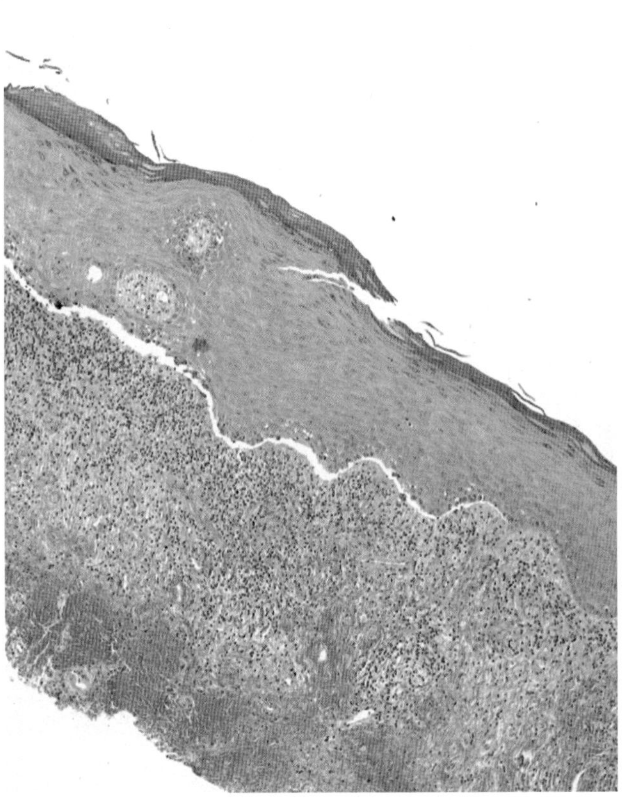

Figure 4.18.1.
Mucous membrane pemphigoid. The entire mucosal epithelium is cleaving from the underlying lamina propria.

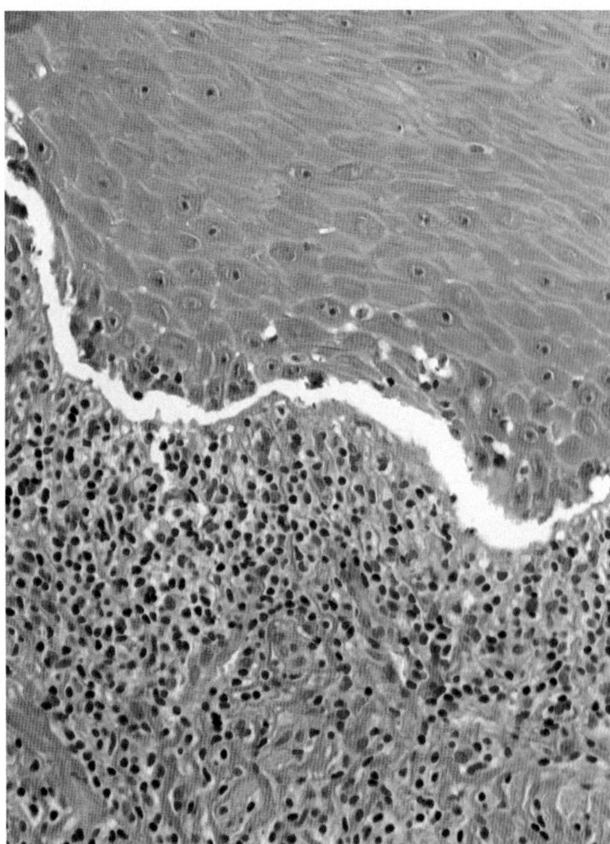

Figure 4.18.2.
Mucous membrane pemphigoid. There is separation of the stratified squamous epithelium from the underlying inflamed lamina propria at the level of the basement membrane.

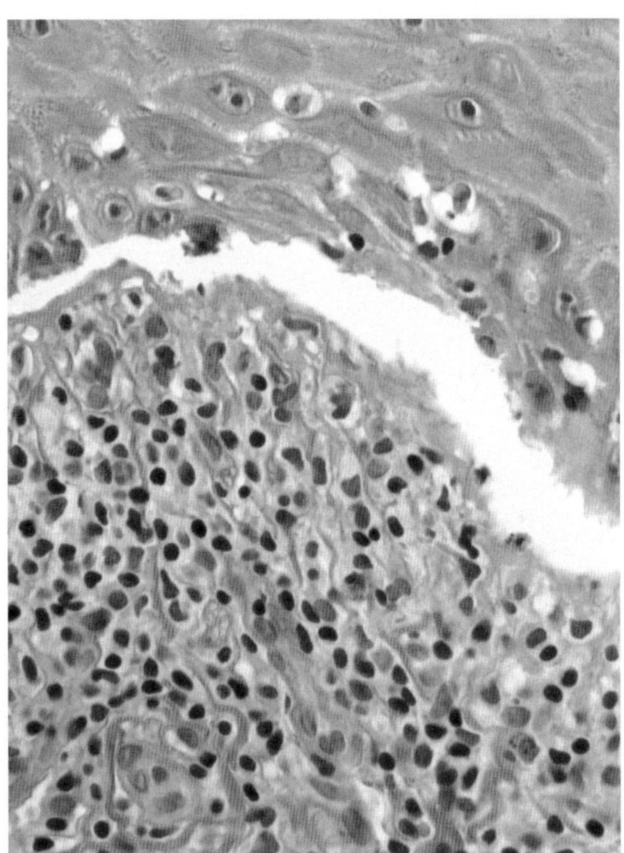

Figure 4.18.3.
Mucous membrane pemphigoid. Subepithelial separation and inflamed lamina propria (higher power).

4.19 Pemphigus Vulgaris

Definition

A chronic blistering and ulcerative dermatologic disease that could be commonly observed initially on the oral mucosa

Presentation

Small to large vesicles that rupture rapidly leaving shallow ulcers. Positive Nikolsky sign (denudation of the surface epithelium following the gentle manipulation of normal-appearing mucosa). Palate, lips, buccal mucosa, tongue, and gingiva. Patients are usually older than 50 years.

Microscopic Findings

- Intraepithelial, suprabasilar vesicle.
- Lesional basal cells resemble a row of bricks.
- Spinous layer falls apart because of acantholysis of the involved keratinocytes resulting in rounded squamous cells within the blister (Tzanck cells).
- Submucosa contains mixed inflammatory infiltrate, including eosinophils.

Special Stains/Immunopathology

Indirect immunofluorescence is positive in 80% to 90% of the patients. This test is performed on tissue fixed in Michel's solution and used in evaluating response to treatment.

Histopathologic Differential

Mucous membrane pemphigoid features sub-, rather than intraepithelial, cleavage and there is an absence of Tzanck cells in the overlying vesicle.

Treatment and Prognosis

Steroids, immunomodulators.

Additional

Half of the patients with pemphigus vulgaris have oral blisters before vesicles show up on the skin.

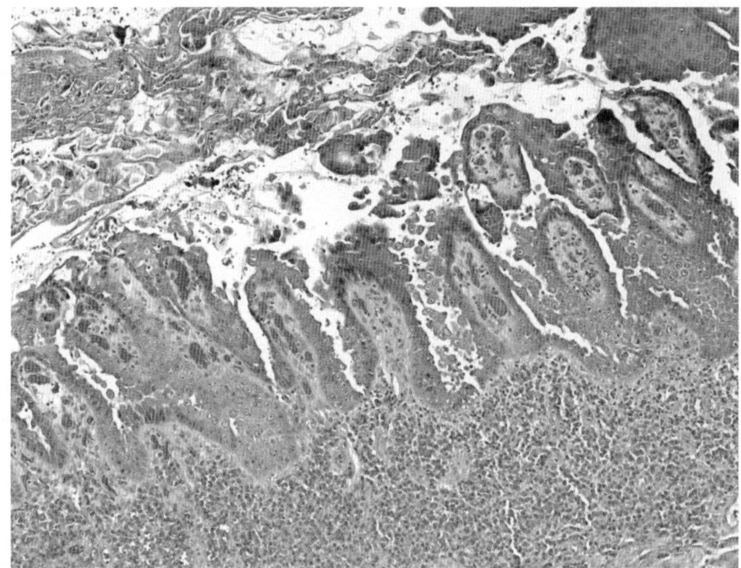

Figure 4.19.1.
Pemphigus vulgaris. Suprabasilar cleavage of the epithelium forms a vesicle over the attached basal cells. There are abundant inflammatory cells in the lamina propria.

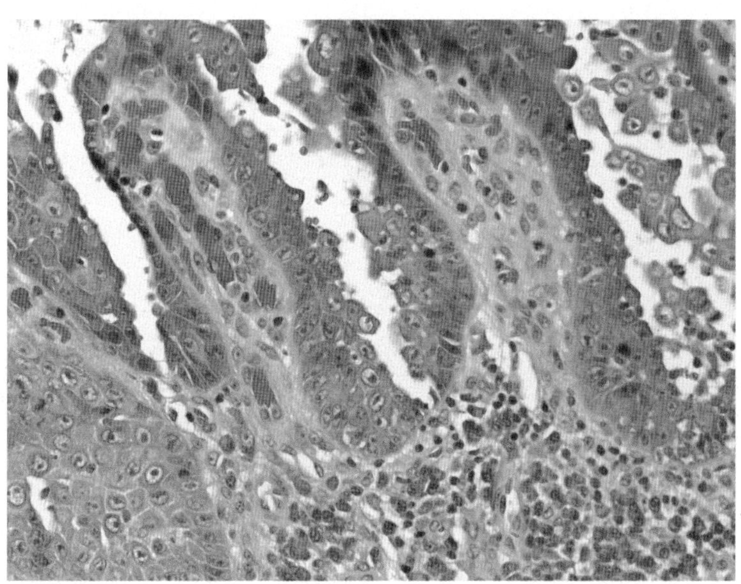

Figure 4.19.2.
Pemphigus vulgaris. Suprabasilar cleavage with rounded Tzanck cells in the vesicle, especially at right. Note the intact basement membrane.

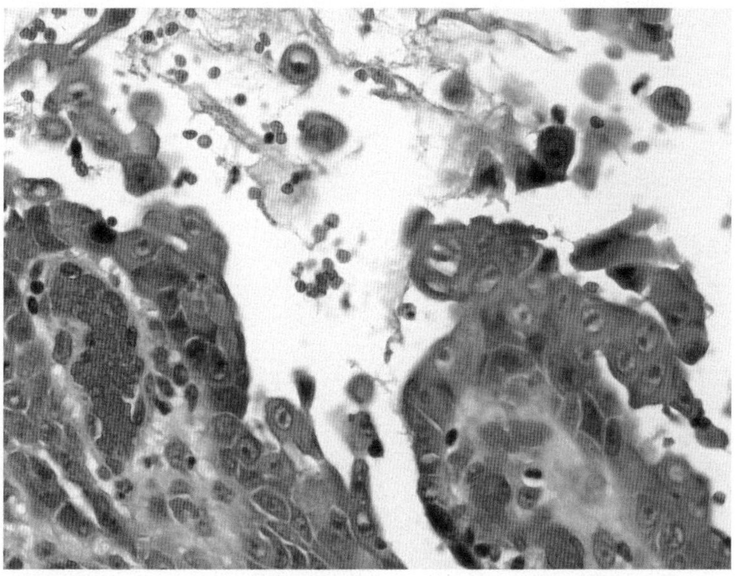

Figure 4.19.3.
Pemphigus vulgaris. Within the vesicle, squamous cells lose their intercellular bridges to form rounded, free-floating Tzanck cells.

4.20 Amalgam Tattoo

Definition

Submucosal pigmented lesion caused by accidental implantation of amalgam particles during placement or removal of a silver amalgam filling

Presentation

Irregular bluish-black macule. Gingiva, alveolar mucosa, and buccal mucosa.

Microscopic Findings

- Multiple black particles in the subepithelial connective tissue accompanied by brown to black staining of the perivascular fibrous connective tissue.
- Lymphocytes, plasma cells, and foreign body giant cells may be seen.

Treatment and Prognosis

No treatment necessary.

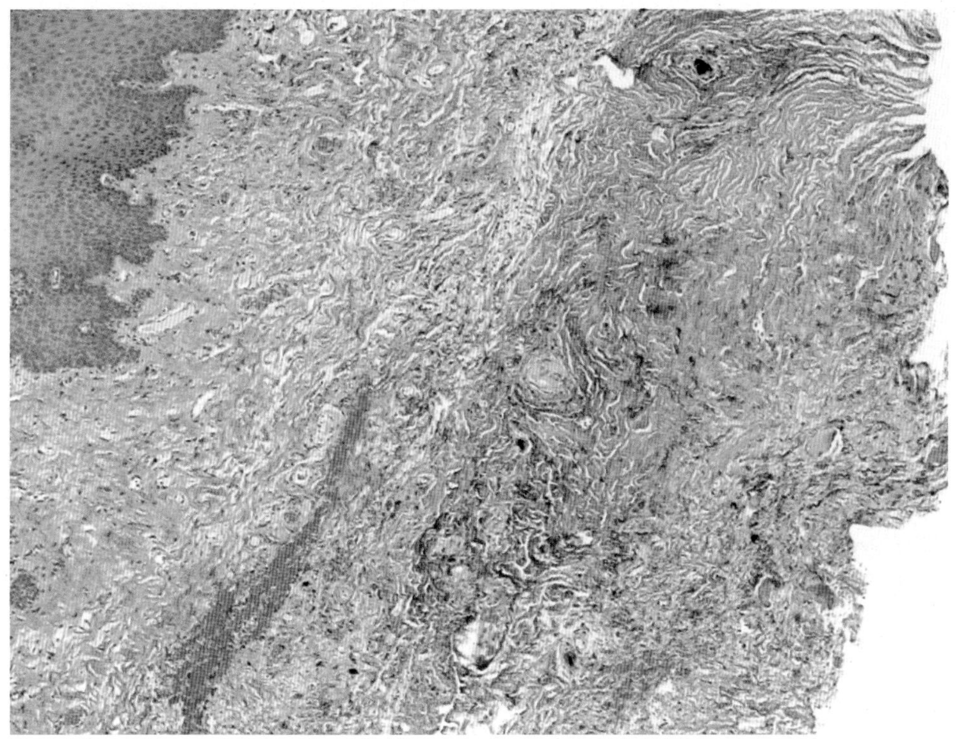

Figure 4.20.1.
Amalgam tattoo. Submucosa contains small black particles and areas of brown stain.

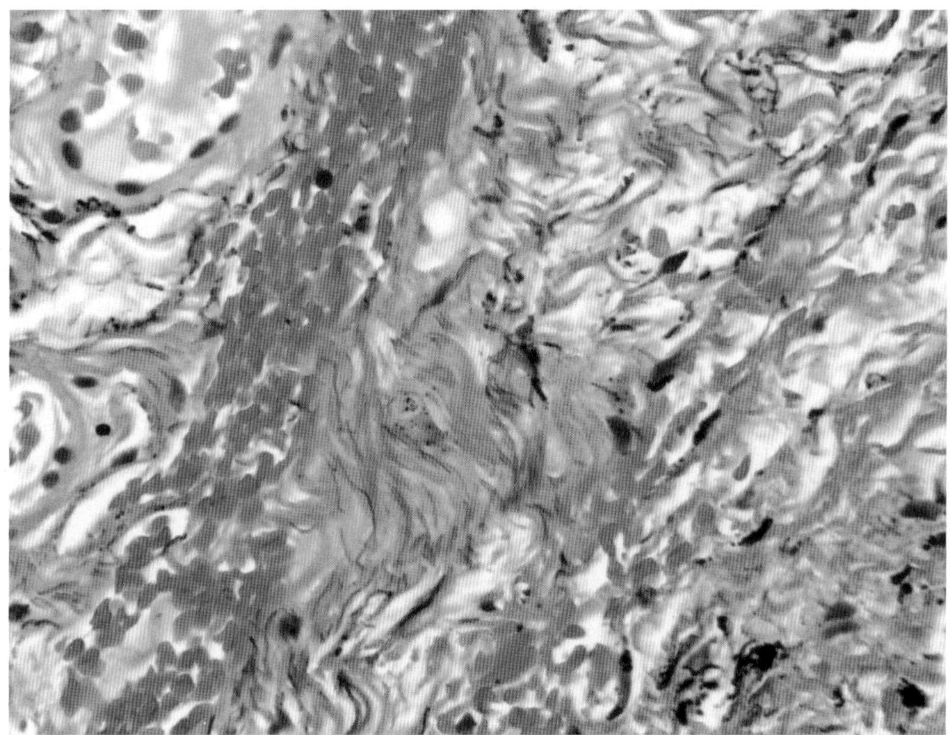

Figure 4.20.2.
Amalgam tattoo. Collagen fibers contain a brown stain, and blackish strands are seen.

4.21 Oral Melanotic Macule

Presentation

Solitary light brown macule, oval to round and usually less than 1 cm in diameter. Vermilion of the lower lip. Also palate, gingiva, or buccal mucosa. Mostly in adult females.

Microscopic Findings

- Circumscribed area of mucosa in which basal epithelial cells contain brown melanin granules
- Melanin-containing subepithelial melanophages
- No increase in the number of melanocytes

Treatment and Prognosis

Excisional biopsy. Malignant transformation has not been reported.

Additional

The most common variant, on the lower lip (labial melanotic macule), may be related to sun exposure.

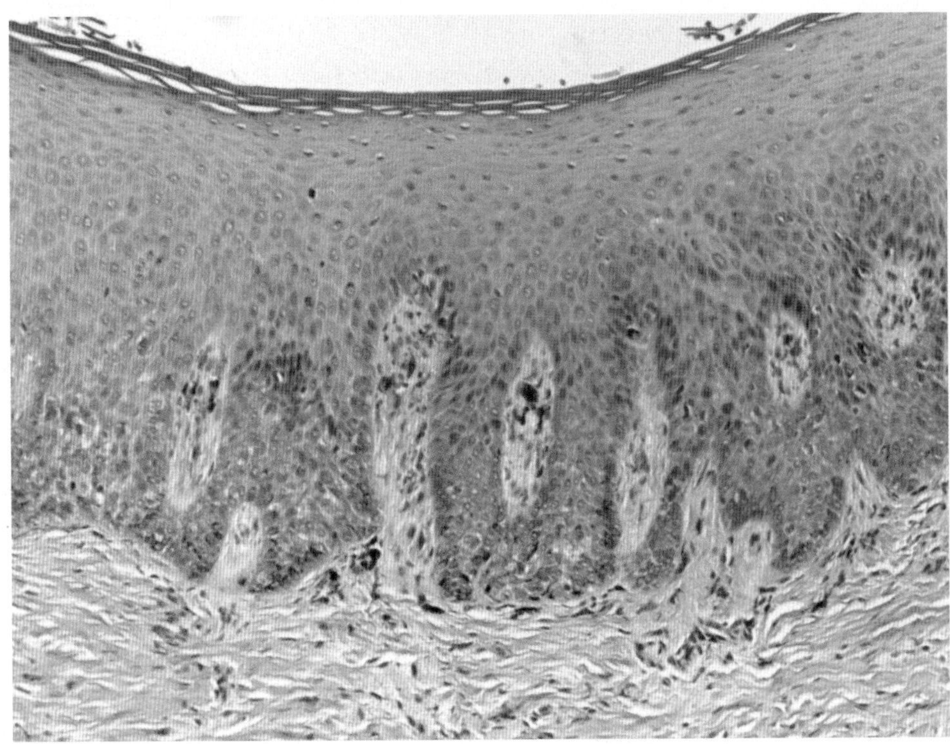

Figure 4.21.1.
Oral melanotic macule. The lesional epithelium shows elongated rete ridges exhibiting melanin-containing basal cells.

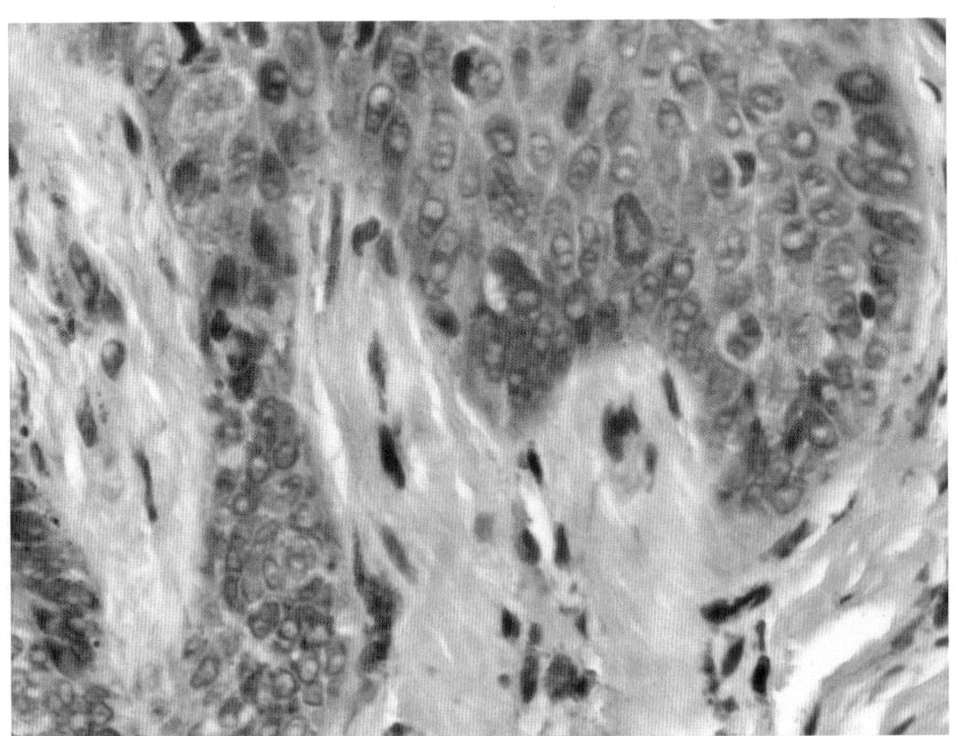

Figure 4.21.2
Oral melanotic macule. Melanophages are seen in the lamina propria.

4.22 Intramucosal Nevus

Definition

The mucosal variant of the common intradermal nevus

Presentation

Brown to black papule or nodule on the palate or gingiva. Mostly in adult females.

Microscopic Findings

Unencapsulated nests of mature nevus cells:

- Superficial cells are epithelioid and contain melanin granules.
- Deeper cells are smaller, less epithelioid, and devoid of melanin.
- Deepest cells are spindled and also devoid of melanin.

Histopathologic Differential

Malignant melanoma is marked by atypical and pleomorphic melanocytes and invasion.

Treatment and Prognosis

Excisional biopsy

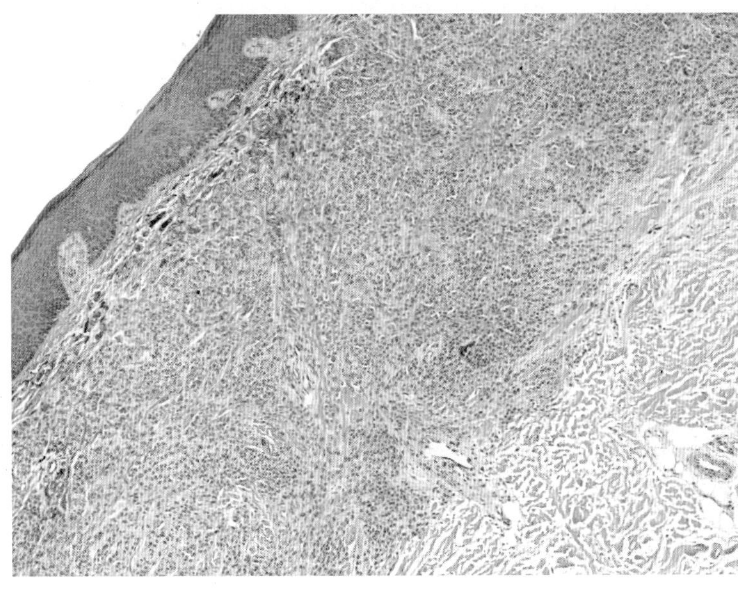

Figure 4.22.1.
Intramucosal nevus. Submucosal thèques of epithelioid cells. Some of the superficial cells contain melanin granules.

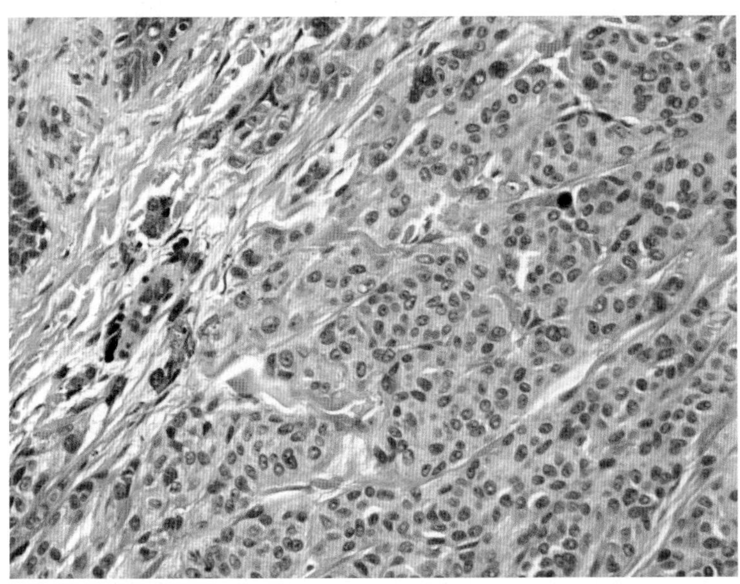

Figure 4.22.2.
Intramucosal nevus. Nests of polygonal, epithelioid nevus cells containing melanin granules.

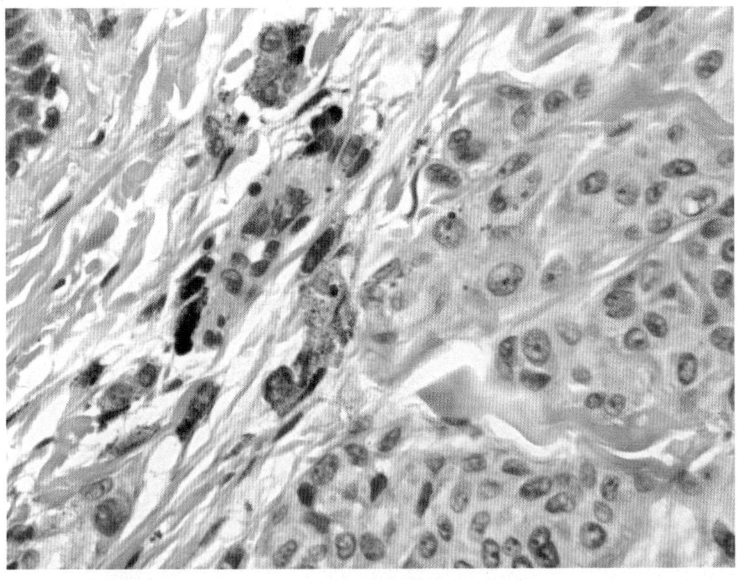

Figure 4.22.3.
Intramucosal nevus. Nests of uniform nevus cells, some containing melanin granules.

4.23 Oral Mucosal Melanoma

Presentation

Irregular brown or black patch or nodule on the palate or gingiva. Mostly in adult males.

Microscopic Findings

- Clusters of atypical, pigmented melanocytes in the lamina propria and deeper tissues
- Nests of frankly malignant melanocytes invading regional tissues

Special Stains/Immunopathology

- Tumor cells are positive for S100, HMB-45, and Melan-A.

Treatment and Prognosis

Radical surgery. The 5-year survival rate for oral melanoma is 20%.

Additional

Melanoma is a rare and highly lethal neoplasm in the oral cavity.

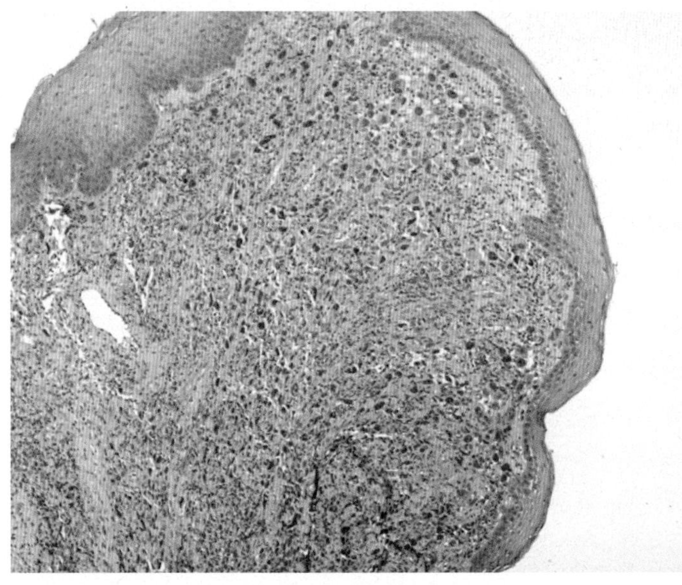

Figure 4.23.1.
Oral mucosal melanoma. The tumor nodule is composed of crowded, hyperchromatic, pleomorphic cells.

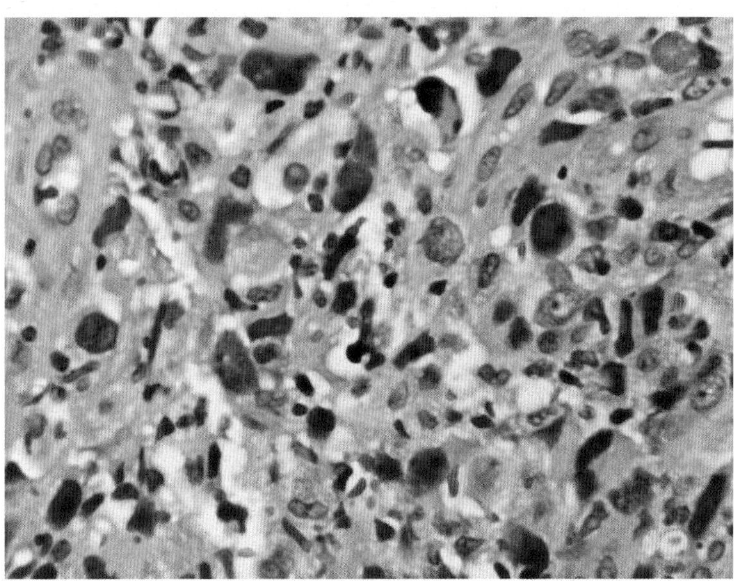

Figure 4.23.2.
Oral mucosal melanoma. Nests of anaplastic epithelioid cells with pleomorphic, hyperchromatic nuclei.

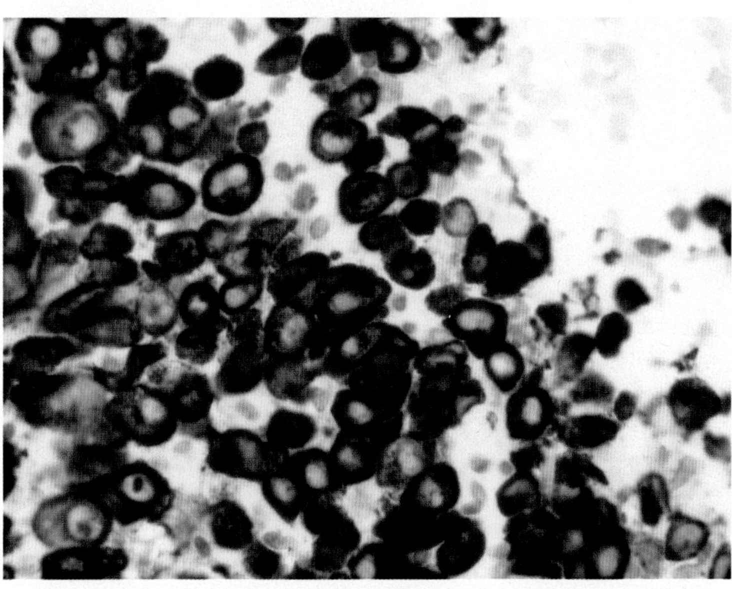

Figure 4.23.3.
Oral mucosal melanoma, HMB-45 stain. Diffuse positivity confirms the cells' melanocytic lineage.

4.24 Sjögren Syndrome and Sarcoidosis

Patients with Sjögren syndrome and sarcoidosis are sometimes referred for labial salivary gland biopsy to confirm their diagnosis.

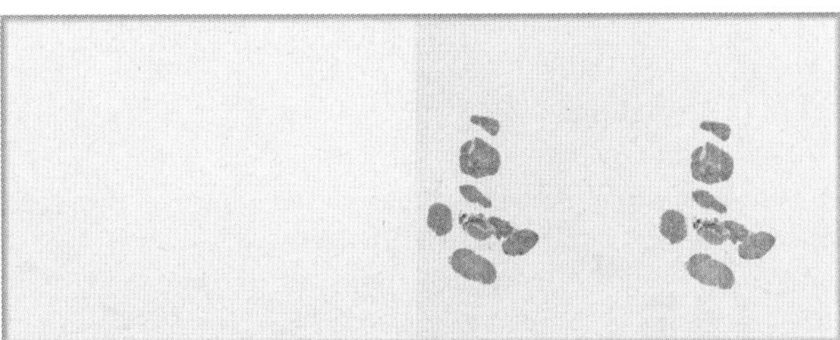

Figure 4.24.1.
Sjögren syndrome. Several minor salivary glands harvested from the lower lip are seen in this whole mount.

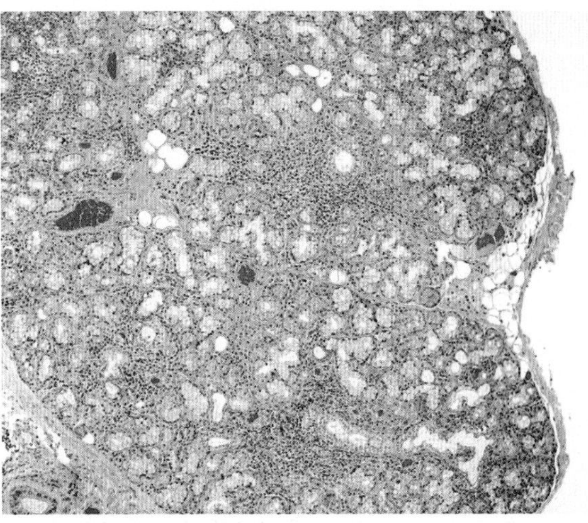

Figure 4.24.2.
Sjögren syndrome. A positive result is more than one focus of 50 or more lymphocytes in a periductal location. This minor salivary gland exhibits three such foci.

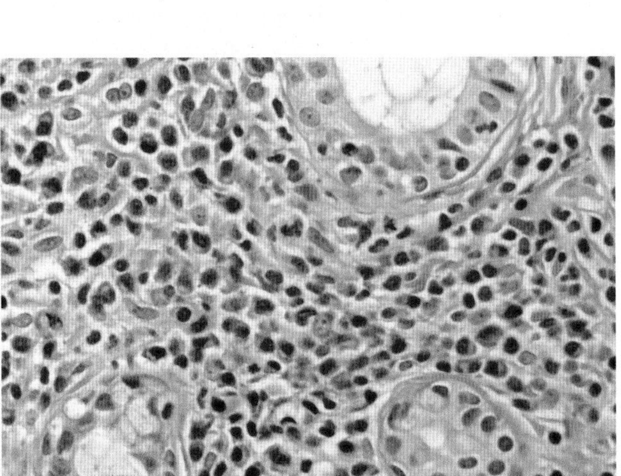

Figure 4.24.3.
Sjögren syndrome. A closer view of periductal lymphocytes (and the occasional plasma cell).

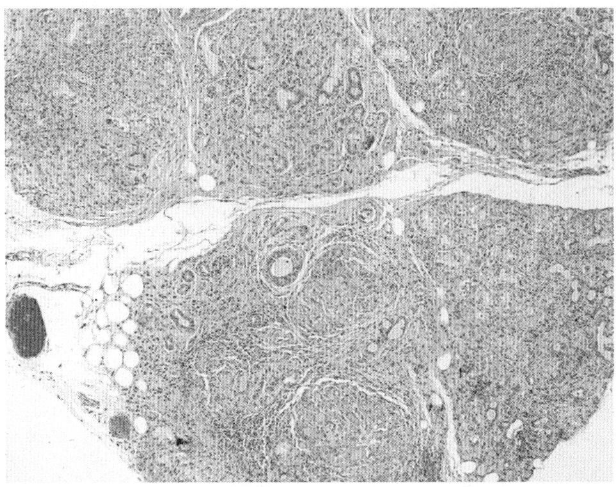

Figure 4.25.1.
Sarcoidosis. Biopsy of a lip nodule discloses epithelioid granulomas within minor salivary glands. The patient was sent in for a diagnostic biopsy to confirm the clinical impression of sarcoidosis.

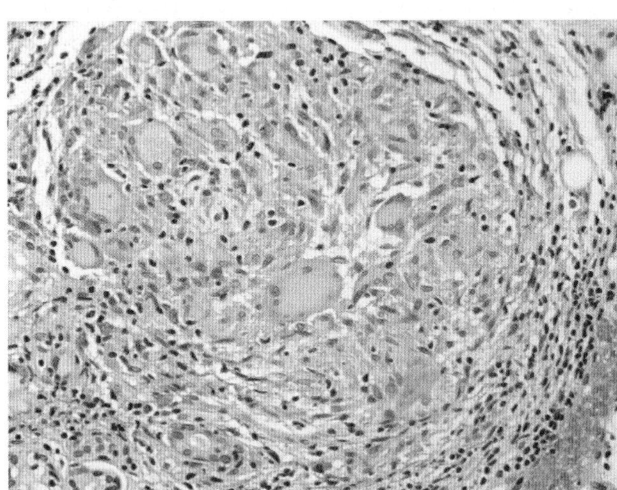

Figure 4.25.2.
Sarcoidosis. Granulomas are surrounded by a sparse lymphoid reaction.

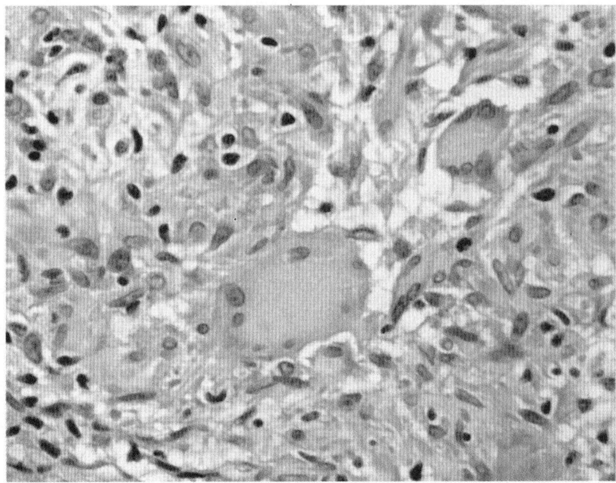

Figure 4.25.3.
Sarcoidosis. Histiocytes and giant cells within the granuloma.

Bibliography and Suggested Reading

4.1

Nasser W, Flechtenmacher C, Holzinger D, et al. Aberrant expression of p53, p16(INK4a) and Ki-67 as basic biomarker for malignant progression of oral leukoplakias. *J Oral Pathol Med.* 2011;40(8)629–635.

4.2

Hsue SS, Wang WC, Chen CH, et al. Malignant transformation in 1458 patients with potentially malignant oral mucosal disorders: a follow-up study based in a Taiwanese hospital. *J Oral Pathol Med.* 2007;36:25–29.

4.3

Summerlin DJ, Dunipace A, Potter R. Histologic effects of smokeless tobacco and alcohol on the pouch mucosa and organs of the Syrian hamster. *J Oral Pathol Med.* 1992;21:105–108.

4.4

Rekha KP, Angadi PV. Verrucous carcinoma of the oral cavity: a clinico-pathologic appraisal of 133 cases in Indians. *Oral Maxillofac Surg.* 2010;14:211–218.

4.5

Laco J, Vosmikova H, Novakova V, et al. The role of high-risk human papillomavirus infection in oral and oropharyngeal squamous cell carcinoma in non-smoking and non-drinking patients: a clinicopathological and molecular study of 46 cases. *Virchows Arch.* 2011;458:179–187.

4.6

Barnes L, Ferlito A, Altavilla G, et al. Basaloid squamous cell carcinoma of the head and neck: clinicopathological features and differential diagnosis. *Ann Otol Rhinol Laryngol.* 1996;105:75–82.

Ide F, Shimoyama T, Horie N, et al. Basaloid squamous cell carcinoma of the oral mucosa: a new case and review of 45 cases in the literature. *Oral Oncol.* 2002;38:120–124.

4.7

Shibuya Y, Umeda M, Yokoo S, et al. Spindle cell squamous carcinoma of the maxilla: report of a case with immunohistochemical analysis. *J Oral Maxillofac Surg.* 2000;58:1164–1169.

4.8

Martin JL. Leukoedema: a review of the literature. *J Natl Med Assoc.* 1992;84:938–940.

4.9

Milo lu O, Göregen M, Akgül HM, et al. The prevalence and risk factors associated with benign migratory glossitis lesions in 7619 Turkish dental outpatients. *Oral Surg Oral Med Oral Pathol Oral Radiol Endod.* 2009;107:e29–e33.

4.10

Woo SB, Lin D. Morsicatio mucosae oris—a chronic oral frictional keratosis, not a leukoplakia. *J Oral Maxillofac Surg.* 2009;67:140–146.

4.11

Piperi E, Omlie J, Koutlas IG, et al. Oral hairy leukoplakia in HIV-negative patients: report of 10 cases. *Int J Surg Pathol.* 2010;18:177–183.

4.12

Philipsen HP, Reichart PA, Takata T, et al. Verruciform xanthoma—biological profile of 282 oral lesions based on a literature survey with nine new cases from Japan. *Oral Oncol.* 2003;39:325–336.

4.13

Henley JD, Summerlin DJ, Tomich CE. Condyloma acuminatum and condyloma-like lesions of the oral cavity: a study of 11 cases with an intraductal component. *Histopathology.* 2004;44:216–221.

Jaju PP, Suvarna PV, Desai RS. Squamous papilloma: case report and review of literature. *Int J Oral Sci.* 2010;2:222–225.

4.14

Chattopadhyay A, Shetty KV. Recurrent aphthous stomatitis. *Otolaryngol Clin North Am.* 2011;44:79–88, v.

4.15

López-Pintor RM, Hernández G, de Arriba L, et al. Oral ulcers during the course of cytomegalovirus infection in renal transplant recipients. *Transplant Proc.* 2009;41:2419–2421.

4.16

Roopashree MR, Gondhalekar RV, Shashikanth MC, et al. Pathogenesis of oral lichen planus—a review. *J Oral Pathol Med.* 2010;39:729–734.

4.17

Aggarwal V, Jain A, Kabi D. Oral lichenoid reaction associated with tin component of amalgam restorations: a case report. *Am J Dermatopathol.* 2010;32:46–48.

4.18

Kourosh AS, Yancey KB. Pathogenesis of mucous membrane pemphigoid. *Dermatol Clin.* 2011;29:479–484.

4.19

Dagistan S, Goregen M, Miloglu O, et al. Oral pemphigus vulgaris: a case report with review of the literature. *J Oral Sci.* 2008;50:359–362.

4.20

Buchner A, Hansen LS. Amalgam pigmentation (amalgam tattoo) of the oral mucosa: a clinicopathologic study of 268 cases. *Oral Surg Oral Med Oral Pathol.* 1980;49:139–147.

4.21

Shen ZY, Liu W, Bao ZX, et al. Oral melanotic macule and primary oral malignant melanoma: epidemiology, location involved, and clinical implications. *Oral Surg Oral Med Oral Pathol Oral Radiol Endod.* 2011;112:e21–e25.

4.22

Buchner A, Merrell PW, Carpenter WM. Relative frequency of solitary melanocytic lesions of the oral mucosa. *J Oral Pathol Med.* 2004;33:550–557.

4.23

Patel SG, Prasad ML, Escrig M, et al. Primary mucosal malignant melanoma of the head and neck. *Head Neck.* 2002;24:247–257.

4.24

Giuca MR, Bonfiqli D, Bartoli F, et al. Sjögren's syndrome: correlation between histopatholgic result and clinical and serologic parameters. *Minerva Stomatol.* 2010;59:149–154.

Teppo H, Revonta M. A follow-up study of minimally invasive lip biopsy in the diagnosis of Sjögren's syndrome. *Clin Rheumatol.* 2007;26:1099–1103.

4.25

Blinder D, Yahatom R, Taicher S. Oral manifestations of sarcoidosis. *Oral Surg Oral Med Oral Pathol Oral Radiol Endod.* 1997;83:458–461.

Marcoval J, Mañá J. Specific (granulomatous) oral lesions of sarcoidosis: report of two cases. *Med Oral Pathol Oral Cir Bucal.* 2010;15:e456—e458.

CHAPTER

5

Soft Tissue Tumors and Reactive Lesions

Irritation fibroma
Giant cell fibroma
Epulis fissuratum
Pyogenic granuloma (lobular capillary hemangioma)
Peripheral ossifying fibroma
Peripheral giant cell granuloma
Lipoma
Solitary fibrous tumor
Traumatic neuroma
Palisaded encapsulated neuroma
Schwannoma
Neurofibroma
Granular cell tumor
Hemangioma
Caliber-persistent artery
Intravascular papillary endothelial hyperplasia
Traumatic ulcerative granuloma with stromal eosinophilia (TUGSE)
Kaposi sarcoma
Lymphangioma
Vascular leiomyoma (angioleiomyoma)
Myofibroma
Leiomyosarcoma
Unusual soft tissue masses

Introduction

The soft tissue tumors of the mouth include tumors of fibroblastic, lipomatous, neurogenic, vascular, and smooth muscle lineage. Most are similar to their counterparts elsewhere in the body. Several of the reactive lesions—epulis fissuratum, peripheral ossifying fibroma, and peripheral giant cell granuloma—are unique to the oral cavity

The most common oral soft tissue biopsies received by the pathology laboratory are irritation fibroma, epulis fissuratum, and the three "P" lesions of the gingiva: pyogenic granuloma, peripheral ossifying fibroma, and peripheral giant cell granuloma. Other frequently submitted biopsies include lipomas, the various neurogenic tumors, granular cell tumors, and hemangiomas.

Most pathologists are familiar with the pseudoepitheliomatous hyperplasia of the granular cell tumor, but other benign soft tissue tumors can present diagnostic challenges, including solitary fibrous tumor and myofibroma. Immunohistochemical stains are helpful in elucidating the nature of these neoplasms.

Malignant soft tissue tumors within the mouth are rare. Kaposi sarcoma in HIV-infected patients was once the most common sarcoma received by the pathology laboratory; it is now, fortunately, rarely seen.

At the end of the chapter are three entities that are often submitted as oral submucosal masses: reactive lymphoid hyperplasia, lymphoma, and foreign body granuloma.

5.1 Irritation Fibroma

Presentation

Firm, exophytic nodule, often in areas associated with chronic trauma, such as the buccal mucosa. Most patients are aged between 30 and 60 years.

Histology

- Mass of dense fibrous connective tissue
- Flattened rete ridges in overlying oral mucosa
- Can be ulcerated or show a hyperkeratotic surface

Histopathologic Differential

- The mucosal epithelium overlying a *giant cell fibroma* shows long, narrow rete ridges; the connective tissue mass contains large stellate fibroblasts.
- A maturing *pyogenic granuloma* has features of inflamed granulation tissue.

Treatment and Prognosis

Excision and removal of the source of irritation

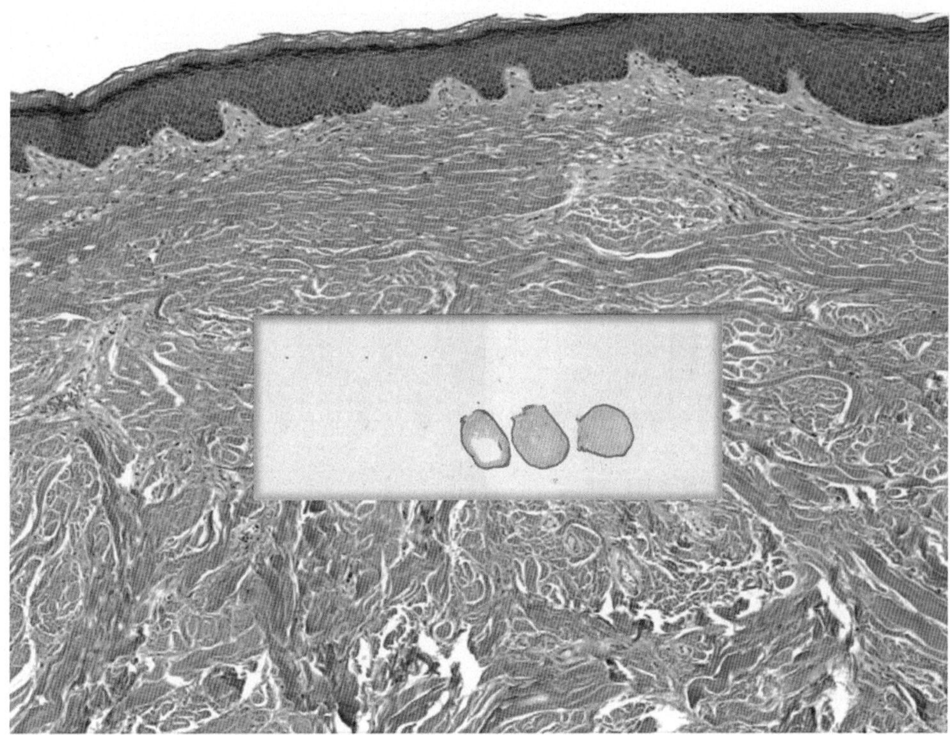

Figure 5.1.1.
Irritation fibroma. A dome-shaped lesion composed of a subepithelial mass of dense fibrous connective tissue.

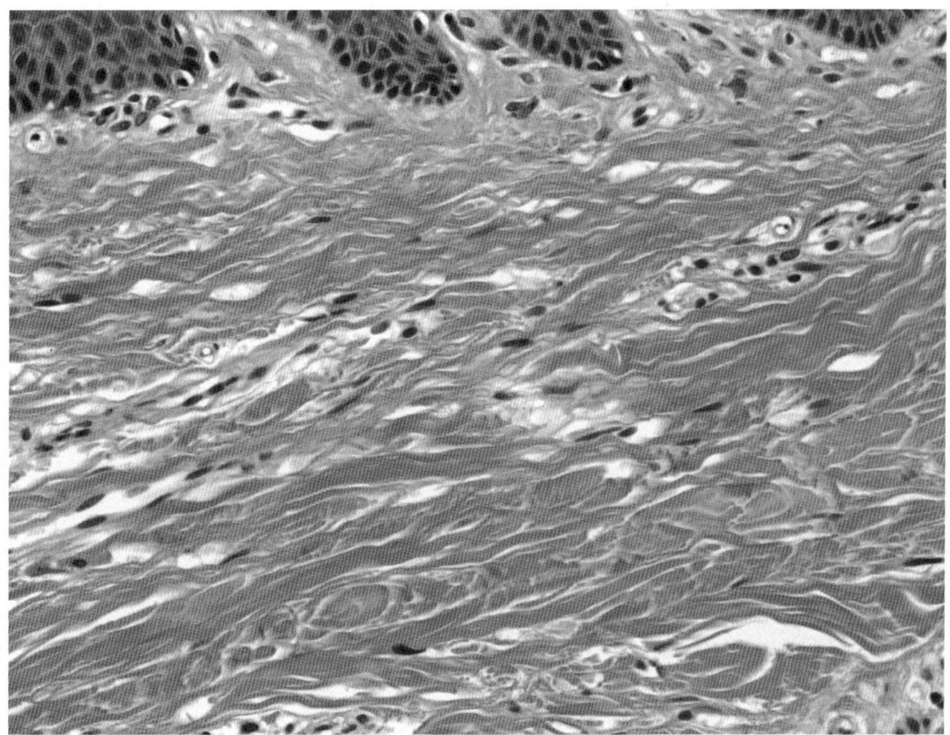

Figure 5.1.2.
Irritation fibroma. Abundant dense collagen bundles and scattered fibroblasts.

5.2 Giant Cell Fibroma

Presentation

Small exophytic mass, mainly of the gingiva. Most patients are younger than 30 years.

Histology

- Small nodule of fibrous connective tissue containing large stellate fibroblasts with single or multiple enlarged nuclei
- Hyperplastic overlying mucosa with narrow, elongated, interconnecting rete ridges

Histopathologic Differential

The mucosal epithelium overlying an *irritation fibroma* is thin or hyperkerantotic and the epithelial–connective tissue interface is flat (no rete ridges). Large, stellate fibroblasts are absent.

Treatment and Prognosis

Excision

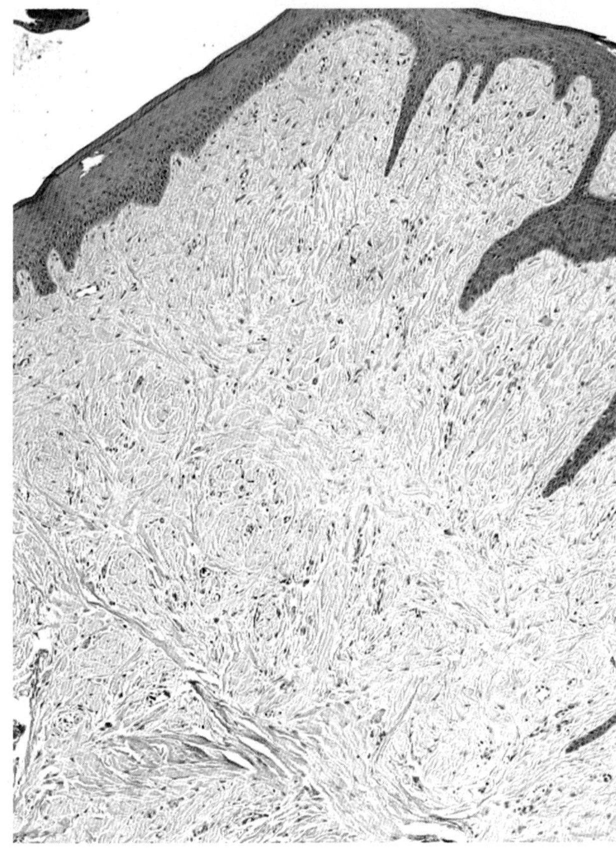

Figure 5.2.1.
Giant cell fibroma. A nodular mass of fibrous connective tissue. The epithelium is hyperplastic, and the rete ridges are thin and elongated.

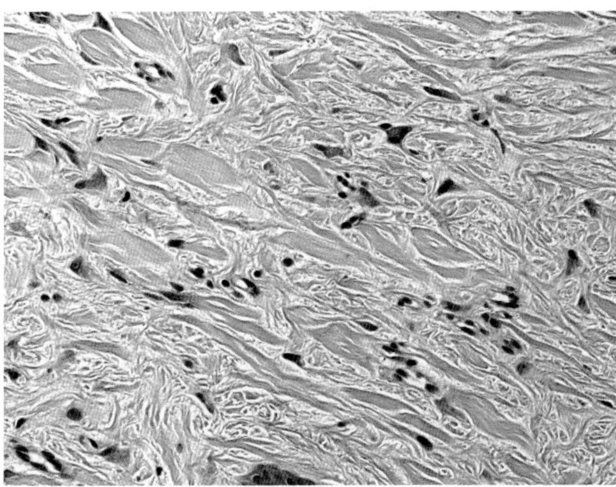

Figure 5.2.2.
Giant cell fibroma. Numerous stellate fibroblasts exhibiting large, hyperchromatic nuclei.

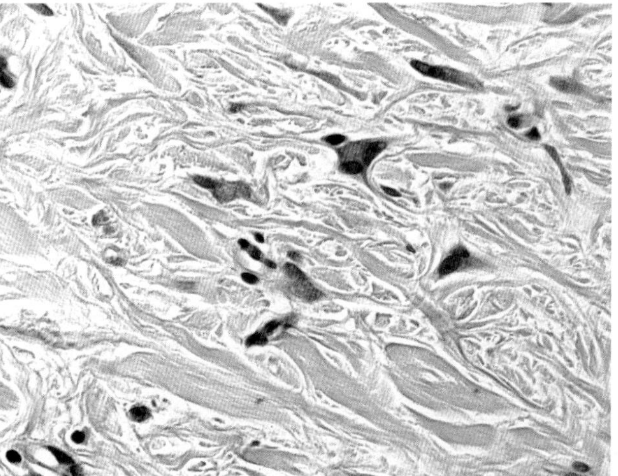

Figure 5.2.3.
Giant cell fibroma. The giant, stellate fibroblasts have multiple nuclei.

5.3 Epulis Fissuratum

Definition

Reactive fibrous tissue overgrowth due to an ill-fitting denture

Presentation

Gingiva and alveolar mucosa

Histology

- Hyperplastic fibrous connective tissue, often inflamed
- Papillary hyperplasia of the overlying mucosa
- Osseous or chondromatous metaplasia is occasionally seen within the fibrous stroma

Treatment and Prognosis

Excision and removal of the source of irritation, generally fabrication of a new denture

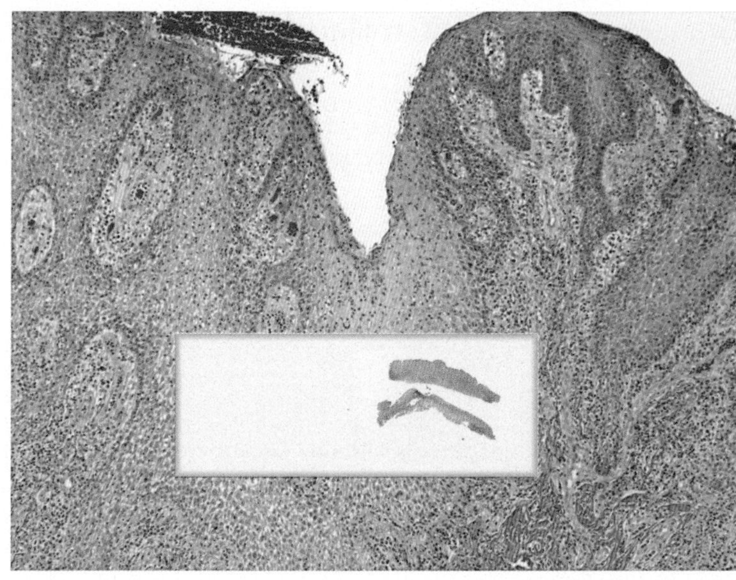

Figure 5.3.1.
Epulis fissuratum. Epithelial and fibrous proliferation with inflammation and edema. The fissure in the epithelium was created by a denture flange.

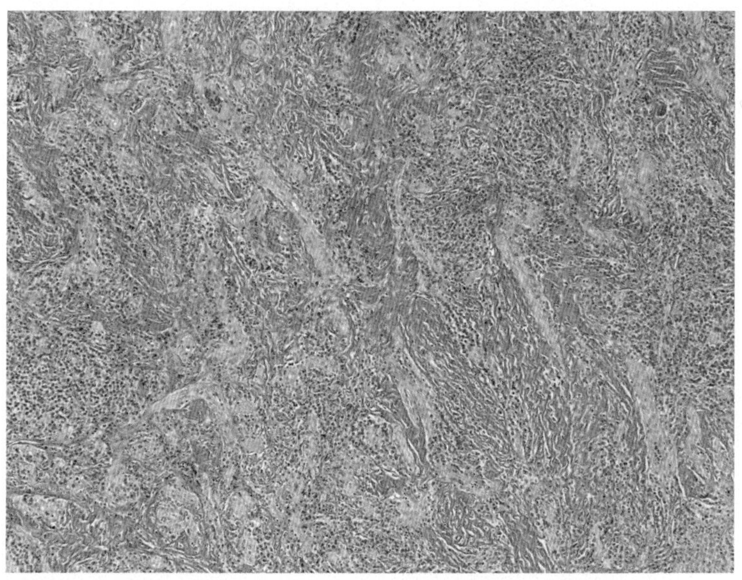

Figure 5.3.2.
Epulis fissuratum. Chronic irritation has resulted in a fibrous hyperplasia that is dense and hyalinized. Inflammation is intense.

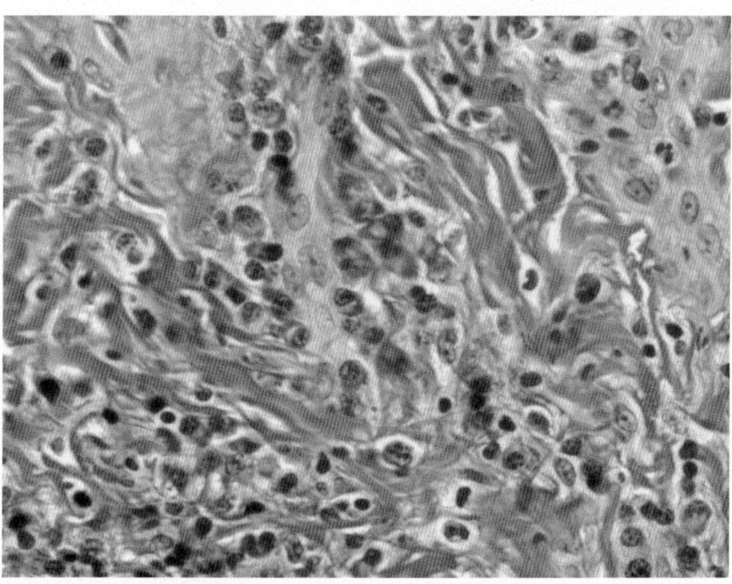

AQ4

Figure 5.3.3.
Epulis fissuratum. The inflammatory component consists of lymphocytes and plasma cells.

5.4 Pyogenic Granuloma (Lobular Capillary Hemangioma)

Presentation

Pedunculated, lobular, ulcerated mass of the gingiva or a mass of tissue arising from a tooth socket after an extraction. In young adults; common in pregnant women.

Histology

- Surface usually ulcerated
- Granulation tissue and proliferation of small vessels toward surface
- Larger, ectatic vessels in lobular aggregates within deeper connective tissue
- Brisk mitoses, but not atypical

Histopathologic Differential

- *Kaposi sarcoma* will contain fascicles of spindle cells with tiny vascular channels containing red blood cells.
- In *traumatic ulcerative granuloma with stromal eosinophilia* (TUGSE), prominent clusters of histiocytes and eosinophils are present in the deeper lesional stroma.

Treatment and Prognosis

Excision with curettage of the underlying tissue together with removal of any source of irritation. Occasional lesions recur.

Additional

A pyogenic granuloma can mature into an *irritation fibroma,* with many lesions exhibiting the characteristics of both.

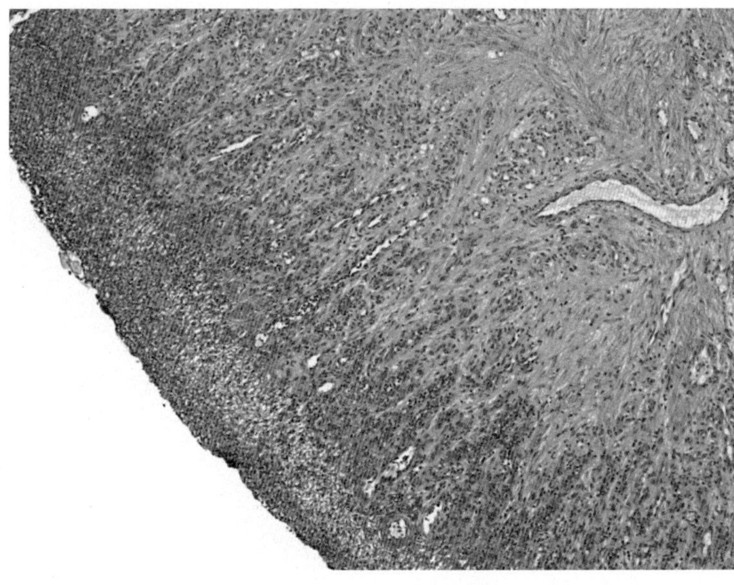

Figure 5.4.1.
Pyogenic granuloma. Fibrin membrane, inflammatory cells, and elongated capillaries in ulcer bed.

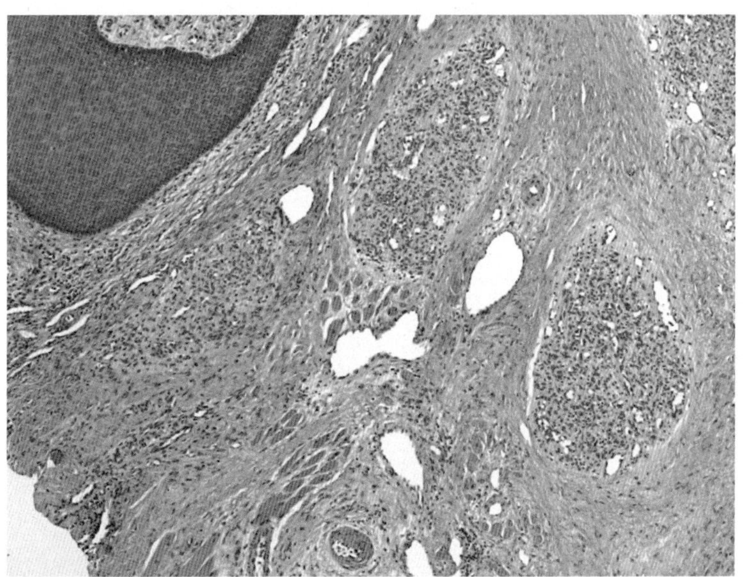

Figure 5.4.2.
Pyogenic granuloma. The deeper stroma contains lobules of endothelial cells and capillaries.

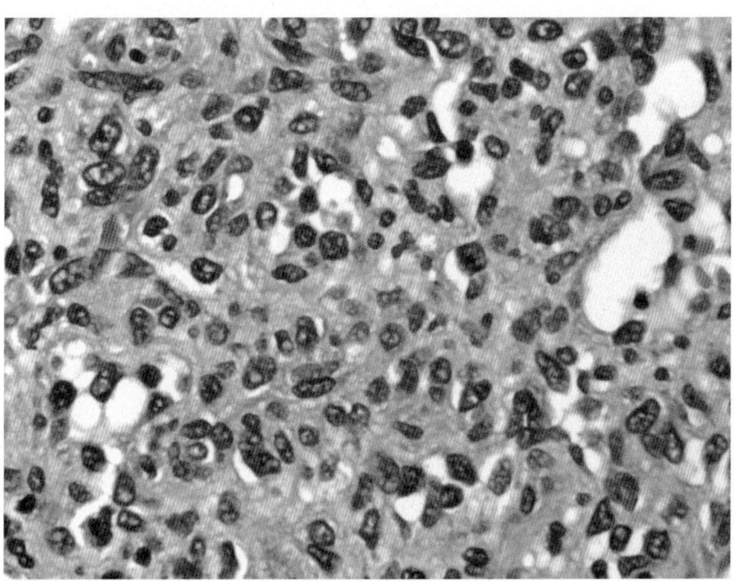

Figure 5.4.3.
Pyogenic granuloma. Capillaries and endothelial cells.

5.5 Peripheral Ossifying Fibroma

Presentation

Exophytic nodule, sometimes ulcerated. Gingiva exclusively. In teenagers, more often in females.

Histology

- Fibroblasts and fibrous connective tissue containing bone or cemental tissue.
- Ulceration of the overlying mucosa is common.

Treatment and Prognosis

Excision with curettage of the underlying tissue together with removal of any source of irritation. Occasional lesions recur.

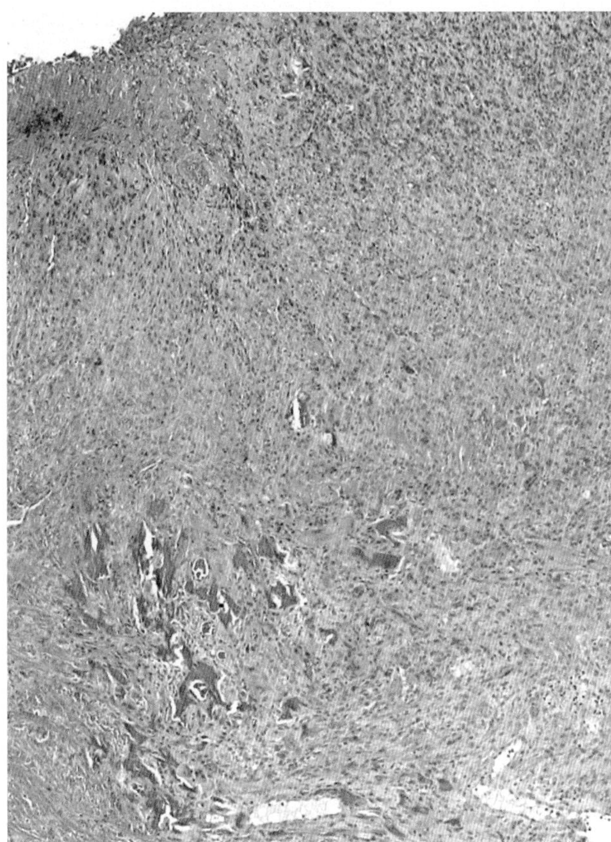

Figure 5.5.1.
Peripheral ossifying fibroma. Ulcerated surface overlying a proliferation of fibroblasts and metaplastic cemento-osseous tissue.

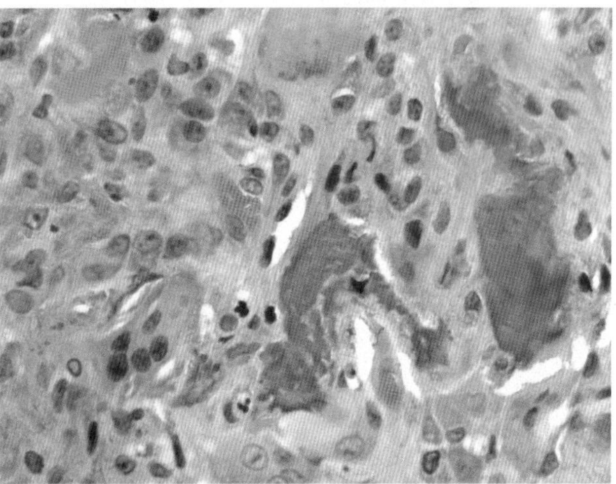

Figure 5.5.2.
Peripheral ossifying fibroma. Metaplastic cemento-osseous tissue set in a cellular, vascular stroma.

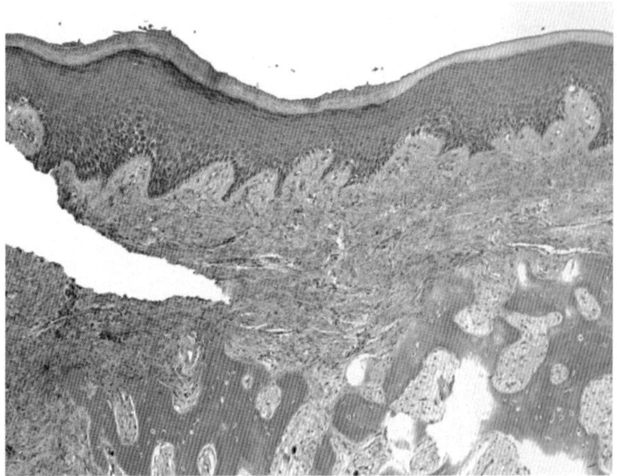

Figure 5.5.3.
Peripheral ossifying fibroma. Osseous trabeculae are seen in the lesional fibrous connective tissue.

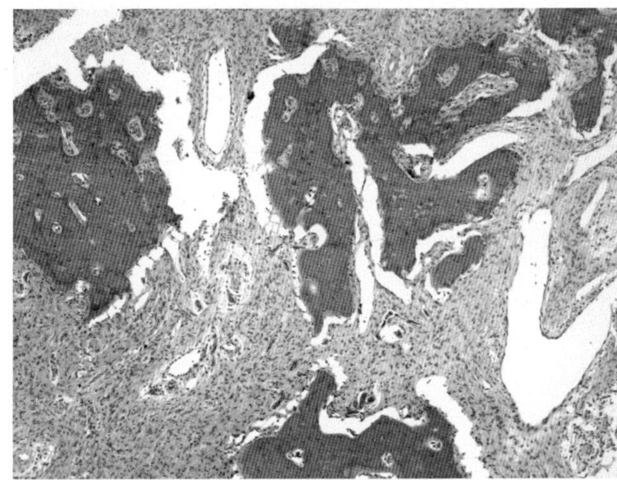

Figure 5.5.4.
Peripheral ossifying fibroma. Fragments of mature bone in a cellular, well-vascularized fibrous tissue.

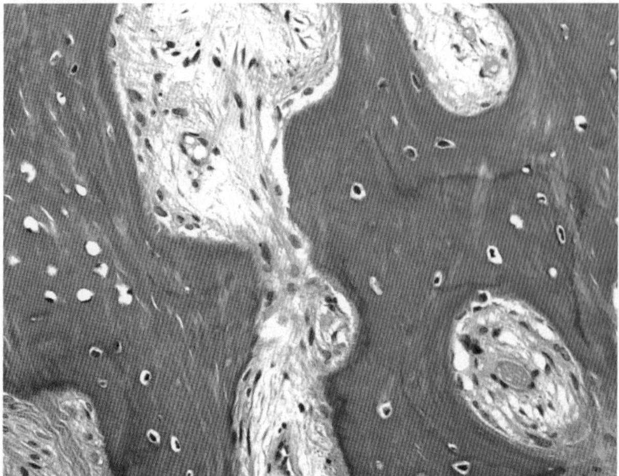

Figure 5.5.5.
Peripheral ossifying fibroma. Trabeculae consist of mature lamellar-bone within a loose fibrous connective tissue stroma.

5.6 Peripheral Giant Cell Granuloma

Presentation

Exophytic purplish nodule, often ulcerated. Gingiva exclusively. Teenagers, often females.

Histology

- Proliferation of plump, spindle cells with normal mitotic figures
- Clusters of multinucleated giant cells
- Rich vascularity with erythrocyte extravasation and hemosiderin deposits

Treatment and Prognosis

Excision with curettage of the underlying tissue together with removal of any source of irritation.

Additional

The histology of the peripheral giant cell granuloma is identical to that of the *brown tumor of bone.* This peripheral (mucosal-based) lesion, however, is not associated with hyperparathyroidism.

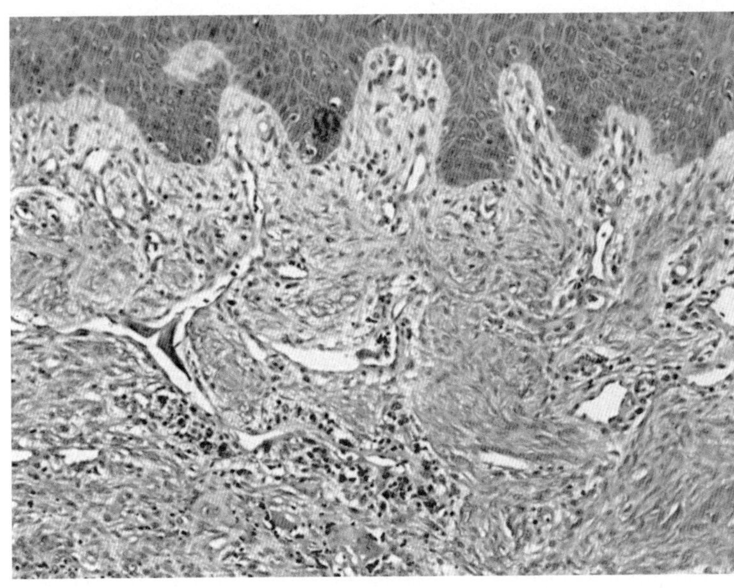

Figure 5.6.1.
Peripheral giant cell granuloma. A poorly circumscribed mass of multinucleated giant cells is seen in the deep submucosa at the lower left.

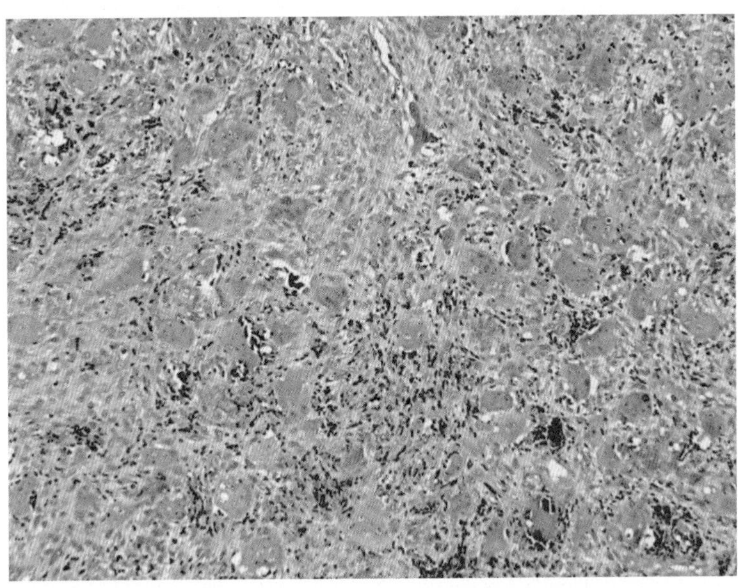

Figure 5.6.2.
Peripheral giant cell granuloma. Multinucleated giant cells set in a loose, hemorrhagic stroma.

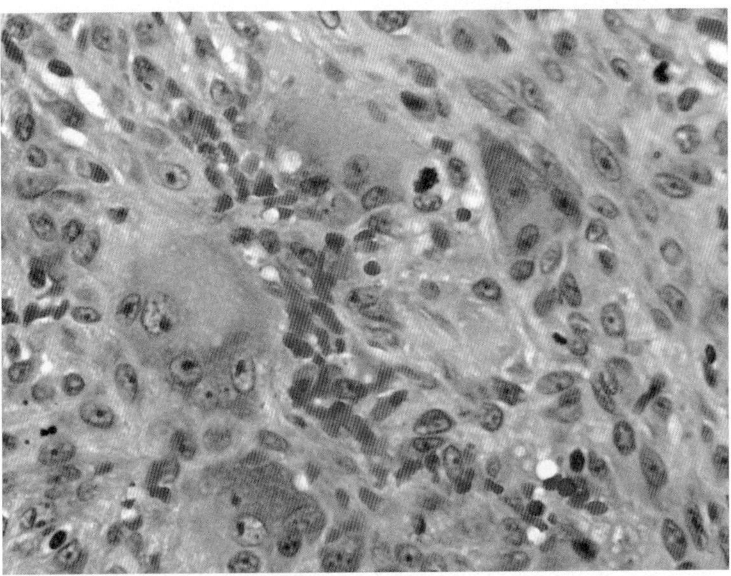

Figure 5.6.3.
Peripheral giant cell granuloma. Multinucleated giant cells, plump stromal cells, and extravasated erythrocytes. Mitotic figures are present within the stromal spindle cells.

5.7 Lipoma

Presentation

Submucosal nodule, frequently with a yellowish tinge. Buccal mucosa and tongue. In older adults; rare in children.

Histology

Most are classic lipomas, consisting of mature adipocytes and variable amounts of fibrous connective tissue.

Treatment and Prognosis

Excision. Does not recur.

Additional

Liposarcomas of the oral cavity are exceedingly rare. Spindle cell lipomas and intramuscular myxoid lipomas have been reported.

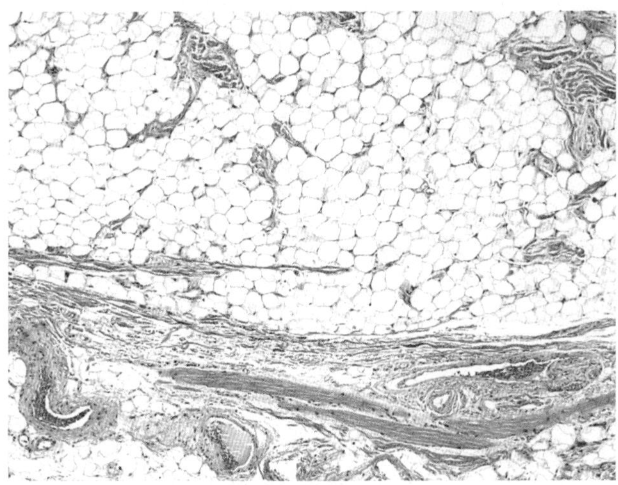

Figure 5.7.1.
Lipoma. Lobules of mature adipose tissue.

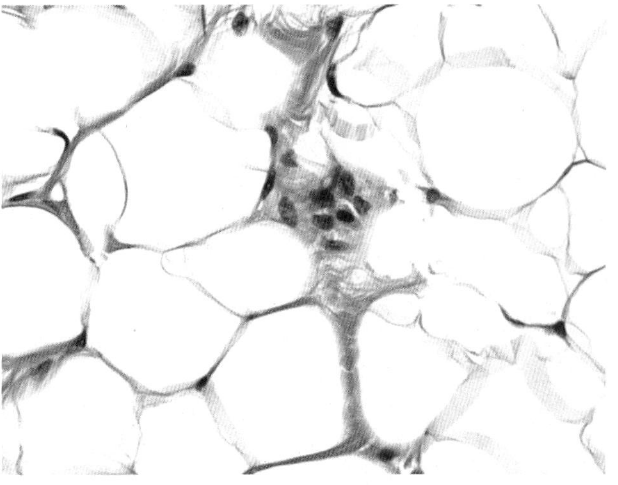

Figure 5.7.2.
Lipoma. Thin fibrous bands separate groups of adipocytes.

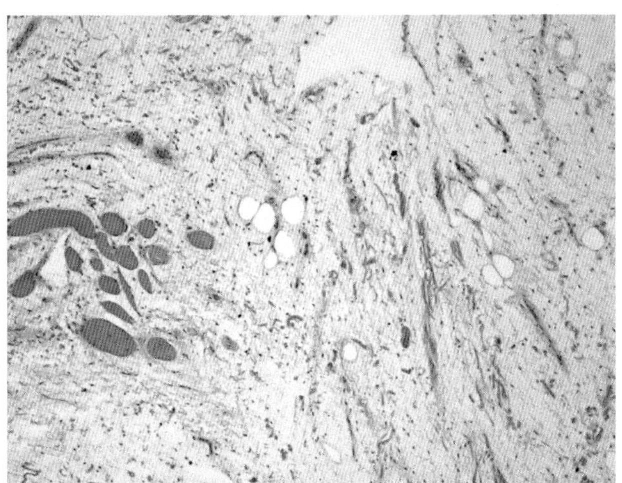

Figure 5.7.3.
Lipoma, intramuscular myxoid. Intramuscular proliferation of myxoid and adipose tissue.

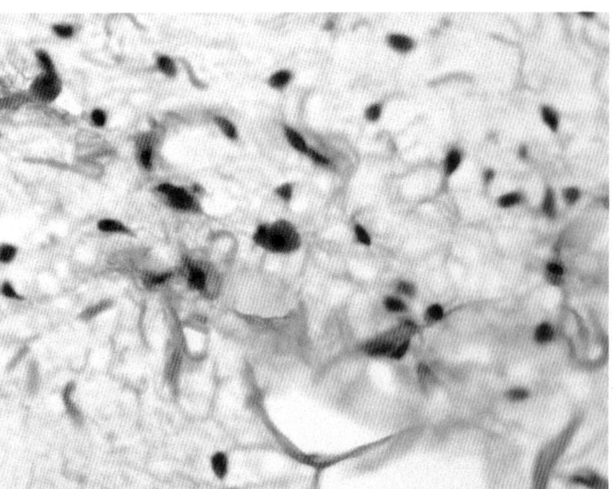

Figure 5.7.4.
Lipoma, intramuscular myxoid. Myxoid tissue, lipocytes, and a solitary mast cell.

5.8 Solitary Fibrous Tumor

Presentation

Slow-growing, painless nodule, usually of buccal mucosa. In adults.

Histology

- Spindle cell proliferation with alternating hyper- and hypocellular areas
- Vessels with hemangiopericytomatous, "staghorn" pattern

Special Stains/Immunopathology

Spindle cells are positive for CD34 and BCL2.

Histopathologic Differential

- *Schwannomas* and *neurofibromas* are positive for S100.
- *Vascular leiomyomas* and *myofibromas* are positive for smooth muscle markers.

Treatment and Prognosis

Complete excision. Usually does not recur.

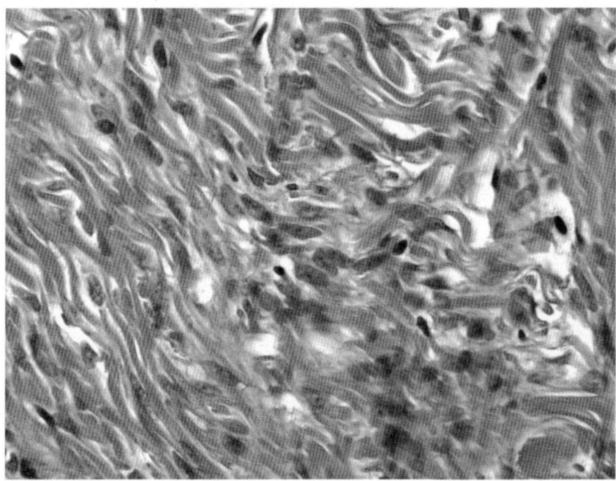

Figure 5.8.1.
Solitary fibrous tumor. Parallel fascicles of spindle cells in one of the more cellular areas.

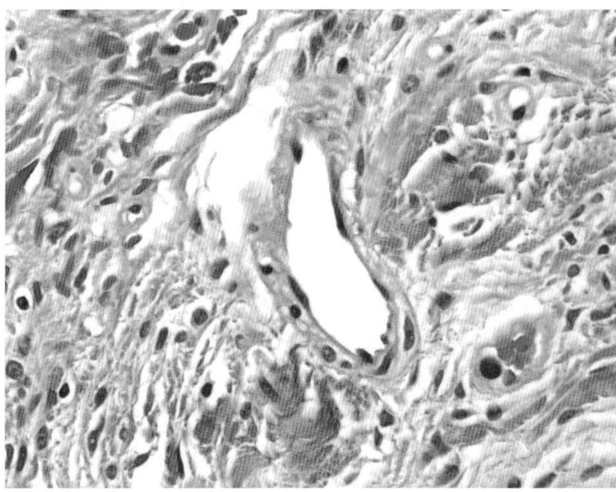

Figure 5.8.2.
Solitary fibrous tumor. Dilated, irregular small vessel in one of the less cellular areas.

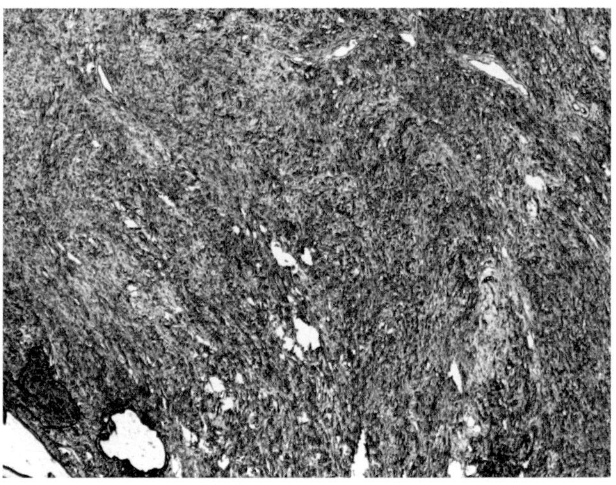

Figure 5.8.3.
Solitary fibrous tumor. CD34-positive staining. Numerous, variably sized staghorn vessels are seen.

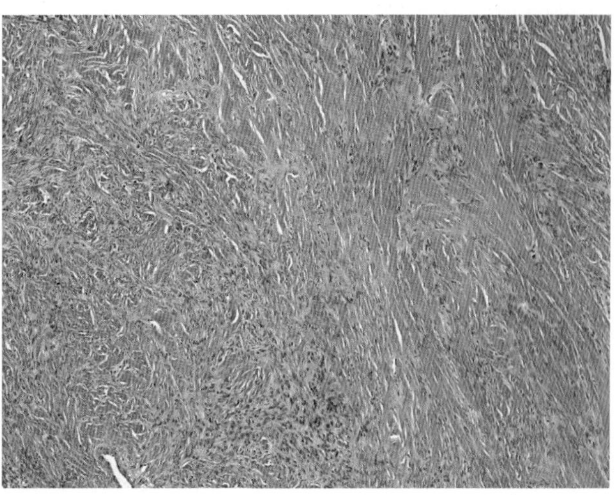

Figure 5.8.4.
Solitary fibrous tumor. This tumor contains distinct hypo- and hypercellular areas within dense bands of fibrous connective tissue.

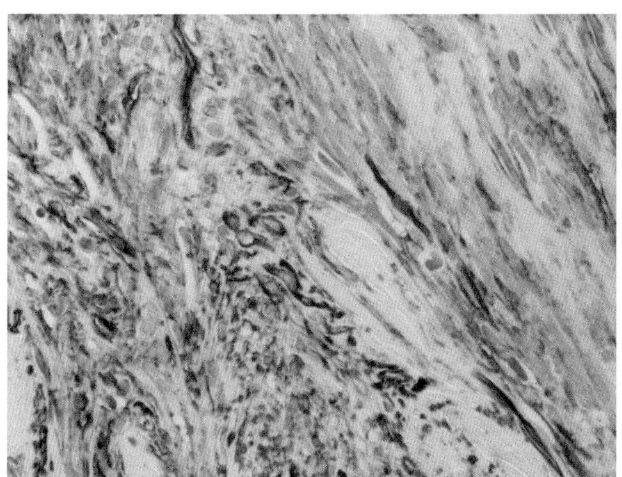

Figure 5.8.5.
Solitary fibrous tumor. The lesional cells are positive for CD34.

5.9 Traumatic Neuroma

Presentation
Painful submucosal nodule often associated with a history of trauma. The mental foramen area of the mandible and lips are the most common sites. In adults; more common in females.

Histology
- Proliferation of intertwined small nerves surrounded by fibrous connective tissue

Histopathologic Differential
- A *neurofibroma* lacks discrete clusters of small nerves.
- *Oral mucosal neuromas* (see Additional) tend to have a thick, onion-skin perineurium.

Treatment and Prognosis
Excision. Does not recur.

Additional
Multiple oral mucosal neuromas in children may suggest the presence of multiple endocrine neoplasia type IIB.

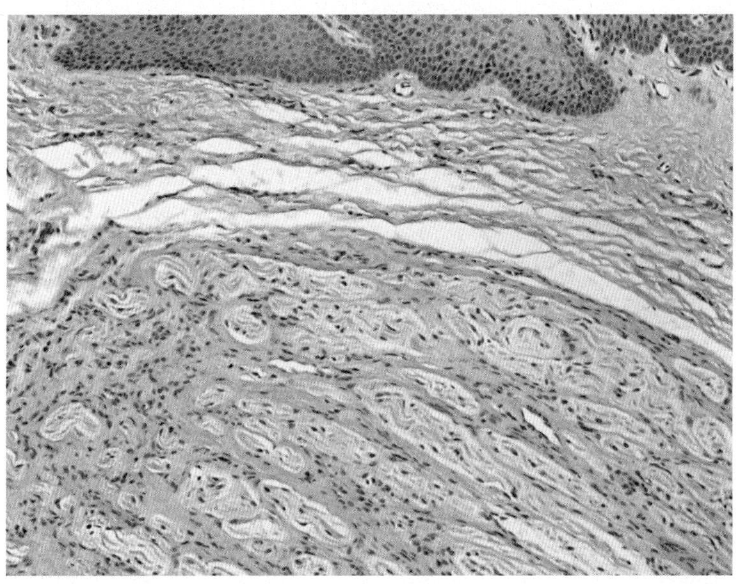

Figure 5.9.1.
Traumatic neuroma. A submucosal proliferation of small neural structures surrounded by fibrous connective tissue.

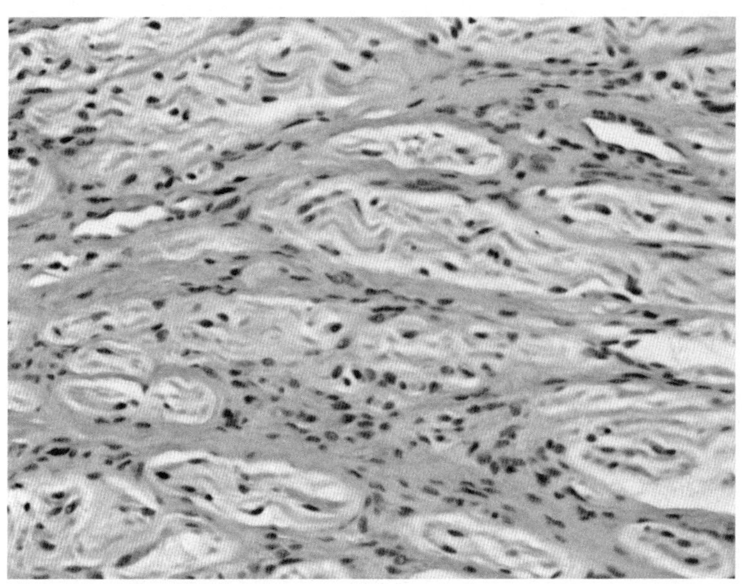

Figure 5.9.2.
Traumatic neuroma. The mass consists of two distinct populations of spindle cells: Schwann cells and perineural fibroblasts.

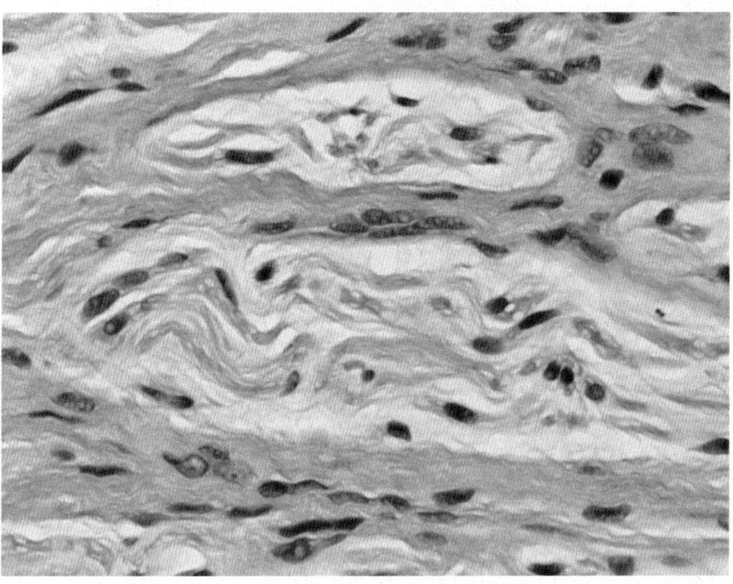

Figure 5.9.3.
Traumatic neuroma. Fascicles of Schwann cells with distinctive, curved nuclei are surrounded by perineural fibroblasts. Small neurites are also seen.

5.10 Palisaded Encapsulated Neuroma

Presentation

Submucosal nodule 1 cm or less, typically on the hard palate or lips. In adults.

Histology

- Circumscribed, generally unilobular
- Mass of spindle-shaped Schwann cells with wavy, pointed nuclei
- Suggestion of nuclear palisading sometimes seen, but generally not in the form of distinct Verocay bodies

Special Stains/Immunopathology

Tumor cells are S100-positive.

Histopathologic Differential

- A *schwannoma* contains Antoni A and B areas and Verocay bodies.
- A *traumatic neuroma* is a less organized proliferation of recognizable small nerves within a fibrous connective tissue.

Treatment and Prognosis

Excision. Does not recur.

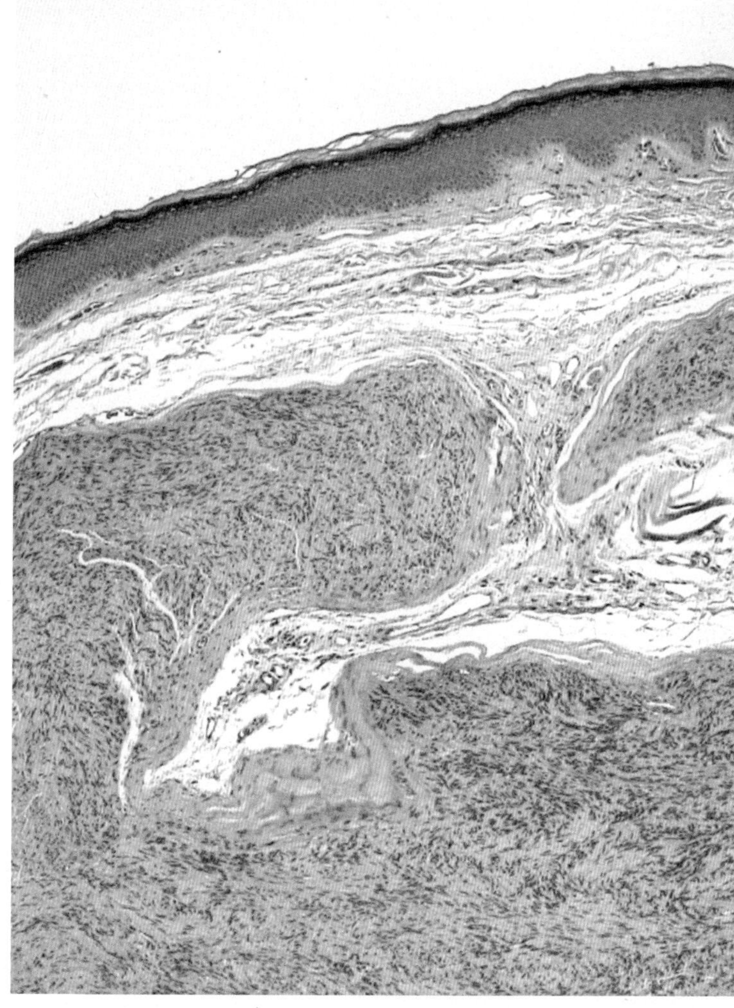

Figure 5.10.1.
Palisaded encapsulated neuroma. A circumscribed subepithelial tumor composed of intertwined bands of spindle cells with scant eosinophilic stroma.

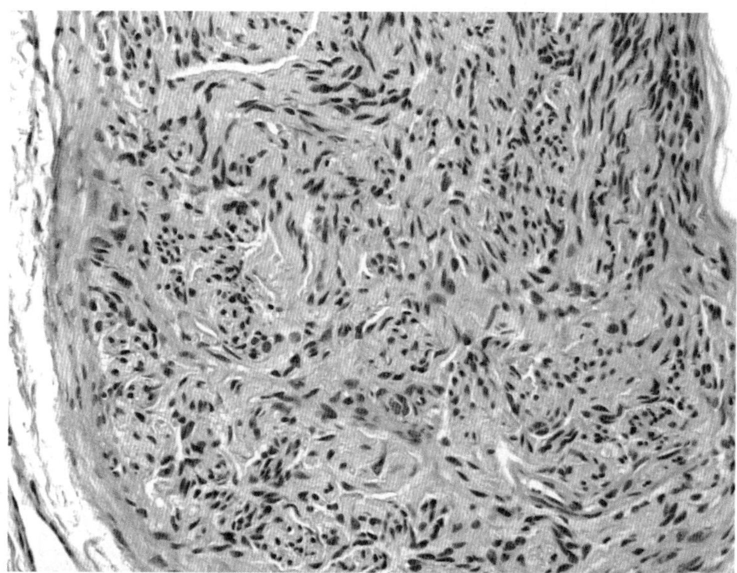

Figure 5.10.2.
Palisaded encapsulated neuroma. A circumscribed mass of Schwann cells with a suggestion of nuclear palisading.

5.11 Schwannoma

Presentation

Submucosal nodule, usually of the tongue. In adults.

Histology

- Circumscribed tumor.
- Lesion consists almost entirely of Schwann cells.
- Loose, myxoid areas alternate with cellular areas containing Verocay bodies (palisading Schwann cell nuclei around a central acellular, eosinophilic core).
- A nerve trunk is sometimes seen outside the main tumor mass.

Special Stains/Immunopathology

Tumor cells are S100-positive.

Histopathologic Differential

A *palisaded encapsulated neuroma* lacks distinct Antoni A and B areas and well-formed Verocay bodies.

Treatment and Prognosis

Excision

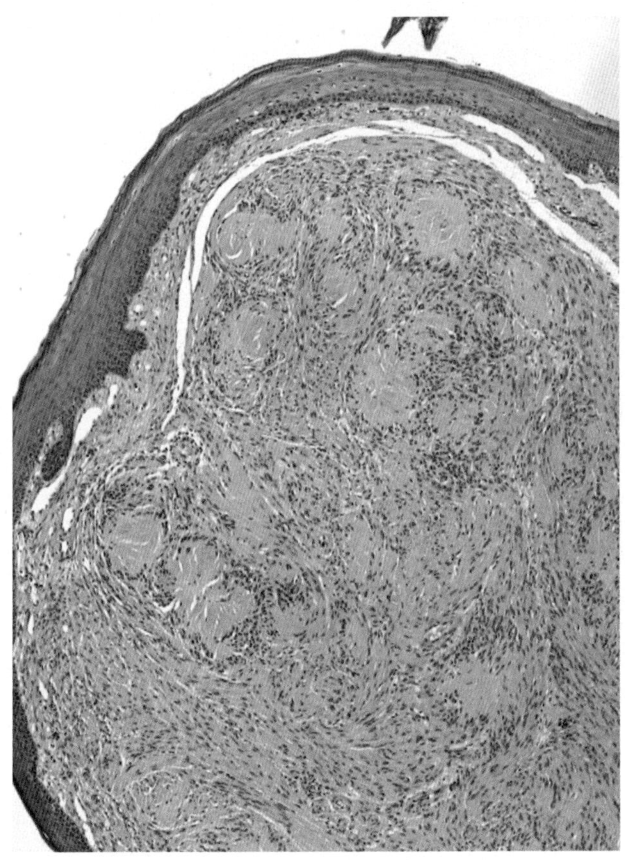

Figure 5.11.1.
Schwannoma. A circumscribed, subepithelial tumor composed of spherical nodules of acellular eosinophilic material surrounded by palisaded nuclei (Verocay bodies).

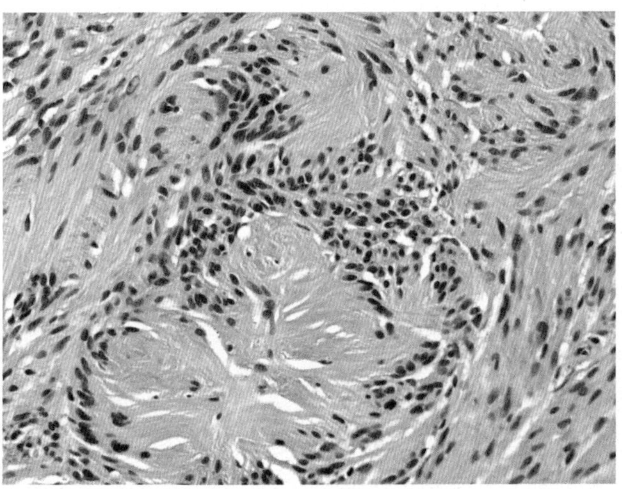

Figure 5.11.2.
Schwannoma. Nodules of eosinophilic material surrounded by palisaded nuclei (Verocay bodies).

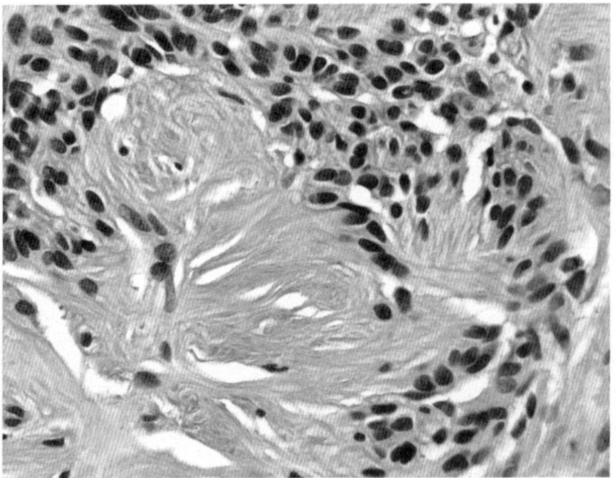

Figure 5.11.3.
Schwannoma. The Verocay body consists of Schwann cell nuclei surrounding a central, acellular core composed of reduplicated basement membrane and cytoplasmic processes.

5.12 Neurofibroma

Presentation

Submucosal nodule. Tongue, buccal mucosa. In young patients.

Histology

- Diffuse, unencapsulated
- A mixture of fibroblasts and spindled Schwann cells with wavy, pointed nuclei
- Fibrous and myxoid stroma with occasional entrapped small nerve trunks or axons
- Scattered mast cells

Special Stains/Immunopathology

Tumor cells are S100-positive.

Histopathologic Differential

- A *palisaded encapsulated neuroma* is circumscribed, not diffuse.
- A *solitary fibrous tumor* is S100-negative.

Treatment and Prognosis

Excision. Evaluation for neurofibromatosis.

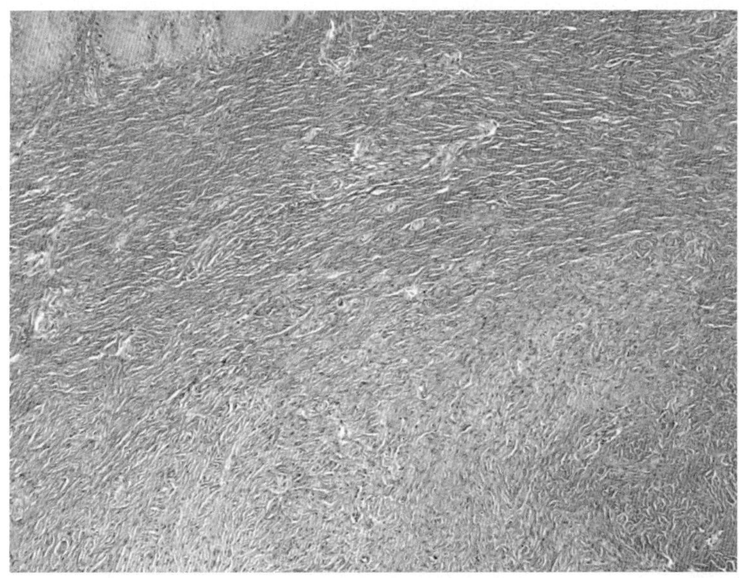

Figure 5.12.1.
Neurofibroma. An unencapsulated, submucosal proliferation of spindle cells blends imperceptibly into the adjacent fibrous connective tissue.

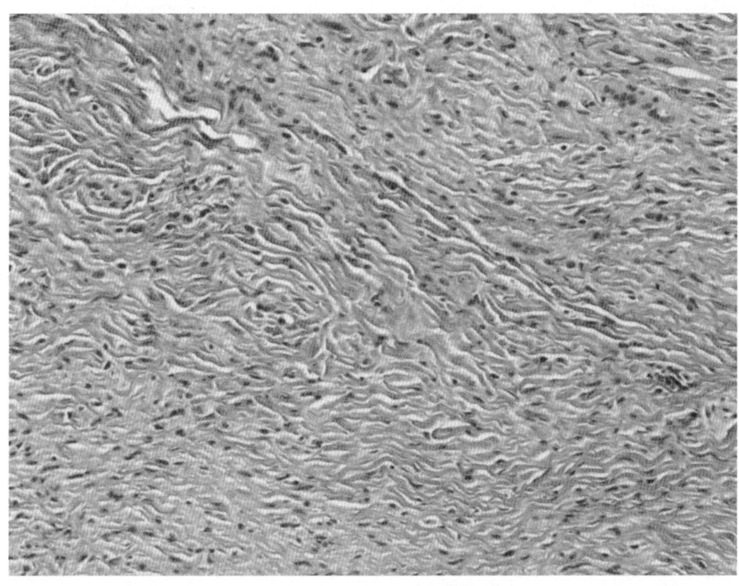

Figure 5.12.2.
Neurofibroma. The spindle cells are elongated and fusiform and growing in many different directions.

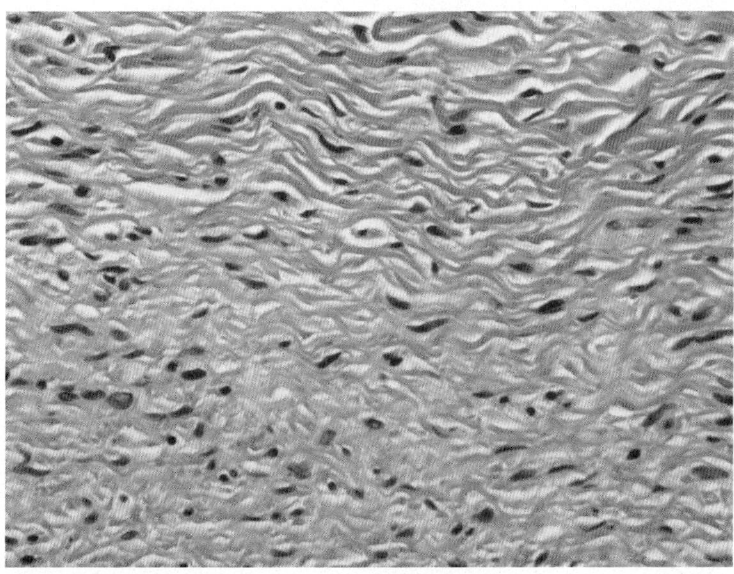

Figure 5.12.3.
Neurofibroma. The wavy, tightly packed cells have the pointed, comma-shaped nuclei typical of Schwann cells.

5.13 Granular Cell Tumor

Presentation

Yellowish submucosal mass, usually of the tongue. In adults, more often in females.

Histology

- Unencapsulated; margins often infiltrative
- Nests of polygonal, eosinophilic cells with granular cytoplasm and vesicular nuclei
- Pseudoepitheliomatous hyperplasia of the overlying mucosa

Special Stains/Immunopathology

Granular cells are S100-positive.

Histopathologic Differential

A *granular cell leiomyoma* will be positive for muscle specific actin and negative for S100.

Treatment and Prognosis

Excision. Does not recur.

Additional

More than half of the granular cell tumors exhibit pseudoepitheliomatous hyperplasia, which can mimic squamous cell carcinoma. This tumor is considered of Schwann cell origin.

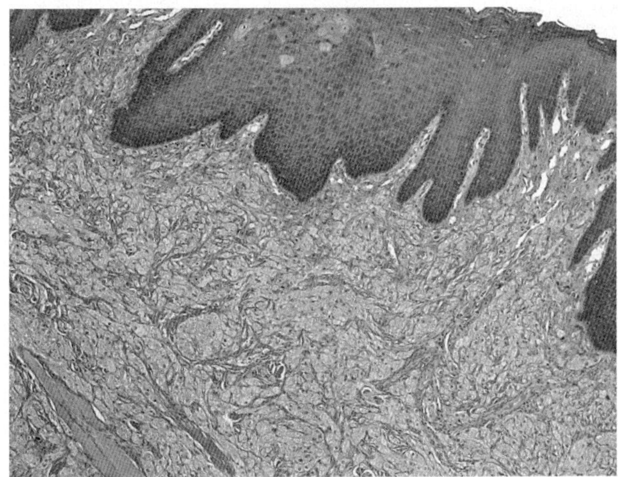

Figure 5.13.1.
Granular cell tumor. The tumor consists of an unencapsulated mass of polygonal, eosinophilic cells.

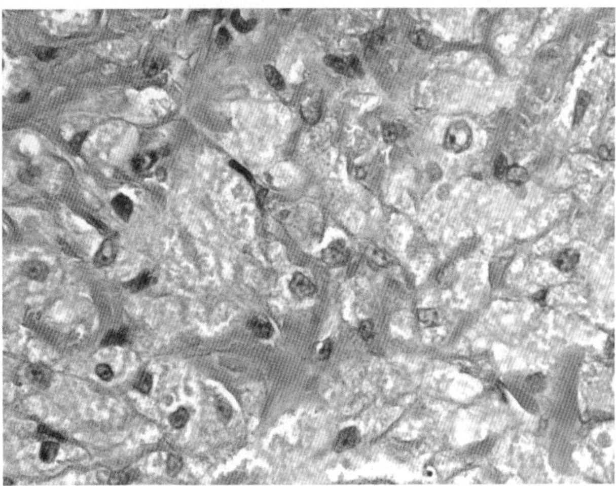

Figure 5.13.2.
Granular cell tumor. The cells have a granular cytoplasm and vesicular nuclei.

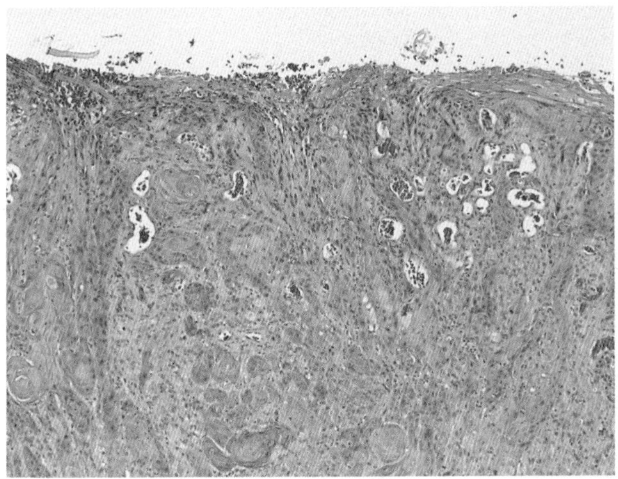

Figure 5.13.3.
Granular cell tumor. Intense pseudoepitheliomatous hyperplasia overlying a large tumor on the dorsum of the tongue.

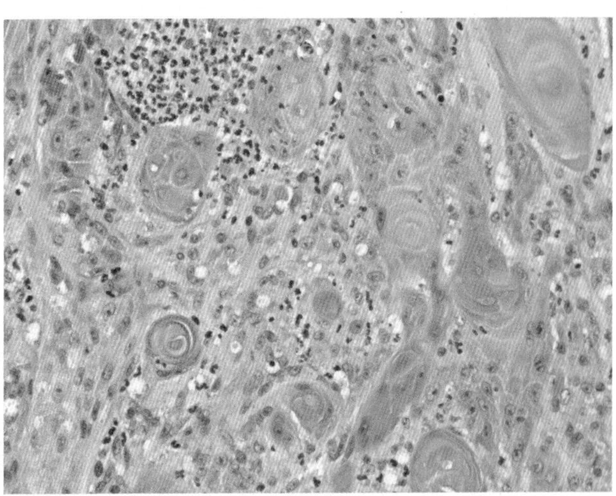

Figure 5.13.4.
Granular cell tumor. An acute inflammatory reaction accompanies the cellular atypia and keratin pearls of the epithelial proliferation.

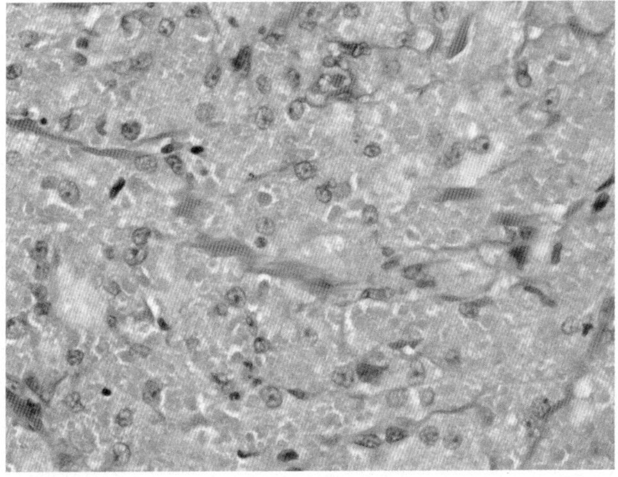

Figure 5.13.5.
Granular cell tumor. Dense sheets of granular cells are seen beneath the proliferating epithelium.

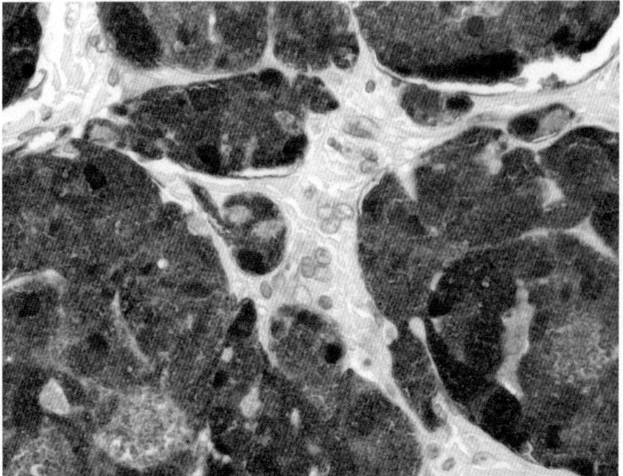

Figure 5.13.6.
Granular cell tumor. S100-positivity confirms the diagnosis.

5.14 Hemangioma

Presentation
Submucosal bluish nodule that blanches on pressure. In children and young adults.

Histology
Small capillary channels or larger, cavernous, endothelial-lined spaces filled with blood

Special Stains/Immunopathology
Tumor cells are positive for factor VIII, CD31, and CD34.

Treatment and Prognosis
Excision or, for larger lesions, sclerosing solutions

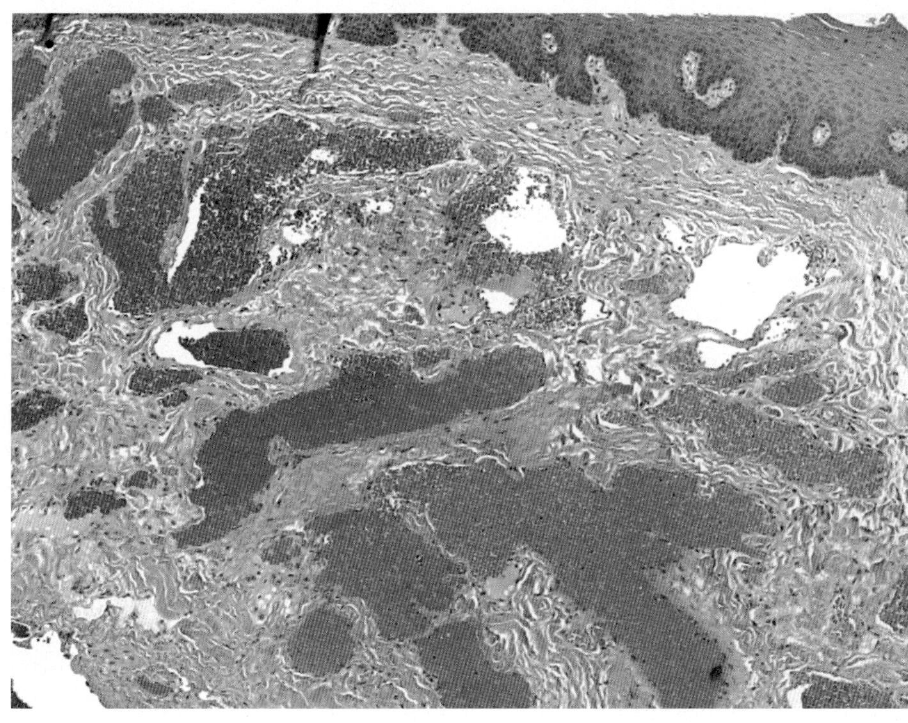

Figure 5.14.1. Hemangioma. Cavernous vascular channels are seen in the fibrous stroma.

5.15 Caliber-Persistent Artery

Definition

A large, thick-walled artery in a superficial submucosal location normally devoid of large vessels

Presentation

Pulsating, linear submucosal nodule of the lip. In older adults.

Histology

Large artery with thick, smooth muscle walls

Treatment and Prognosis

No treatment is necessary; however, excision is often attempted in the mistaken clinical impression of a mucocele or hemangioma. Extensive bleeding is usually encountered.

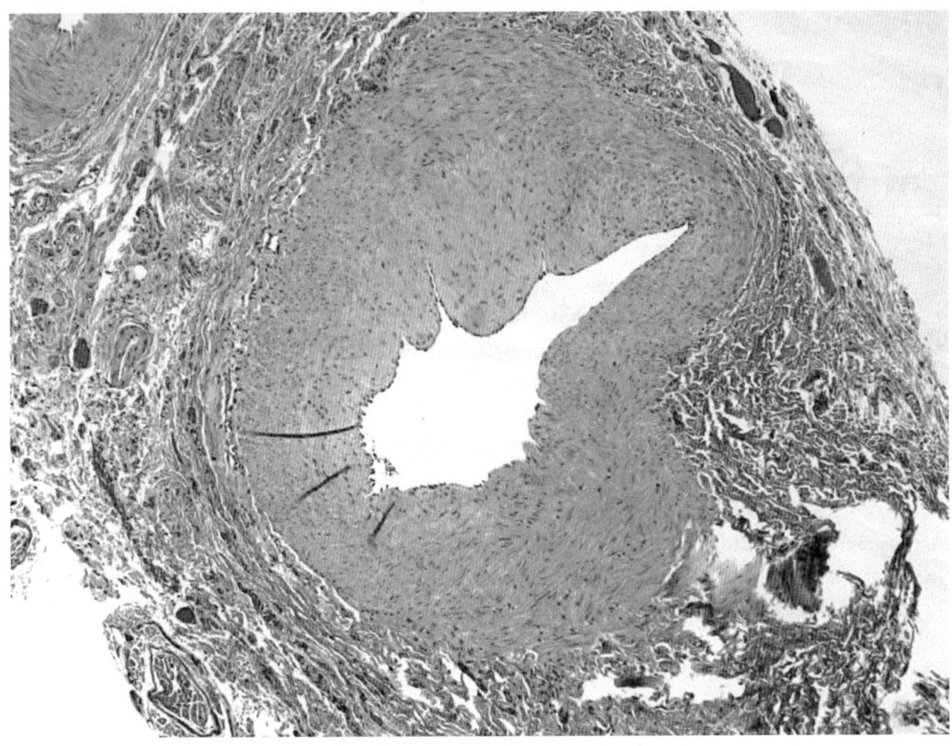

Figure 5.15.1. Caliber-persistent artery. A large artery with thick, muscular walls located just beneath the mucosal epithelium.

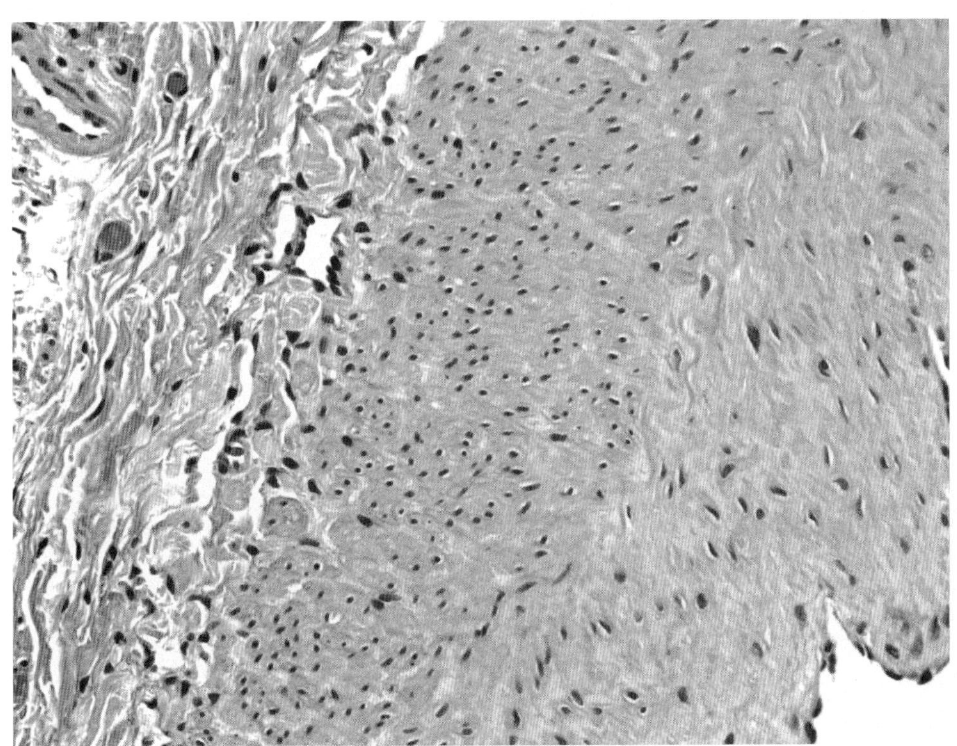

Figure 5.15.2. Caliber-persistent artery. Wall of a large artery.

5.16 Intravascular Papillary Endothelial Hyperplasia

Definition

Rare reaction within a thrombosed vessel that can histologically mimic angiosarcoma

Presentation

Reddish, hard nodule in the buccal mucosa, lip, or tongue

Histology

- Large vessel with thrombus in various stages of organization
- Papillary structures composed of endothelial cells and fibrous connective tissue

Special Stains/Immunopathology

Elastin stain for residual elastic fibers within the artery wall

Histopathologic Differential

An *angiosarcoma* invades tissue and virtually never occurs within a vessel. The endothelial cells lining its interanastamosing channels are pleomorphic and show numerous atypical mitotic figures. Angiosarcomas can be accompanied by necrosis.

Treatment and Prognosis

None

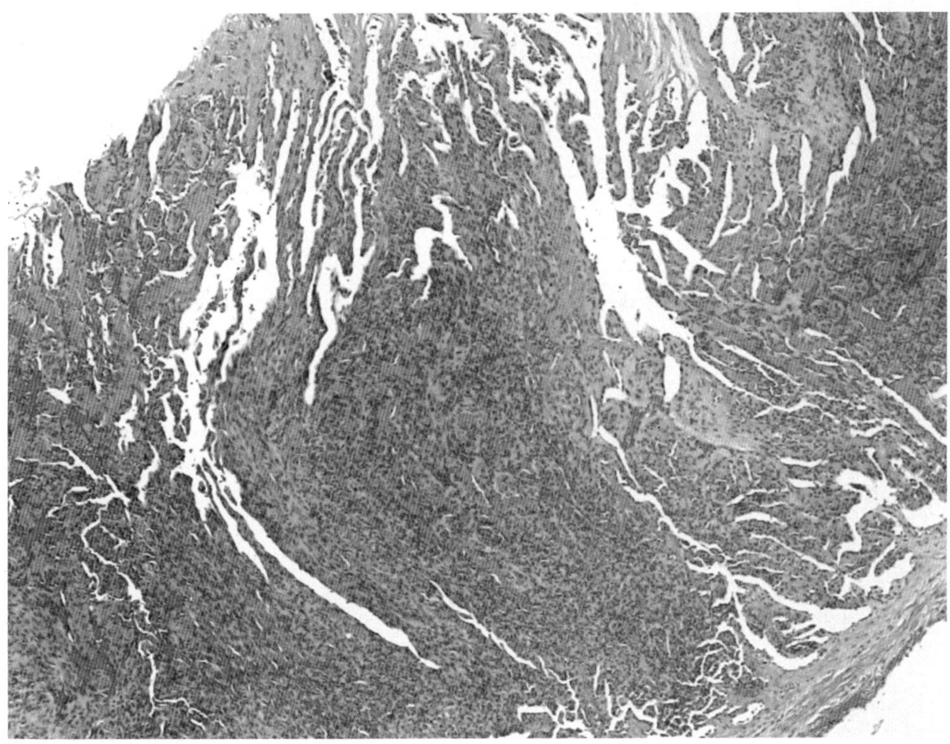

Figure 5.16.1
Intravascular papillary endothelial hyperplasia. Hemorrhage, organization, and papillary formations.

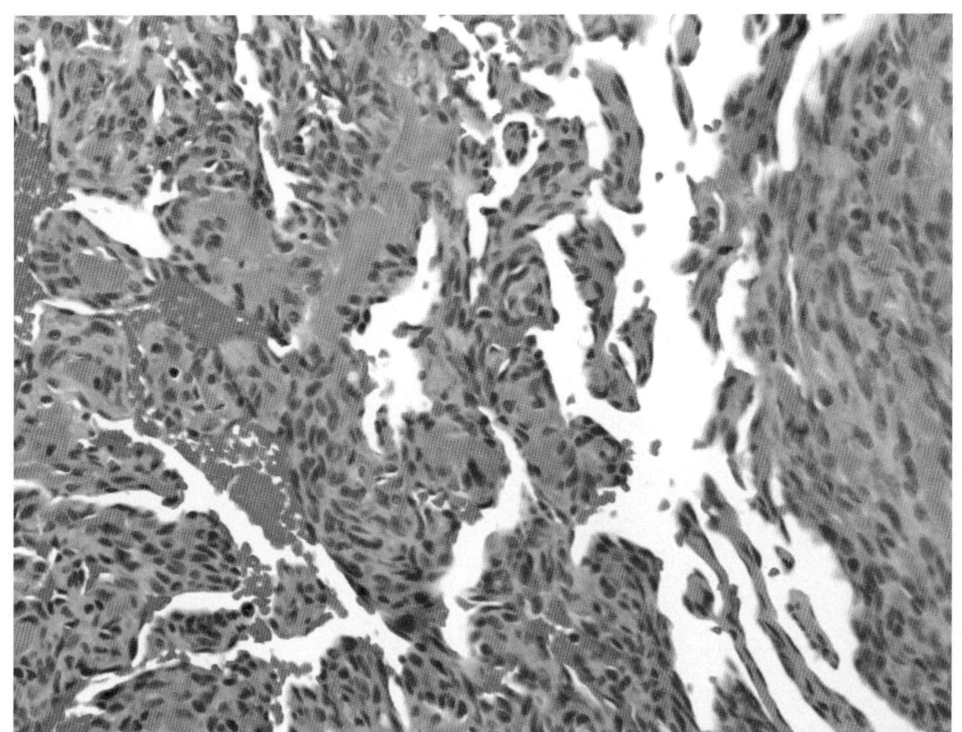

Figure 5.16.2.
Intravascular papillary endothelial hyperplasia. Endothelial cells are flattened and bland and line elongated, fibrovascular papillae.

5.17 Traumatic ulcerative granuloma with stromal eosinophilia (TUGSE)

Definition

A chronic ulcer in an area of crush trauma that can be clinically mistaken for an ulcerated squamous cell carcinoma

Presentation

Deep, flat ulcer with a slightly raised border or ulcerated nodule. Tongue, buccal mucosa.

Histology

- Ulcer covered by fibrin membrane.
- Underlying granulation tissue contains lymphocytes, plasma cells, abundant neutrophils, and sheets of mononuclear cells with enlarged, pale nuclei. A prominent infiltrate of eosinophils is also seen.

Treatment and Prognosis

Incisional biopsy or excision. Often regresses after biopsy

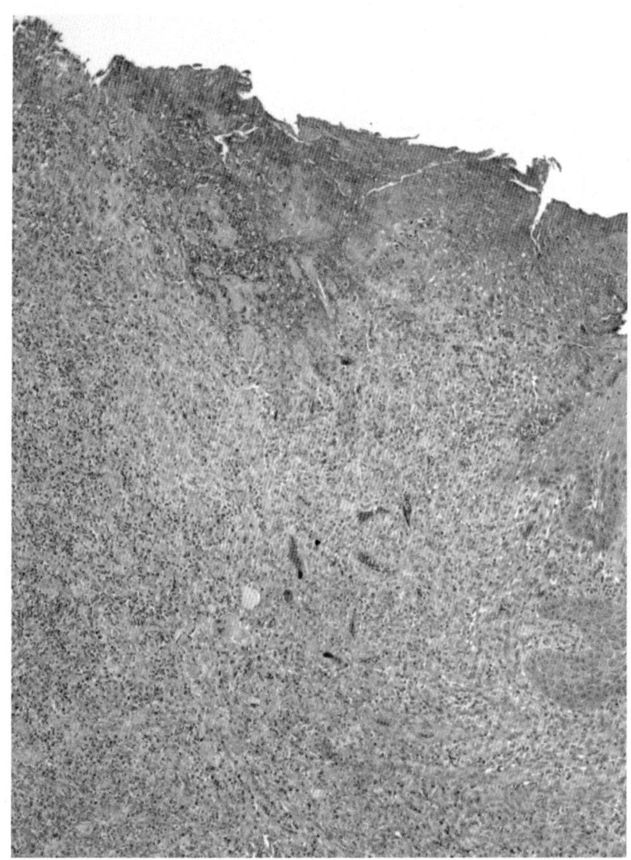

Figure 5.17.1.
Traumatic ulcerative granuloma with stromal eosinophilia. Ulcerated lesion with dense cellular proliferation and numerous small vessels.

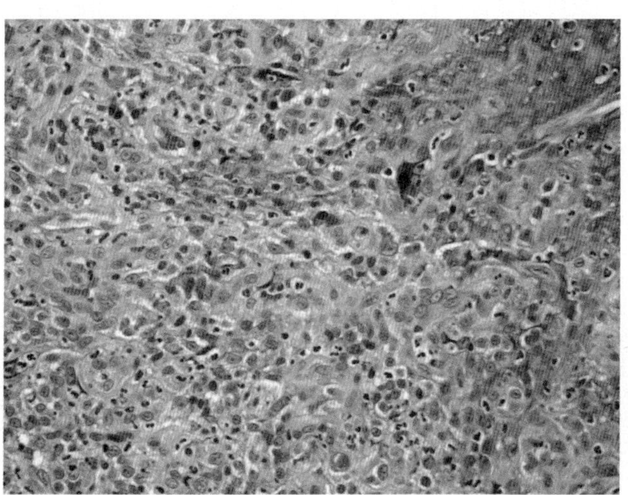

Figure 5.17.2.
Traumatic ulcerative granuloma with stromal eosinophilia. Cellular, fibroblastic granulation tissue with scattered inflammatory cells.

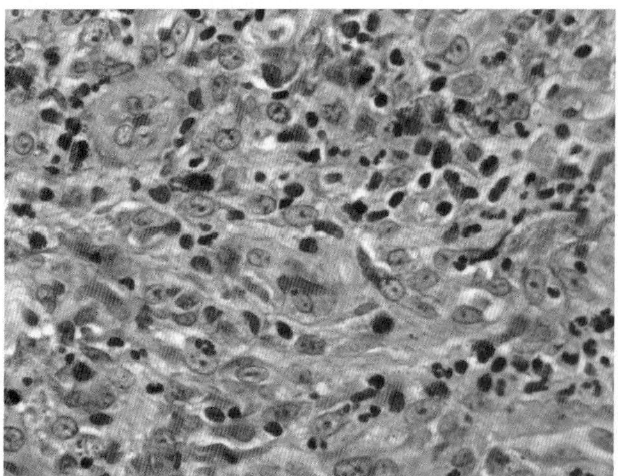

Figure 5.17.3.
Traumatic ulcerative granuloma with stromal eosinophilia. Cellular granulation tissue containing abundant eosinophils and atypical mononuclear cells.

5.18 Kaposi Sarcoma

Presentation

A papular or nodular red or purple lesion seen on the palate, gingiva, or tongue of HIV-infected or otherwise immunocompromised patients. We will discuss only the HIV-associated oral lesions induced by infection with Human Herpes Virus-8 (HHV-8).

Histology

- Fascicles of mildly atypical spindle cells.
- Slit-like vascular channels containing red blood cells, hyaline droplets, and hemosiderin deposits.
- Some tumors show more cellular atypia and an increase in mitoses.

Special Stains/Immunopathology

Endothelial cells react with HHV-8 antibodies.

Histopathologic Differential

- A *pyogenic granuloma* has numerous endothelial-lined vessels with an ulcerated surface covered by a fibrin membrane.

Treatment and Prognosis

Excision, vinblastine, and retrovirals

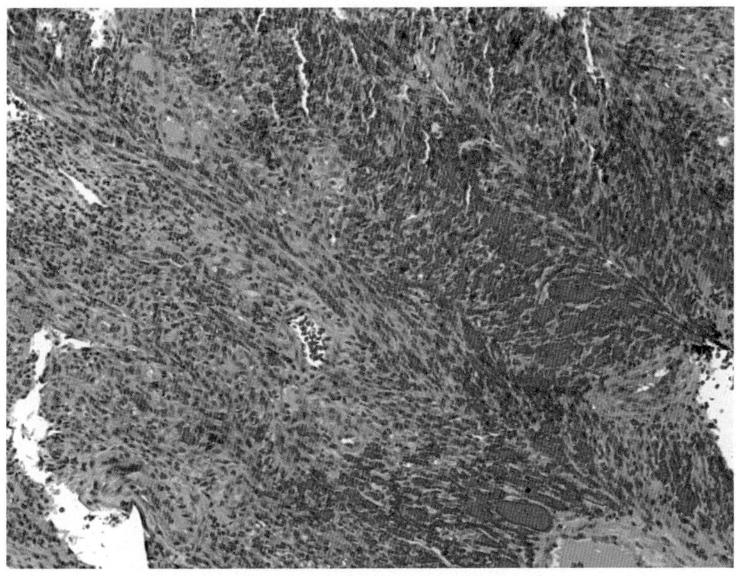

Figure 5.18.1
Kaposi sarcoma. The tumor is composed of fascicles of spindle cells and abundant hemorrhage.

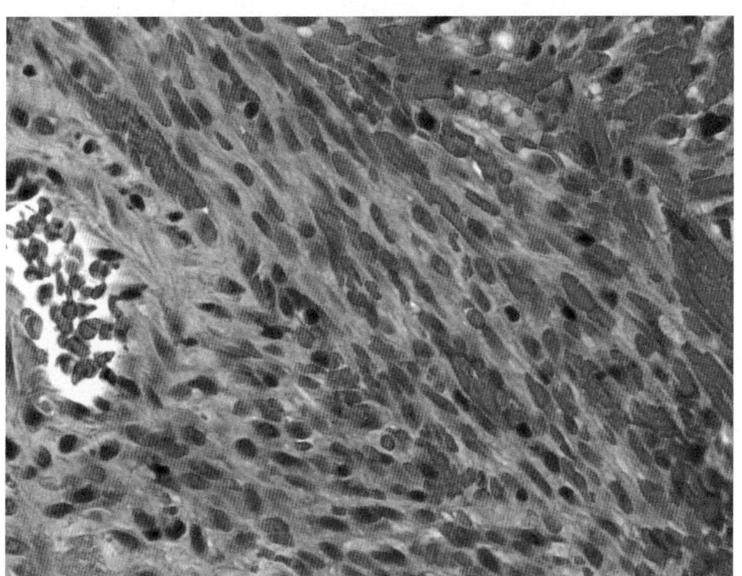

Figure 5.18.2.
Kaposi sarcoma. Fascicles of closely packed spindle cells and extravasated erythrocytes. The spindle cells form vascular slits, and the nuclei exhibit mild atypia.

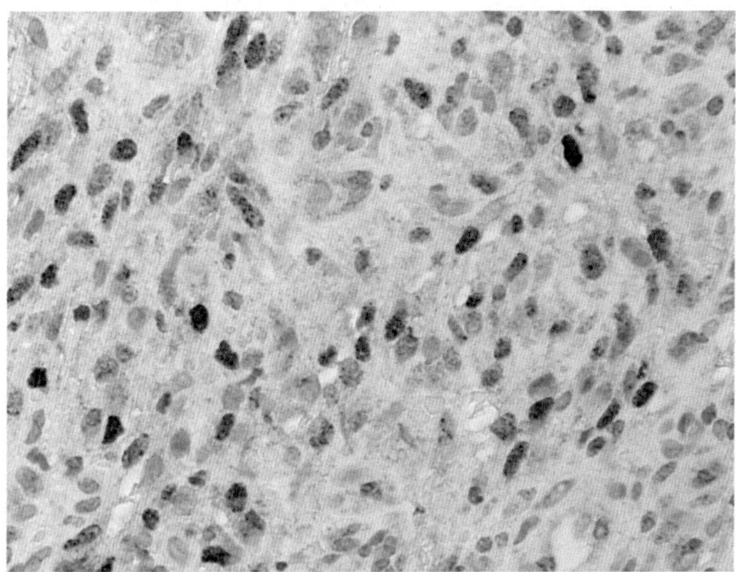

Figure 5.18.3.
Kaposi sarcoma. Nuclei are positive for HHV-8.

5.19 Lymphangioma

Definition

Benign, hamartomatous, often developmental proliferation of lymphatic vessels. Large cavernous lymphangiomas of the neck are usually present at birth. Discussion below is limited to the smaller intraoral lesions.

Presentation

Pebbly surfaced nodule, usually anterior tongue. In infants and children; much less common in adults.

Histology

- An unencapsulated tumor
- Lymph-filled endothelial-lined channels in the submucosa
- Small capillaries sometimes seen admixed with the lymph channels

Treatment and Prognosis

Excision

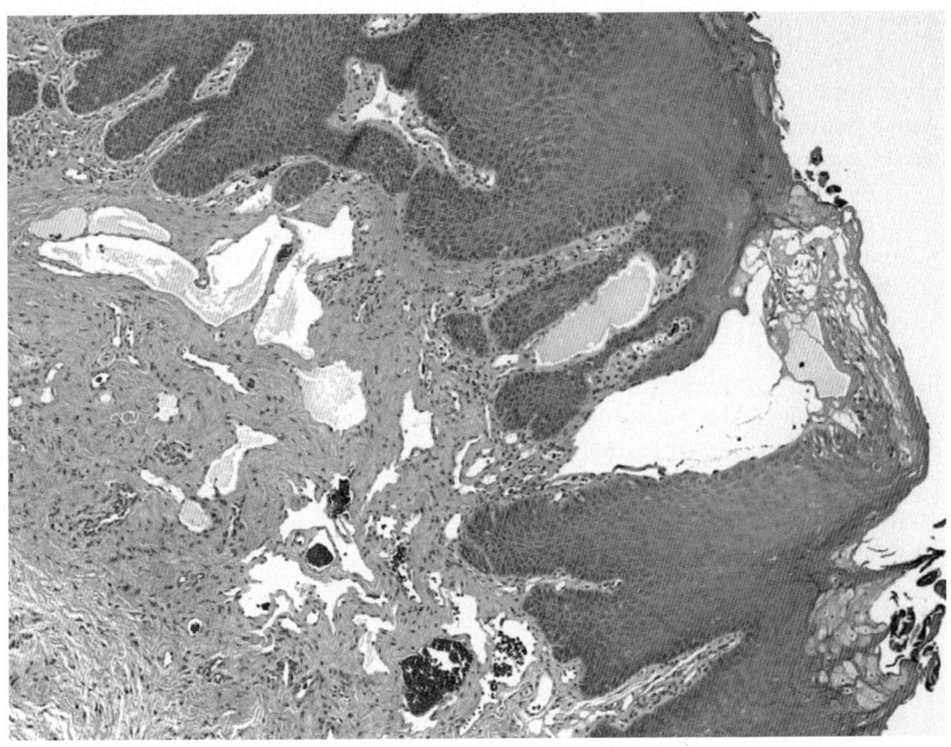

Figure 5.19.1. Lymphangioma. Poorly circumscribed collection of dilated vascular channels, some of which extend upward between the rete pegs.

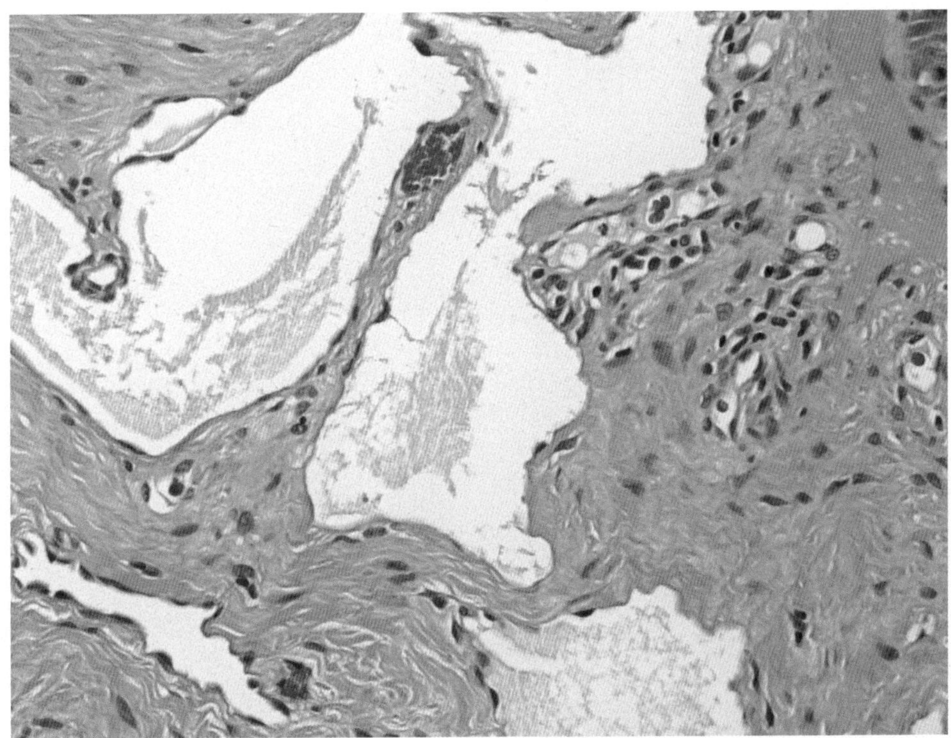

Figure 5.19.2. Lymphangioma. Lymph-filled lymphatic channels lined with a single layer of flattened endothelial cells.

5.20 Vascular Leiomyoma (Angioleiomyoma)

Presentation

A slow-growing nodule that can be tender to palpation. Most common in the lips, tongue, and buccal mucosa. In adults.

Histology

- Well-delineated nodular proliferation of thick-walled vessels with attached nests of spindle cells.
- Nuclei of spindle cells are elongated, cigar-shaped, with blunted edges.

Special Stains/Immunopathology

Tumor cells are positive for smooth muscle actin (SMA), muscle-specific actin (MSA), and desmin. They are negative for S100.

Treatment and Prognosis

Excision. Does not recur.

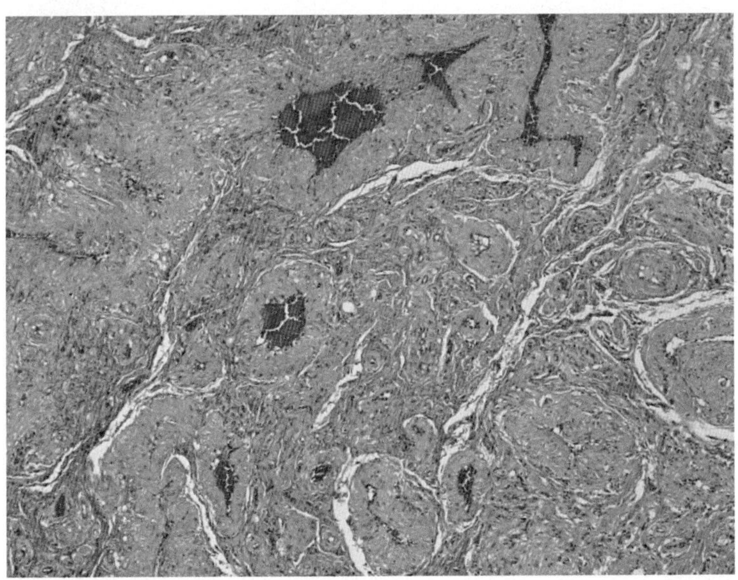

Figure 5.20.1.
Vascular leiomyoma. A large submucosal nodule of smooth muscle containing irregular, thick-walled vessels.

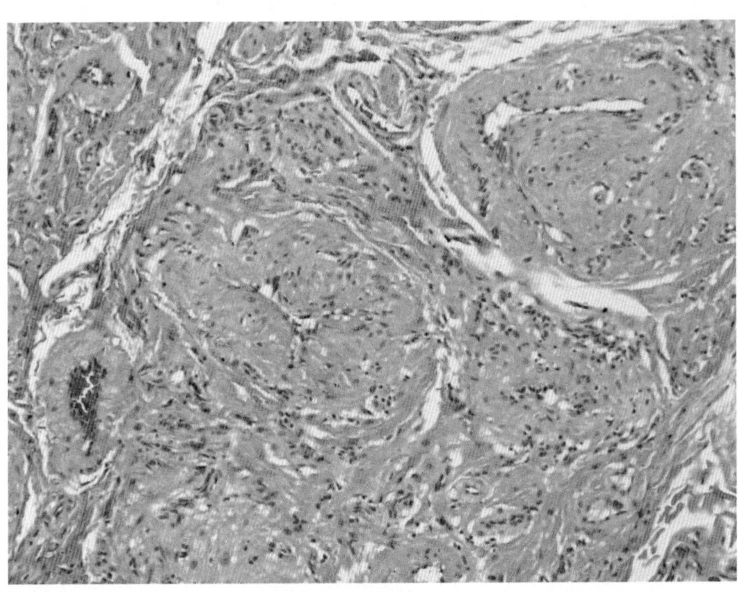

Figure 5.20.2.
Vascular leiomyoma. Numerous thick-walled vessels with partially patent lumina surrounded by smooth muscle.

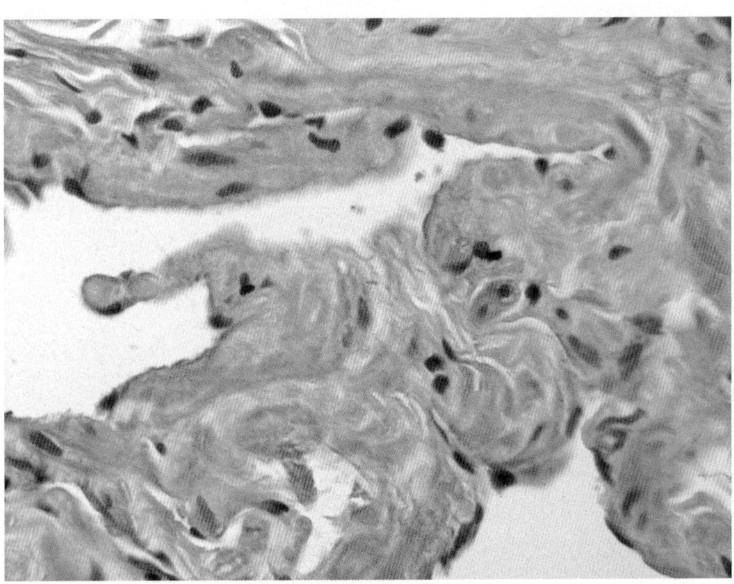

Figure 5.20.3.
Vascular leiomyoma. An irregular proliferation of smooth muscle surrounds distorted vascular channels.

5.21 Myofibroma

Presentation

Submucosal nodule or nodules. Tongue and buccal mucosa. Multiple tumors (myofibromatosis)—in infants and children; solitary tumors—in children and adolescents, occasionally adults.

Histology

- Circumscribed, multinodular lesion with biphasic pattern
- Hypercellular areas of spindled myofibroblasts with hypocellular periphery
- Irregular, staghorn-shaped vessels within the hypercellular areas
- Infiltration of regional skeletal muscle

Special Stains/Immunopathology

Tumor cells are positive for SMA. They are negative for desmin and S100.

Histopathologic Differential

A *leiomyoma* is desmin-positive.
A *leiomyosarcoma* has cellular and nuclear atypia.
A *schwannoma* or *neurofibroma* is S100-positive.

Treatment and Prognosis

Excision. Does not recur if completely removed.

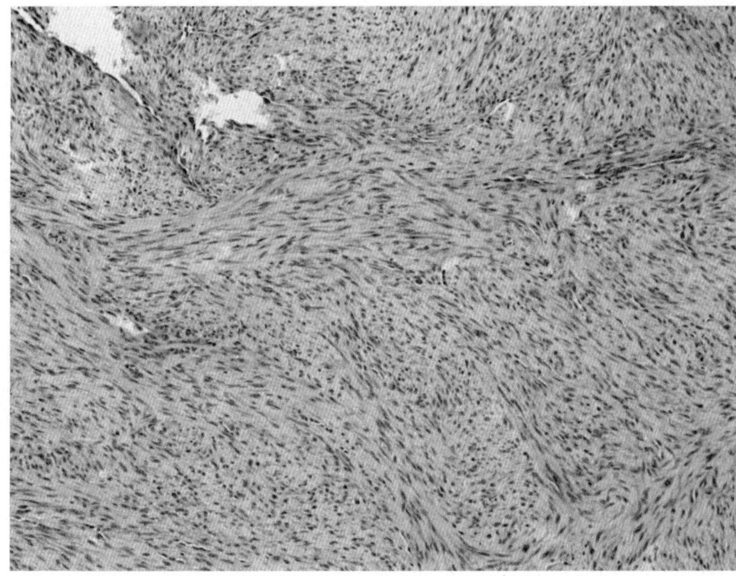

Figure 5.21.1.
Myofibroma. Fascicles of loosely arranged spindle cells with faintly eosinophilic cytoplasm.

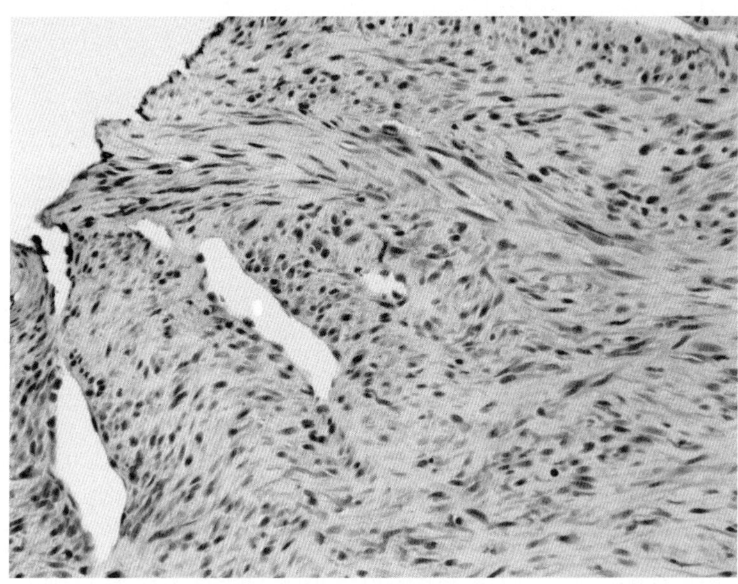

Figure 5.21.2.
Myofibroma. Fascicles of spindle cells surround irregularly shaped endothelial-lined vascular channels.

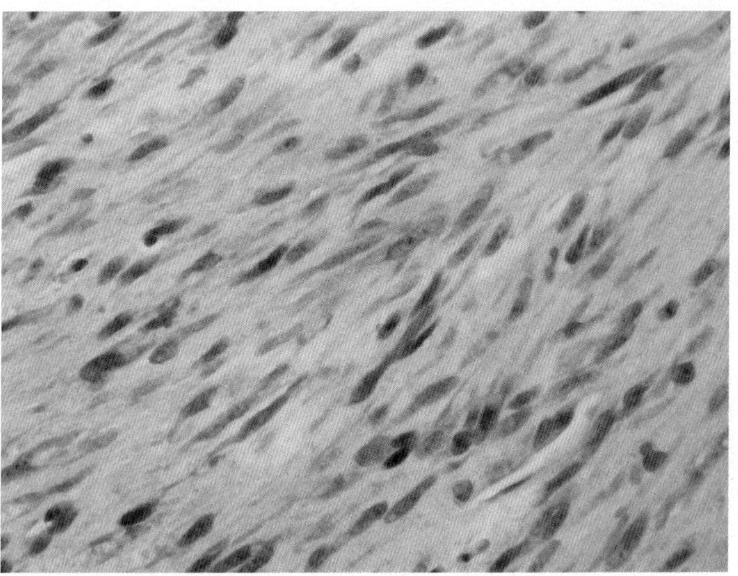

Figure 5.21.3.
Myofibroma. The lightly eosinophilic spindle cells have elongated, hyperchromatic, bipolar nuclei resembling myofibroblasts. This tumor was SMA-positive and -negative for desmin and S100.

5.22 Leiomyosarcoma

Presentation

Enlarging mass of maxillary or mandibular alveolar mucosa. Can be painful and ulcerated. In wide age range.

Histology

- Infiltrating fascicles of spindle cells with elongated, blunted nuclei and eosinophilic cytoplasm
- Degree of pleomorphism and number of mitoses variable

Special Stains/Immunopathology

The tumor cells are positive for SMA, MSA, and desmin.

Histopathologic Differential

The overlying epithelium of a *spindle cell carcinoma* shows dysplastic changes. It is positive for epithelial markers and negative for SMA and MSA.

Treatment and Prognosis

Wide surgical excision

Additional

Epithelioid variant has been reported in oral cavity.

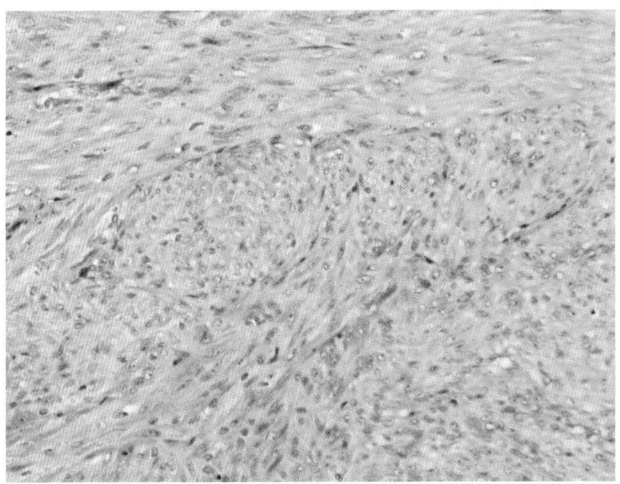

Figure 5.22.1.
Leiomyosarcoma. Intersecting, crisscrossing fascicles of spindle cells.

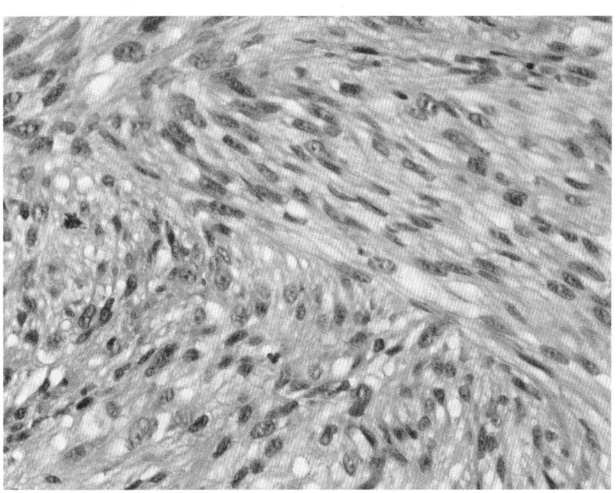

Figure 5.22.2.
Leiomyosarcoma. Individual tumor cells have elongated, blunted nuclei.

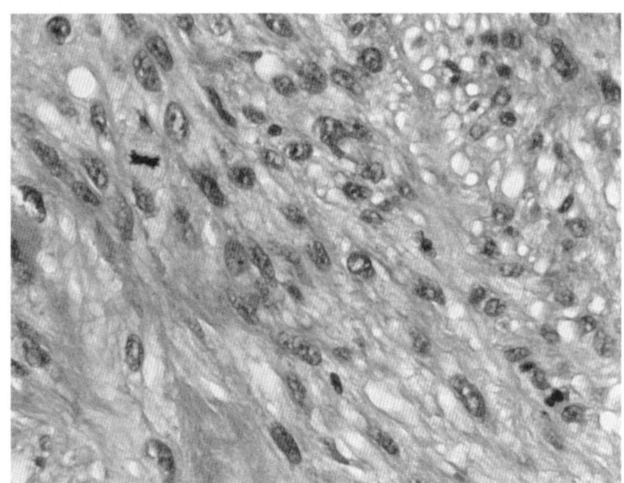

Figure 5.22.3.
Leiomyosarcoma. An atypical mitotic figure is seen.

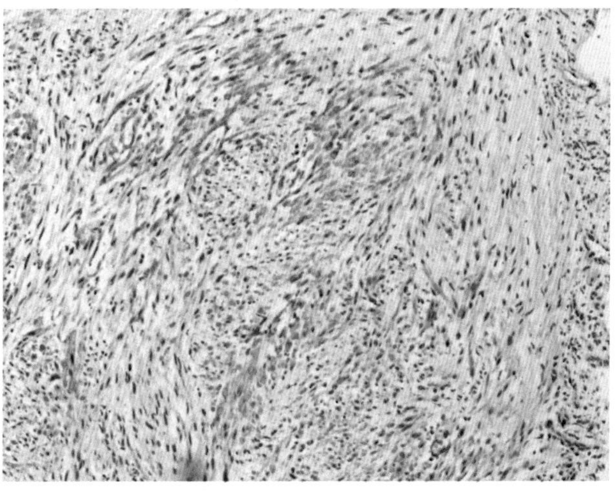

Figure 5.22.4
Leiomyosarcoma, low grade. The tumor is reactive for smooth muscle actin.

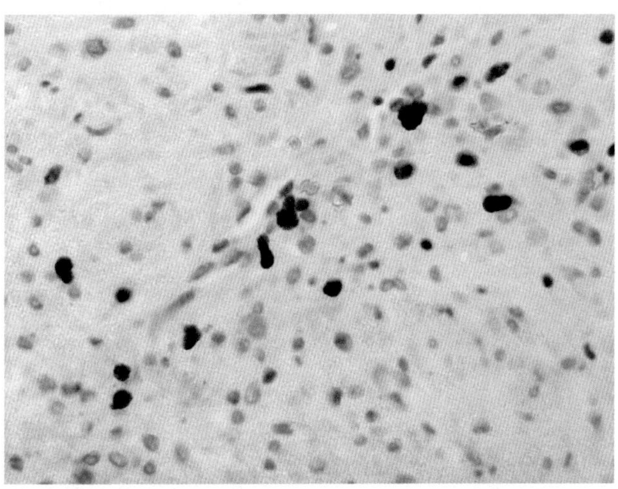

Figure 5.22.5.
Leiomyosarcoma. Ki67 proliferative index is about 25%.

5.23 Unusual soft tissue masses

The following intraoral soft tissue masses are regularly submitted for pathologic evaluation:

Reactive lymphoid hyperplasia

- These present as exophytic, movable submucosal nodules located bilaterally in the lateral posterior tongue, or solitary lesions on the palate and buccal mucosa. They are about 1 cm in diameter and are asymptomatic.
- The buccal mucosal lesion is usually related to drainage from a chronically infected tooth.
- The nodules are composed of non-neoplastic lymphocytes, expanded germinal centers containing lymphoid cells with numerous mitoses and tingible body macrophages.

Lymphoma

- Intraoral lymphomas present as large, boggy, reddish to purplish submucosal masses, which are sometimes ulcerated. These develop in the posterior hard palate, posterior maxillary and mandibular gingiva and buccal vestibule of either jaw. The patients are usually older individuals. Lesions can be either primary in these locations or part of systemic disease.
- The tumors are mostly B cell lymphomas and are composed of large neoplastic lymphoid cells admixed with normal lymphocytes. The tumor cells have irregular nuclei and resemble immunoblasts and rarely plasmablasts. Mitotic figures and stromal sclerosis may be seen.

Foreign body granuloma

The most common granulomatous intraoral soft tissue lesion is the foreign body granuloma. Occasionally, granulomas associated with sarcoidosis, Crohn's disease and, rarely, fungi may be seen.

Foreign body granulomas are found most often in the gingiva, lips, buccal mucosa and floor of mouth. Materials identified in these lesions are:

- Dental amalgam particles and dust, silica from other dental materials, injected dermal fillers of all sorts and other materials not easily identified.
- These masses are most often less than 2 cm in diameter. Complete excision is curative.

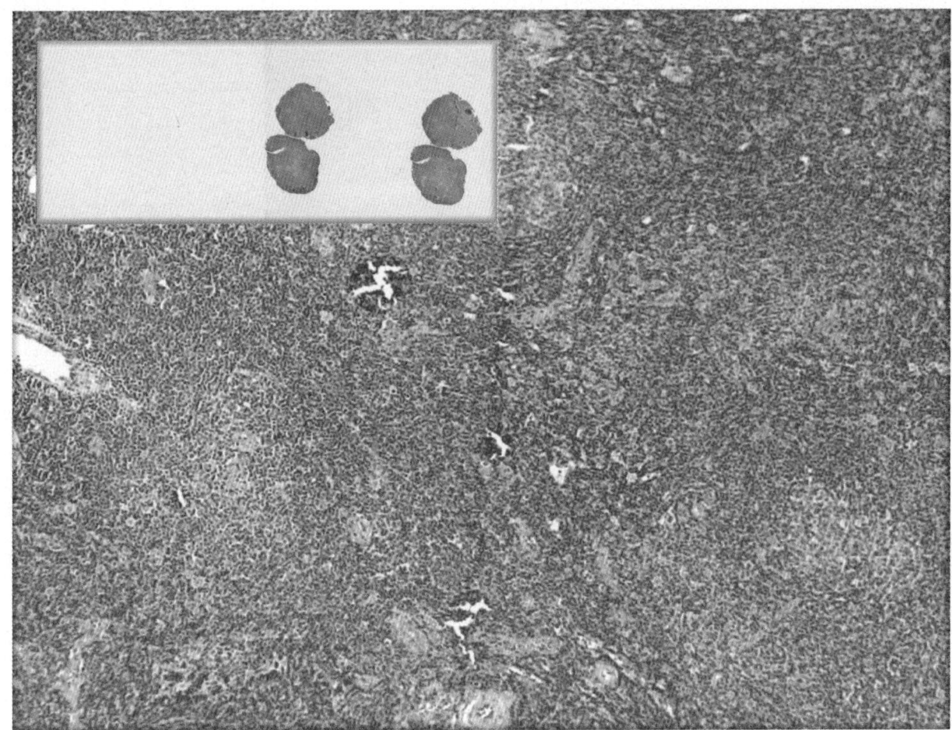

Figure 5.23.1.
Reactive lymphoid hyperplasia. Germinal centers are seen in this lymphoid proliferation that presented as a mass in the buccal mucosa.

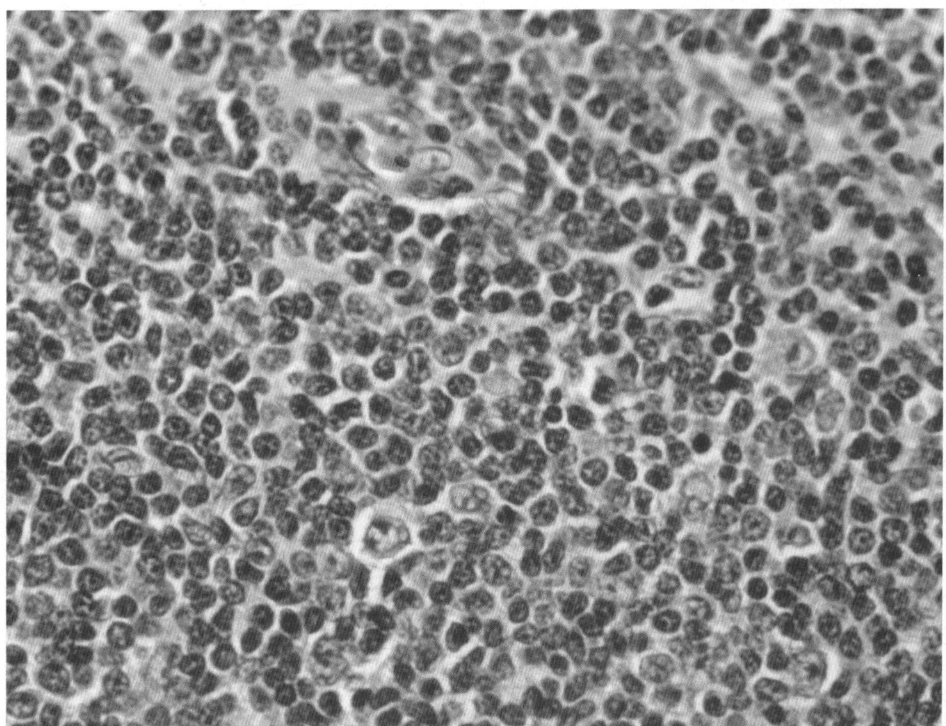

Figure 5.23.2.
Reactive lymphoid hyperplasia. Normal-appearing lymphocytes and a tingible body macrophage. The lymphocytic proliferation was polyclonal and stained with lambda and kappa antibodies. The patient had no other lymphoid masses.

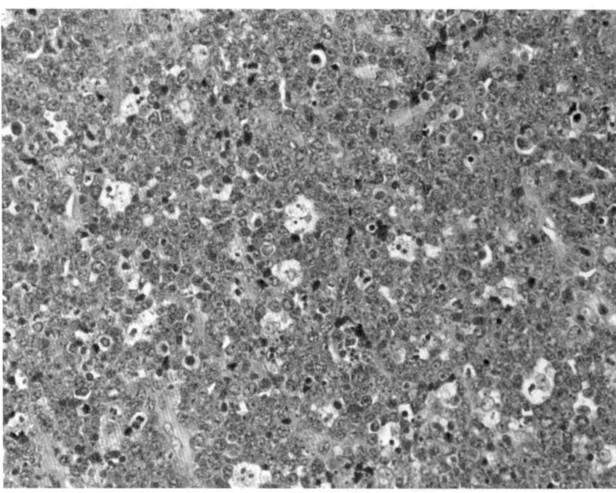

Figure 5.23.3.
Burkitt lymphoma. Scattered histiocytes containing nuclear debris within sheets of atypical lymphocytes produce a starry-sky pattern.

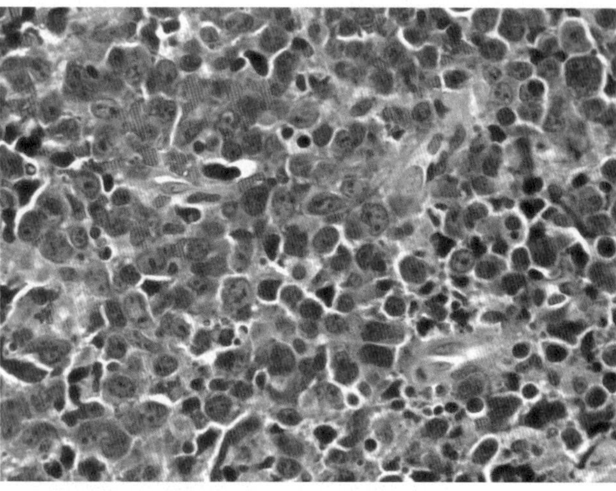

Figure 5.23.4.
Diffuse large B-cell lymphoma. A diffuse proliferation of atypical lymphocytes with angular, pleomorphic nuclei.

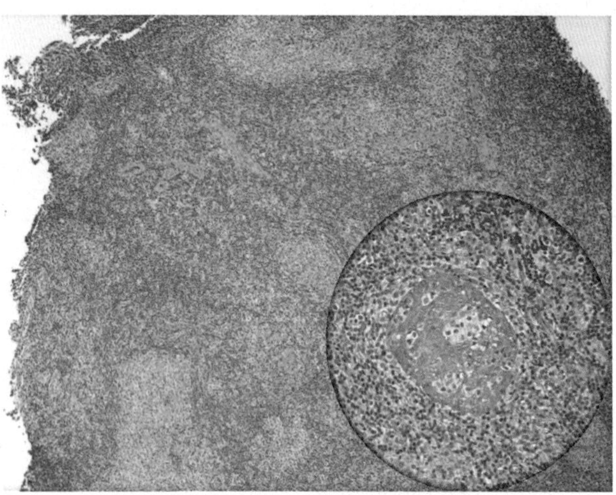

Figure 5.23.5.
MALT (marginal zone) lymphoma. Atypical lymphocytic proliferation containing numerous follicles and scattered epimyoepithelial islands (inset).

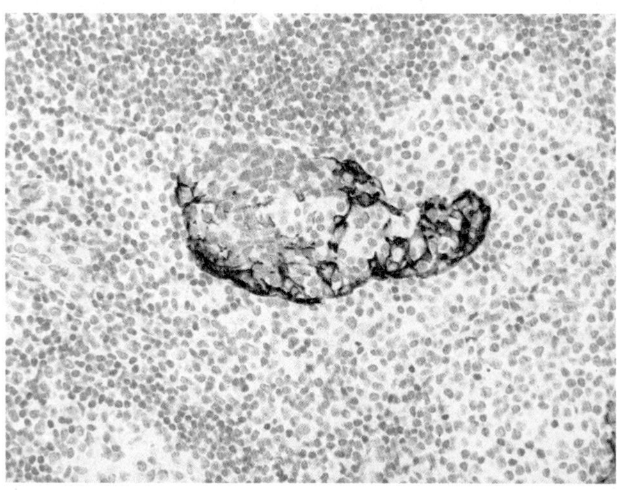

Figure 5.23.6.
MALT (marginal zone) lymphoma. CK18 stains the epithelial cells of the epimyoepithelial islands.

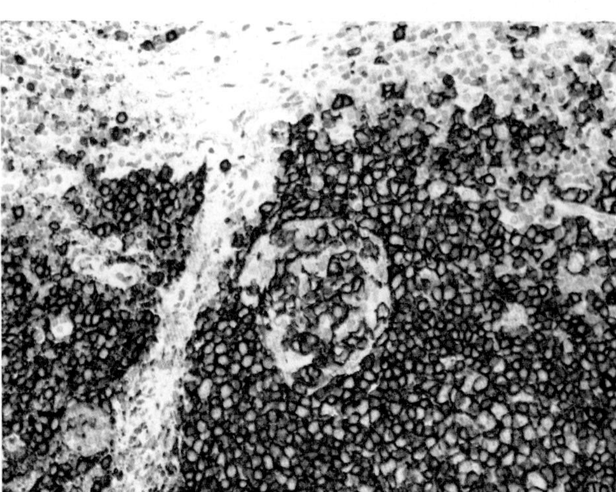

Figure 5.23.7.
MALT (marginal zone) lymphoma. CD20 stains the neoplastic B cells surrounding and within the epimyoepithelial islands.

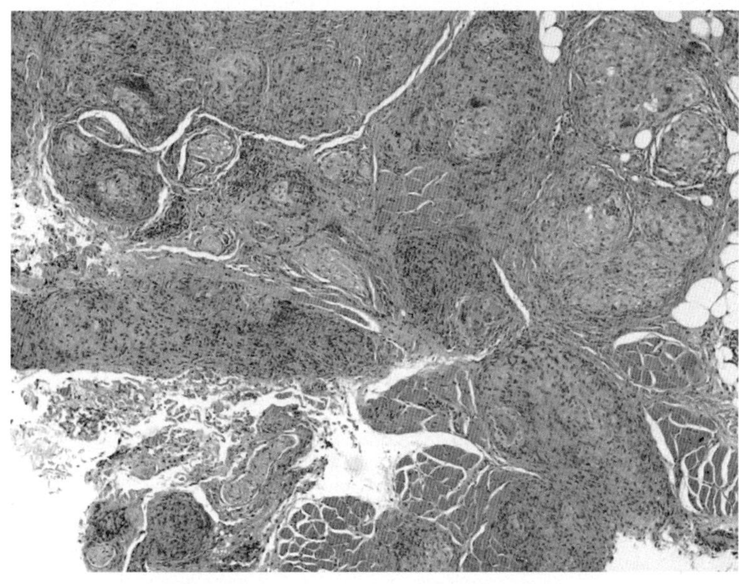

Figure 5.23.8.
Foreign body granuloma. The most common granulomatous lesion seen in the oral cavity. Glass particles, dental amalgams, or, rarely, dermal fillers can induce this reaction.

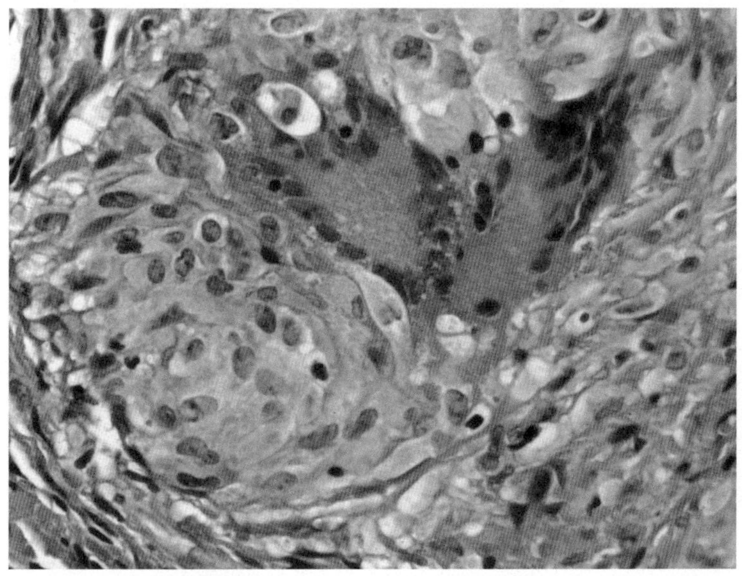

Figure 5.23.9.
Foreign body granuloma. The granuloma is composed of epithelioid histiocytes and giant cells.

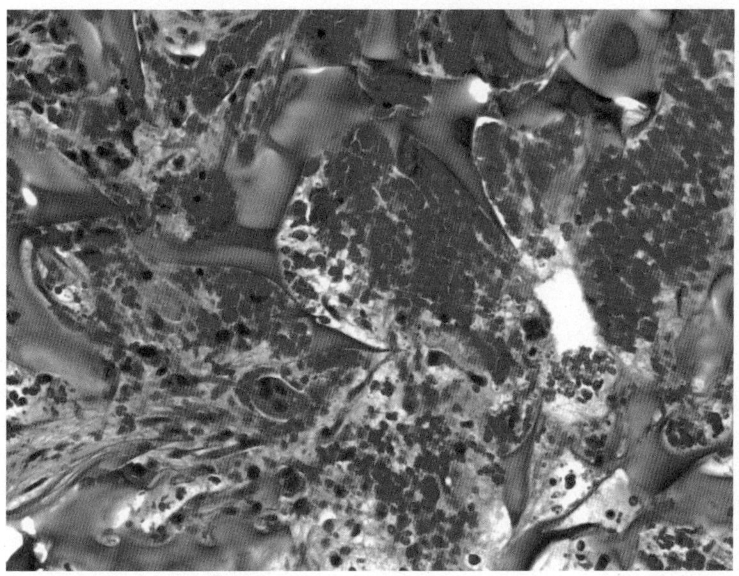

Figure 5.23.10.
Foreign body granuloma. This giant cell reaction was induced by an absorbable hemostatic agent (Gelfoam) placed into the surgical site.

Bibliography and Suggested Reading

5.1–5.2

Shapira M, Akrish S. A 6-year-old girl with a lesion on the tongue: giant cell fibroma of tongue. *Pediatr Ann.* 2011;40:71–74.

5.3– 5.6

Buchner A, Shnaiderman A, Vared M. Pediatric localized reactive gingival lesions: a retrospective study from Israel. *Pediatr Dent.* 2010;32:486–492.

Buchner A, Shnaiderman-Shapiro A, Vered M. Relative frequency of localized reactive hyperplastic lesions of the gingiva: a retrospective study of 1675 cases from Israel. *J Oral Pathol Med.* 2010;39:631–638.

5.7

Furlong MA, Fanburg-Smith JC, Childers EL. Lipoma of the oral and maxillofacial region: site and subclassification of 125 cases. *Oral Surg Oral Med Oral Pathol Oral Radiol Endod.* 2004;98:441–450.

Garavaglia J, Gnepp DR. Intramuscular (infiltrating) lipoma of the tongue. *Oral Surg Oral Med Oral Pathol.* 1987;63:348–350.

Manor E, Sion-Vardy N, Joshua BZ, et al. Oral lipoma: analysis of 58 new cases and review of the literature. *Ann Diagn Pathol.* 2011;15(4):257–261.

5.8

Alawi F, Stratton D, Freedman PD. Solitary fibrous tumor of the oral soft tissues: a clinicopathologic and immunohistochemical study of 16 cases. *Am J Surg Pathol.* 2001;25:900–910.

O'Regan EM, Vanguri V, Allen CM, et al. Solitary fibrous tumor of the oral cavity: clinicopathologic and immunohistochemical study of 21 cases. *Head Neck Pathol.* 2009;3:106–115.

5.9–5.10

Koutlas IG, Scheithauer BW. Palisaded encapsulated ("solitary circumscribed") neuroma of the oral cavity: a review of 55 cases. *Head Neck Pathol.* 2010;4:15–26.

5.11–5.12

Zachariades N, Mezitis M, Vairaktaris E, et al. Benign neurogenic tumors of the oral cavity. *Int J Oral Maxillofac Surg.* 1987;16:70–76.

5.13

Bhattacharyya I, Summerlin DJ, Cohen DM, et al. Granular cell leiomyoma of the oral cavity. *Oral Surg Oral Med Oral Pathol Oral Radiol Endod.* 2006;102:353–359.

5.15

Piccione MJ, Manganaro AM, Almony JS. Caliber-persistent labial artery: diagnosis and treatment—case report. *J Oral Maxillofac Surg.* 2010;68:1987–1989.

5.16

De Courten A, Küffer R, Samson J, et al. Intravascular papillary endothelial hyperplasia of the mouth: report of six cases and literature review. *Oral Dis.* 1999;5:175–178.

5.17

Eleni G, Panagiotis S, Andreas K, et al. Traumatic ulcerative granuloma with stromal eosinophilia: a lesion with alarming histopathologic presentation and benign clinical course. *Am J Dermatopathol.* 2011;33:192–194.

5.18

Lumerman H, Freedman PD, Kerpel SM, et al. Oral Kaposi's sarcoma: a clinicopathologic study of 23 homosexual and bisexual men from the New York metropolitan area. *Oral Surg Oral Med Oral Pathol.* 1988;65:711–716.

Ramírez-Amador V, Martínez-Mata G, González-Ramírez I, et al. Clinical, histological and immunohistochemical findings in oral Kaposi's sarcoma in a series of Mexican AIDS patients: comparative study. *J Oral Pathol Med.* 2009;38:328–333.

5.19

Kalpidis CD, Lysitsa SN, Kolokotronis AE, et al. Solitary superficial microcystic lymphatic malformation (lymphangioma circumscriptum) of the gingiva. *J Periodontol.* 2006;77:1797–1801.

5.20

Gaitan Cepeda LA, Quezada Rivera D, Tenorio Rocha F, et al. Vascular leiomyoma of the oral cavity: clinical, histopathological and immunohistochemical characteristics. Presentation of five cases and review of the literature. *Med Oral Pathol Oral Cir Bucal.* 2008;13:E483–E488.

5.21

Brasileiro BF, Martins-Filho PR, Piva MR, et al. Myofibroma of the oral cavity: a rare spindle cell neoplasm. *Med Oral Patol Oral Cir Bucal.* 2010;15:e596–e600.

Vered M, Allon I, Buchner A, et al. Clinico-pathologic correlations of myofibroblastic tumors of the oral cavity, II: myofibroma and myofibromatosis of the oral soft tissues. *J Oral Pathol Med.* 2007;36:304–314.

5.22

Yan B, Li Y, Pan J, et al. Primary oral leiomyosarcoma: a retrospective clinical analysis of 20 cases. *Oral Dis.* 2010;16:198–203.

5.23

Kolokotronis A, Dimitrakopoulos I, Asimaki A. Follicular lymphoid hyperplasia of the palate: report of a case and review of the literature. *Oral Surg Oral Med Oral Pathol Oral Radiol Endod.* 2003;96:172–175.

Menasce LP, Shanks JH, Banerjee SS, et al. Follicular lymphoid hyperplasia of the hard palate and oral mucosa: report of three cases and a review of the literature. *Histopathology.* 2001;39:353–358.

5.24

Mlotha J, Naidoo S. Oro-facial manifestations of Burkitt's lymphoma: an analysis of 680 cases from Malawi. *SADJ.* 2011;66:77–79.

Vega F, Lin P, Medeiros LJ. Extranodal lymphomas of the head and neck. *Ann Diagn Pathol.* 2005;9:340–350.

5.25

Akrish S, Dayan D, Taicher S, et al. Foreign body granulomas after injection of bio-alcamid for lip augmentation. *Am J Otolaryngol.* 2009;30:356–359.

da Costa Miguel MC, Nonaka CF, dos Santos JN, et al. Oral foreign body granuloma: unusual presentation of a rare adverse reaction to permanent injectable cosmetic filler. *Int J Oral Maxillofac Surg.* 2009;38:385–387.

CHAPTER

6

Bone Pathology

Proliferative periostitis
Bisphosphonate-associated osteonecrosis
Nasopalatine duct cyst
Surgical ciliated cyst
Simple (traumatic) bone cyst
Aneurysmal bone cyst
Central giant cell granuloma
Fibrous dysplasia
Cemento-osseous dysplasia
Ossifying fibroma
Juvenile trabecular ossifying fibroma
Osteoblastoma
Osteochondroma
Synovial chondromatosis
Osteosarcoma
Chondrosarcoma
Metastatic tumors

Introduction

Except for the odontogenic cysts and tumors and the occasional central giant cell granuloma, most of the biopsies received from the jaws will be one of the four benign fibro-osseous lesions: fibrous dysplasia, cemento-osseous dysplasia, ossifying fibroma, and juvenile ossifying fibroma. All share a frustratingly similar histopathologic mix of fibrous, fibroblastic, and osseous tissues.

The first entity, fibrous dysplasia, is generally a clinical and radiographic diagnosis. Even if biopsied, it is often not treated at all unless bony recontouring is required for cosmetic reasons.

Cemento-osseous dysplasia also generally requires no treatment; indeed, in its florid, multi-quadrant form, intervention is to be avoided, since the biopsy procedure itself can set up an infection in devascularized, slow-to-heal bone.

Ossifying fibroma, on the other hand, is a true tumor with real growth potential. It requires surgical intervention, generally enucleation. The juvenile ossifying fibroma, which is more aggressive, may require resection.

A comparison of the benign fibro-osseous lesions in chart form can be found on page 216.

6.1 Proliferative Periostitis (Garre's Osteomyelitis; Periostitis Ossificans)

Definition

A localized periosteal bony proliferation, generally in a young person with a carious, infected tooth

Presentation

Swelling of the inferior and buccal cortex of the mandible adjacent to a carious, infected tooth, a bone fracture, or an infected dental cyst. The average age of the patient is 13 years.

Radiographic Appearance

Thin, radiopaque layers of bone running parallel to the cortex

Microscopic Findings

Parallel, incremental layers or retiform pattern of woven bone trabeculae and loose fibrous tissue

Treatment and Prognosis

After removal of the source of inflammation, the bone will generally recontour within 6 to 12 months.

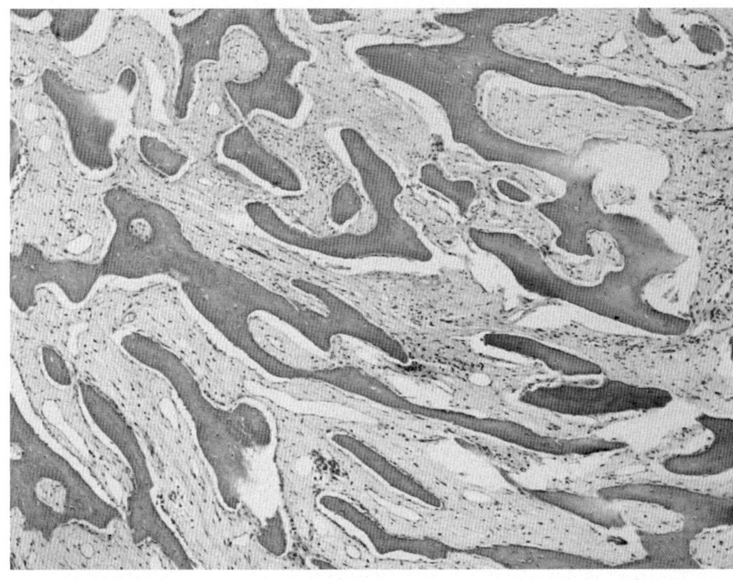

Figure 6.1.1.
Proliferative periostitis. Thin, parallel bony trabeculae with intervening well-vascularized fibrous stroma.

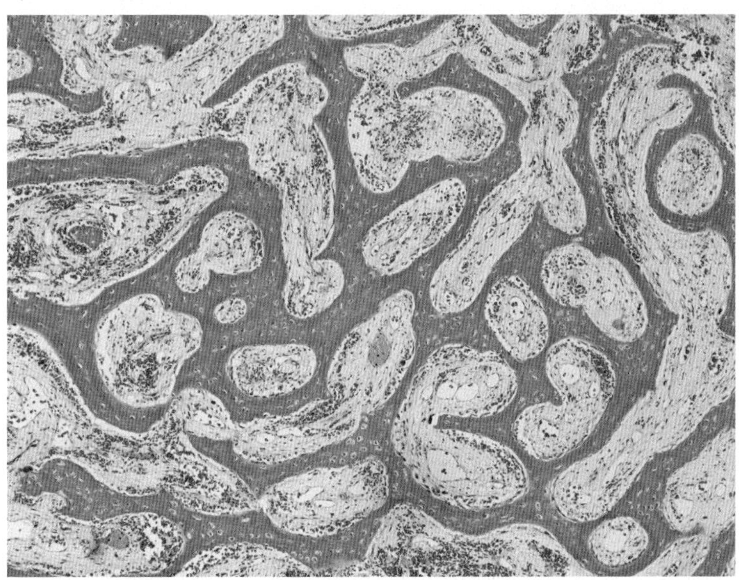

Figure 6.1.2.
Proliferative periostitis. Retiform, interconnecting, delicate osseous trabeculae set in a well-vascularized, loose fibrous connective tissue stroma.

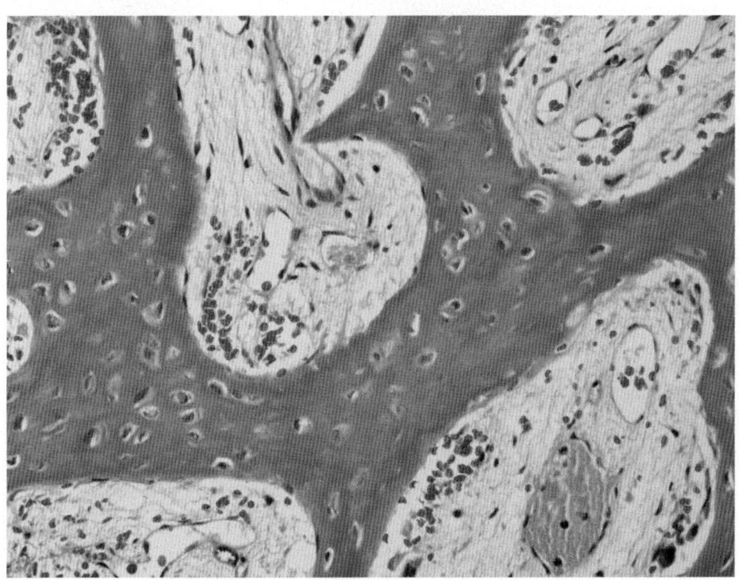

Figure 6.1.3.
Proliferative periostitis. Interconnecting trabeculae set in a well-vascularized, loose connective tissue stroma.

6.2 Bisphosphonate-Associated Osteonecrosis

Definition

A rare bone necrosis characterized by the presence of exposed, necrotic bone for several months following dental extraction or other jaw surgery

Presentation

Painful, exposed necrotic bone; purulent drainage and fistulas. History of intravenous or long-term oral bisphosphonate use (typically in patients with multiple myeloma or metastatic breast carcinoma) followed by tooth extraction or other jaw surgery. More common in the mandible.

Radiographic Appearance

Mottled radiolucency with sequestra (sclerotic bone fragments with a surrounding radiolucency); persistent extraction sockets

Microscopic Findings

- Necrotic bone (empty lacunae devoid of osteocytes).
- Bony trabeculae with resorptive lacunae filled with neutrophils and bacterial colonies.
- Actinomycotic bacterial colonies (sulfur granules) are often seen.

Treatment and Prognosis

The condition is difficult to treat. Generally a combination of surgical debridement and antibiotics is used.

Additional

The microscopic findings of bisphosphonate-associated osteonecrosis are also found in the bacterial osteomyelitis resulting from an infected tooth or fractured mandible.

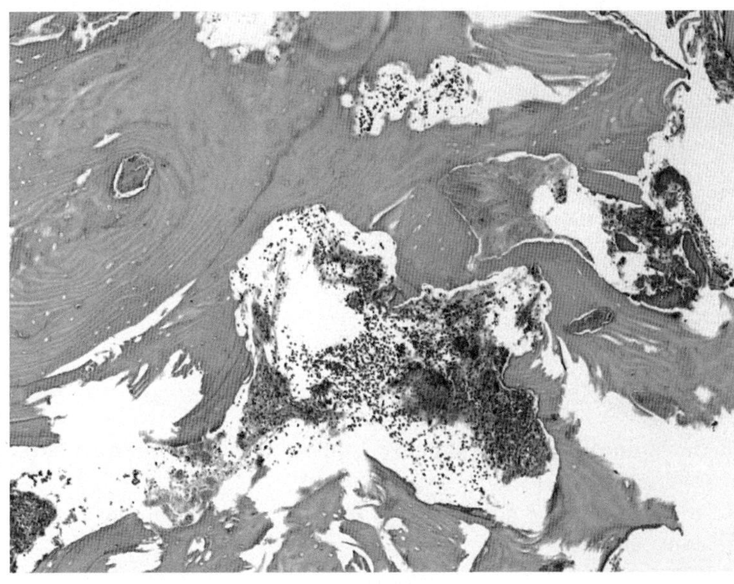

Figure 6.2.1.
Bisphosphonate-associated osteonecrosis. Necrotic bone trabeculae with resorptive lacunae containing bacterial colonies and clusters of inflammatory cells.

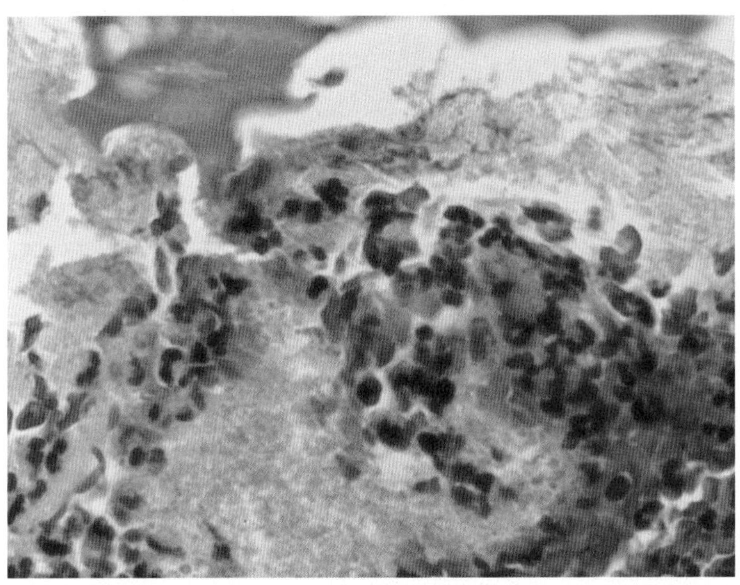

Figure 6.2.2.
Bisphosphonate-associated osteonecrosis. The combination of necrotic bone and acute and chronic inflammatory cells is also found in bacterial osteomyelitis.

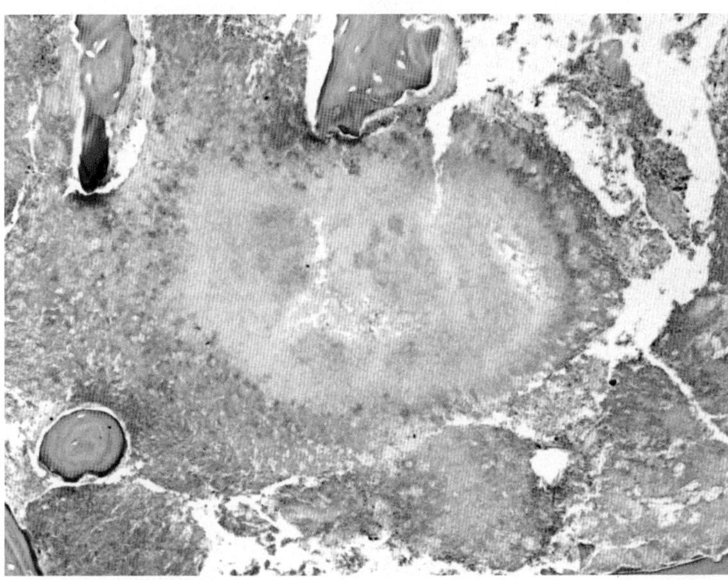

Figure 6.2.3.
Bisphosphonate-associated osteonecrosis. Tangled masses of filamentous bacteria make up an actinomycotic colony, often seen in this lesion.

6.3 Nasopalatine Duct Cyst

Definition
Developmental cyst of the anterior palate in the area of the embryonic nasopalatine canal

Presentation
Swelling of the midline anterior palate with drainage and pain. Can also be an incidental radiographic finding.

Radiographic Appearance
Heart-shaped radiolucency posterior to the upper incisor teeth

Microscopic Findings
- The cyst lining can be stratified squamous epithelium, respiratory epithelium with mucous cells and cilia, or a combination.
- Small nerve trunks, arteries, veins, and mucous glands are often seen in the fibrous cyst wall.
- Foci of chronic inflammatory cells.

Treatment and Prognosis
Enucleation. Recurrence is rare.

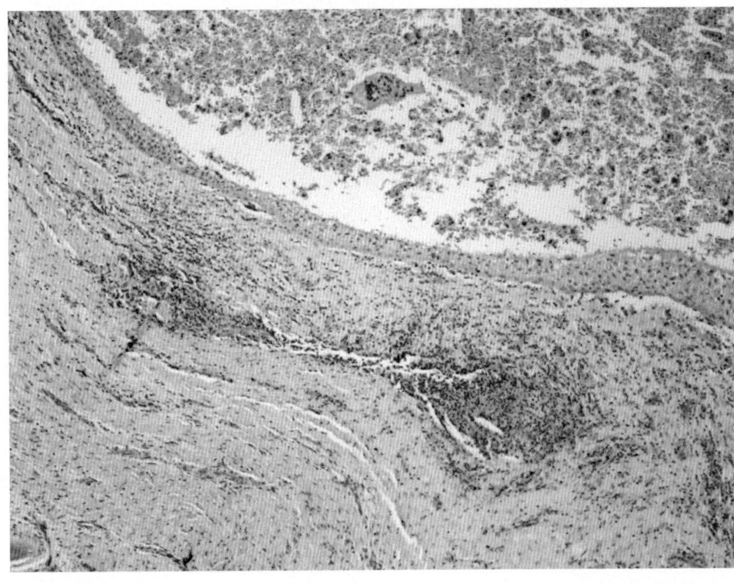

Figure 6.3.1.
Nasopalatine duct cyst. Stratified squamous epithelium lines this portion of the fibro-collagenous, inflamed cyst wall. Small vessels and nerves, a relatively common finding, are not present in this example.

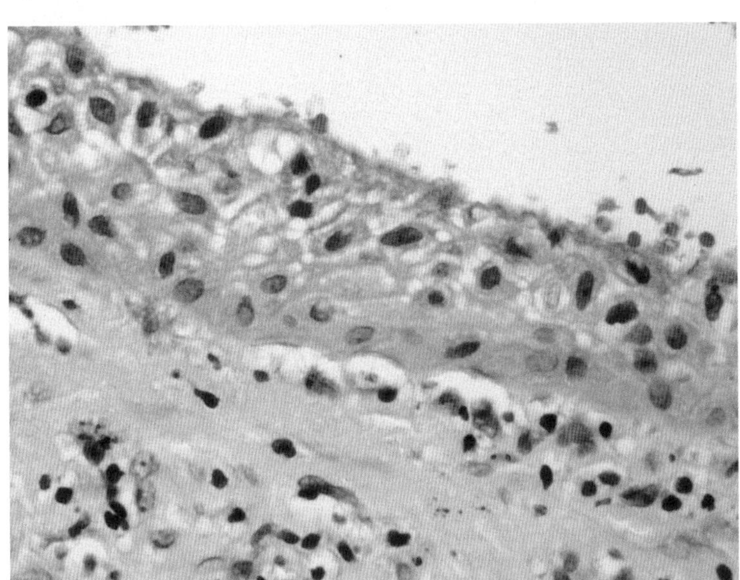

Figure 6.3.2. Nasopalatine duct cyst. A close-up of the inflamed cyst wall and edematous stratified squamous lining.

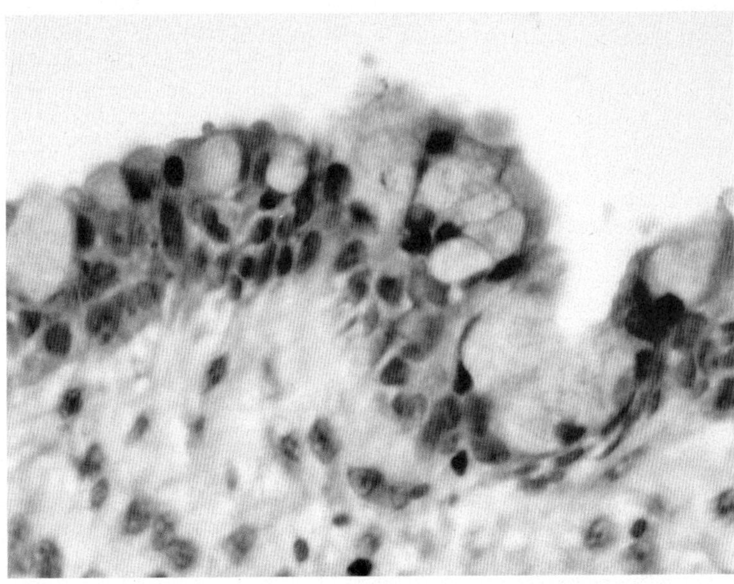

Figure 6.3.3. Nasopalatine duct cyst. Scattered mucous goblet cells are often encountered in the cyst lining.

6.4 Surgical Ciliated Cyst

Definition

A cystic structure resulting from a portion of sinus mucosa becoming entrapped in the adjacent bone during a surgical procedure

Presentation

Patients have a history of a surgical procedure involving the maxilla. The symptoms vary and depend on the nature of the cyst's expansion. Can also be an incidental radiographic finding.

Radiographic Appearance

Radiolucency within maxilla

Microscopic Findings

Fibro-collagenous cyst lined by the same respiratory-type epithelium found lining the normal maxillary sinus

Treatment and Prognosis

The cyst is excised and does not recur.

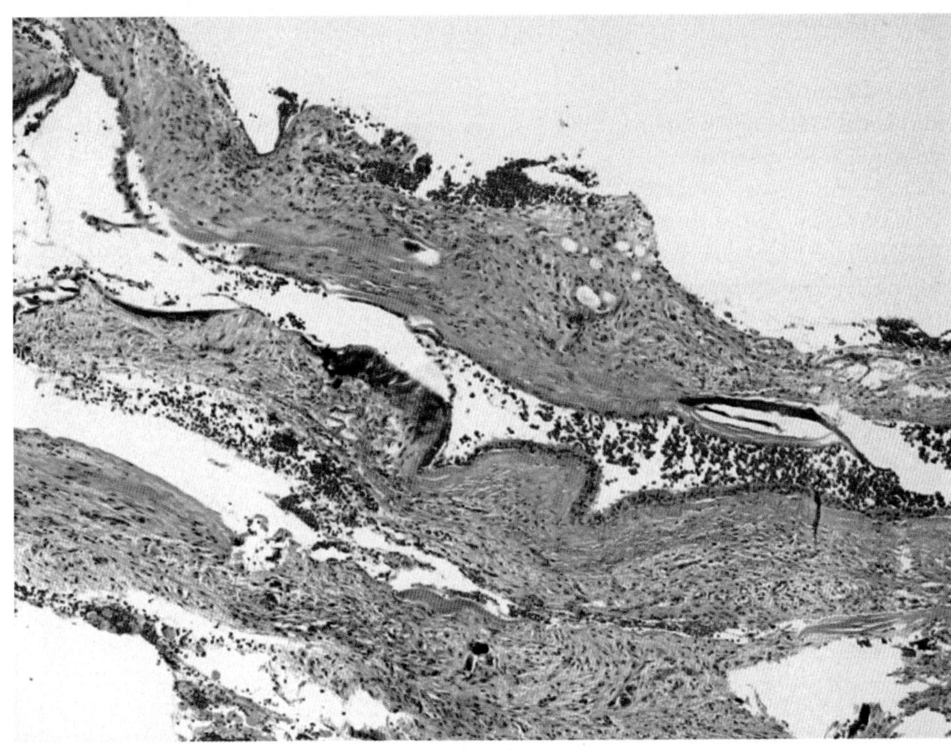

Figure 6.4.1.
Surgical ciliated cyst. A collapsed, epithelial-lined, cystic structure is evident at scanning power.

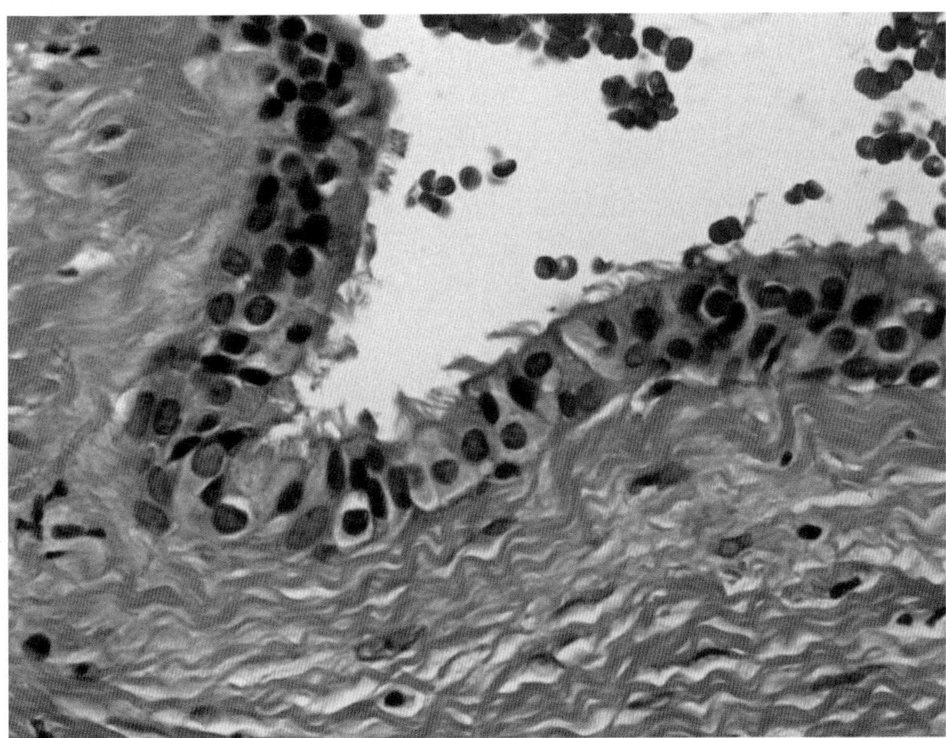

Figure 6.4.2.
Surgical ciliated cyst. Higher power of the lining reveals ciliated respiratory epithelium.

6.5 Simple (Traumatic) Bone Cyst

Presentation

Incidental radiographic finding. Most patients are males and younger than 20 years. More common in the mandible.

Radiographic Appearance

Well-defined unilocular radiolucency; superior margin of mandibular lesions can show scalloping between tooth roots.

Microscopic Findings

Empty bone cavity lined by loose fibrous connective tissue, sometimes with slender calcifications, fibrin, and foci of hemorrhage. No epithelial lining.

Treatment and Prognosis

Biopsy only. The bony cavity usually fills in within 6 months after biopsy.

Additional

Despite the name, often there is no history of trauma. Simple bone cysts can be seen in patients with florid cemento-osseous dysplasia.

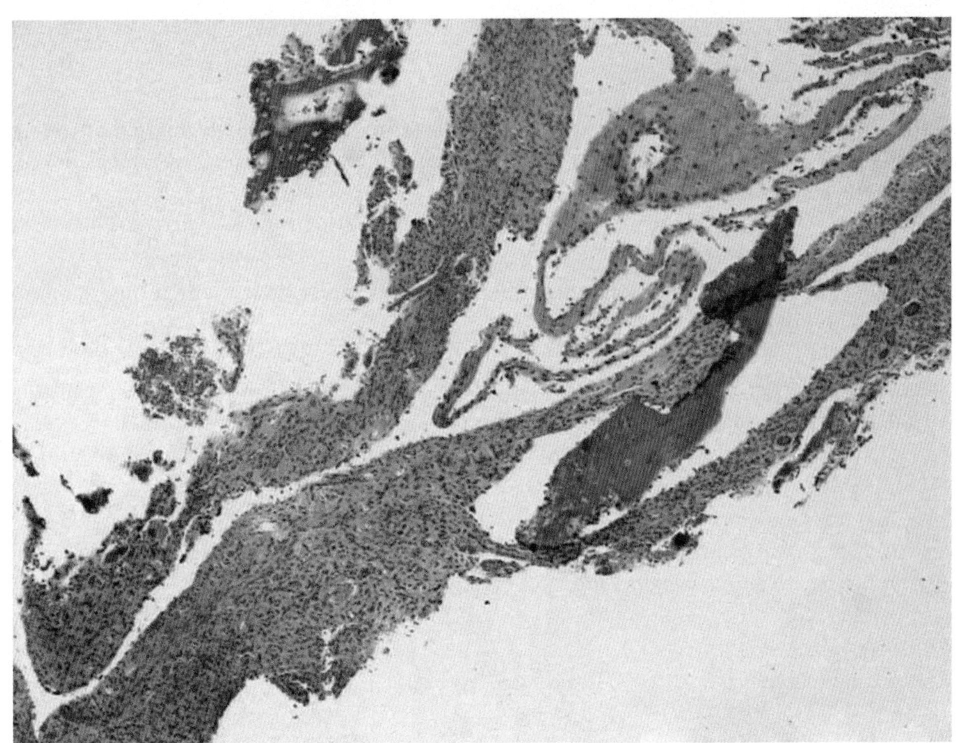

Figure 6.5.1.
Simple (traumatic) bone cyst. Fragments of fibrous connective tissue and bone represent the scrapings from the walls of an empty bony cavity.

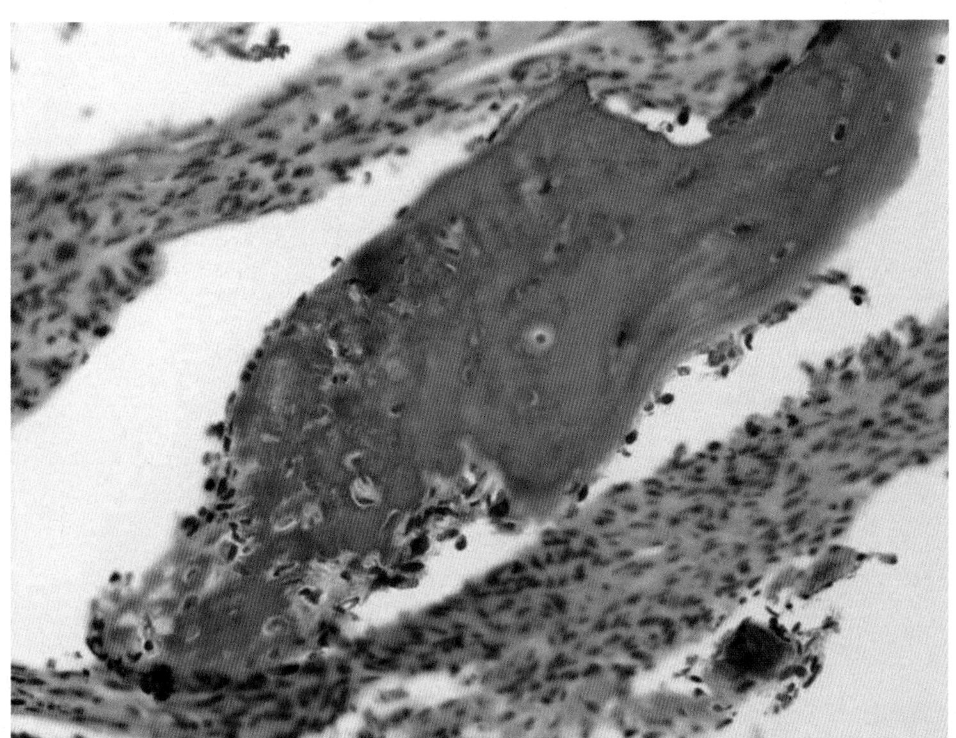

Figure 6.5.2.
Simple (traumatic) bone cyst. The fibrous tissue is cellular and the bone viable.

6.6 Aneurysmal Bone Cyst

Presentation

Painful swelling of the jaw with rapid onset. Usually posterior mandible in children or young adults. Often in association with other bone pathology: fibro-osseous lesions, central giant cell granuloma, osteoblastoma.

Radiographic Appearance

Unilocular or multilocular radiolucency. "Blow out" deformity of the cortex (pronounced expansion and thinning).

Microscopic Findings

- Large non-endothelial-lined blood-filled spaces
- Granulation tissue with foci of multinucleated giant cells, hemorrhage, and hemosiderin
- Reactive woven bone trabeculae

Histopathologic Differential

A *central giant cell granuloma* does not have cavernous blood-filled spaces.

Treatment and Prognosis

Enucleation, curettage, or surgery. Recurrence has been reported.

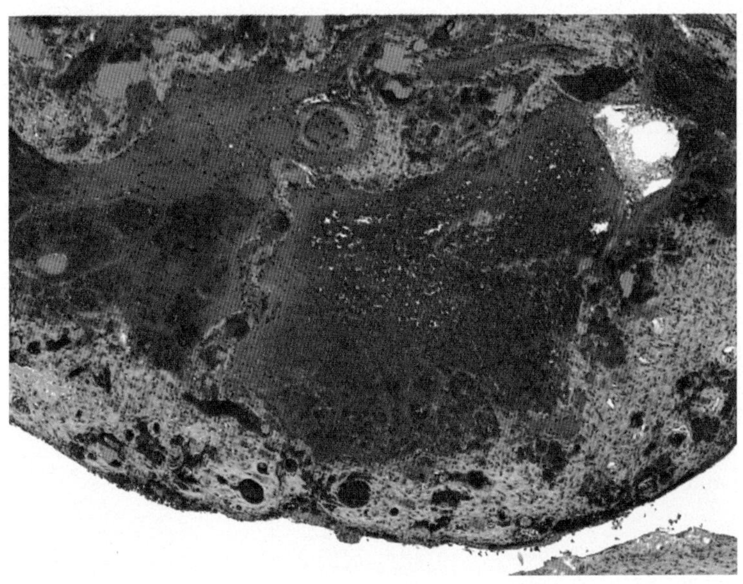

Figure 6.6.1.
Aneurysmal bone cyst. Numerous non-endothelial-lined blood-filled spaces are seen in the fibrovascular stroma.

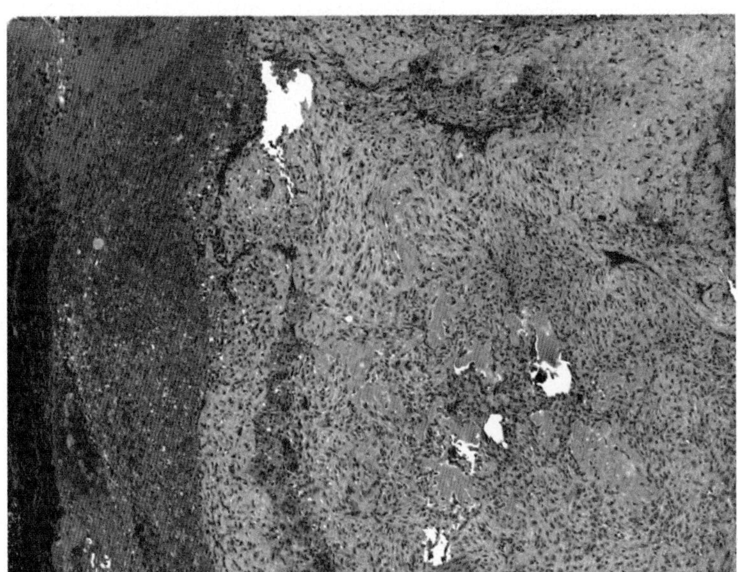

Figure 6.6.2.
Aneurysmal bone cyst. Spindle cells produce metaplastic osteoid or woven bone.

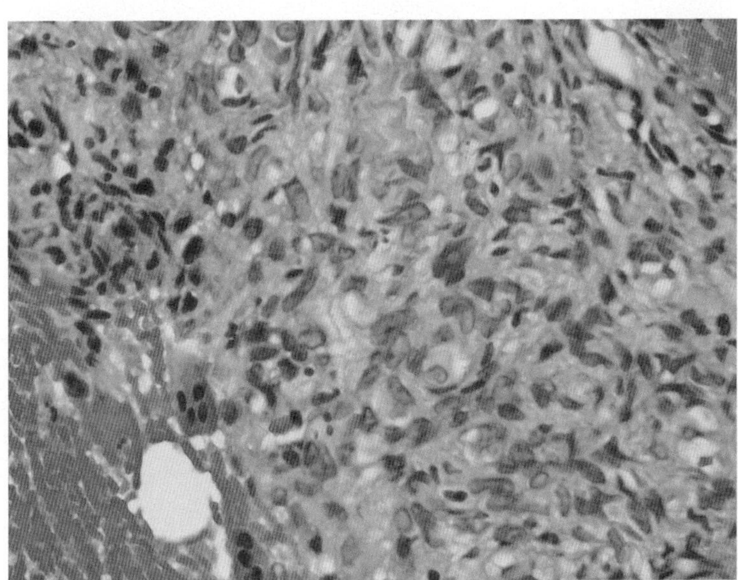

Figure 6.6.3.
Aneurysmal bone cyst. The granulation tissue adjoins a pool of blood and contains inflammatory and multinucleated giant cells.

6.7 Central Giant Cell Granuloma

Presentation

Asymptomatic swelling; larger lesions can be painful and produce paresthesia. Anterior location common; more frequent in the mandible. Children and young adults; especially females.

Radiographic Appearance

Unilocular or multilocular radiolucency. Larger lesions can destroy the bony cortex and cause tooth resorption.

Microscopic Findings

- Cellular fibrous connective tissue containing plump spindle cells, clusters of multinucleated giant cells, and foci of hemorrhage and hemosiderin.
- Reactive woven bone trabeculae are seen.
- Numerous normal mitoses can be seen in the lesional spindle cells.

Histopathologic Differential

An *aneurysmal bone cyst* has a similar histology, but also contains cavernous blood-filled spaces.

The histology of a *brown tumor* is also identical, which should prompt the pathologist to advise evaluation for hyperparathyroidism, especially in patients older than 30 years.

Cherubism must be excluded in a child with multiple central giant cell granulomas.

Treatment and Prognosis

Curettage, radical surgery, and/or injection of corticosteroids, calcitonin, and interferon. Recurrence has been reported.

Additional

Some reports indicate that lesions with large, uniformly spaced giant cells set in a cellular fibrous stroma are more aggressive in biologic behavior and likely to recur.

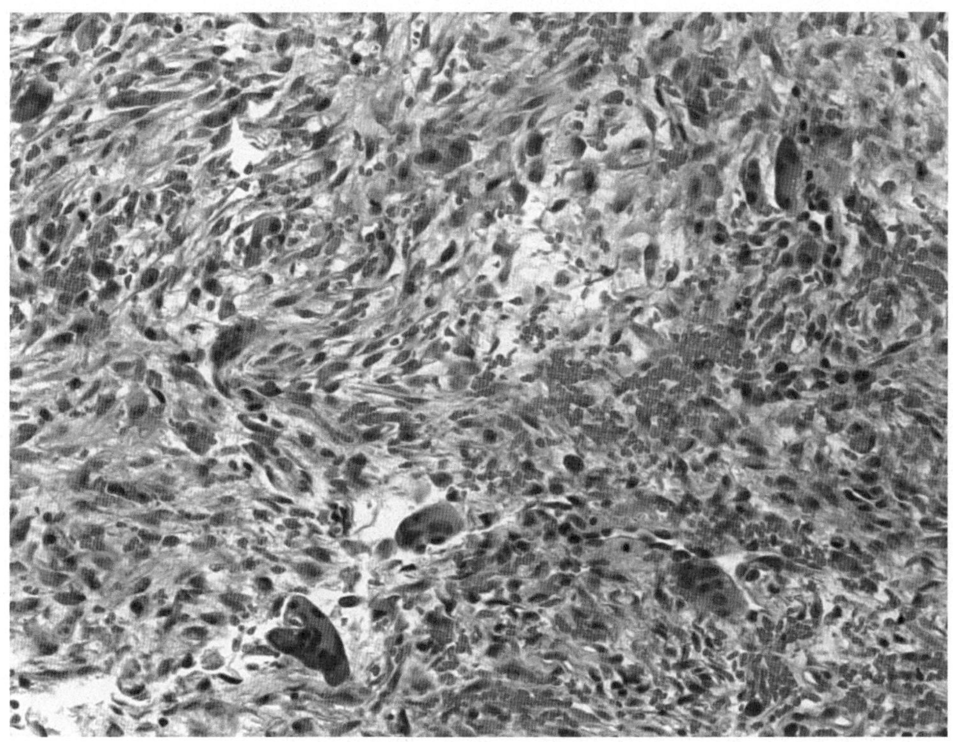

Figure 6.7.1.
Central giant cell granuloma. The cellular, loose, fibrous stroma contains clusters of multinucleated giant cells and abundant hemorrhage.

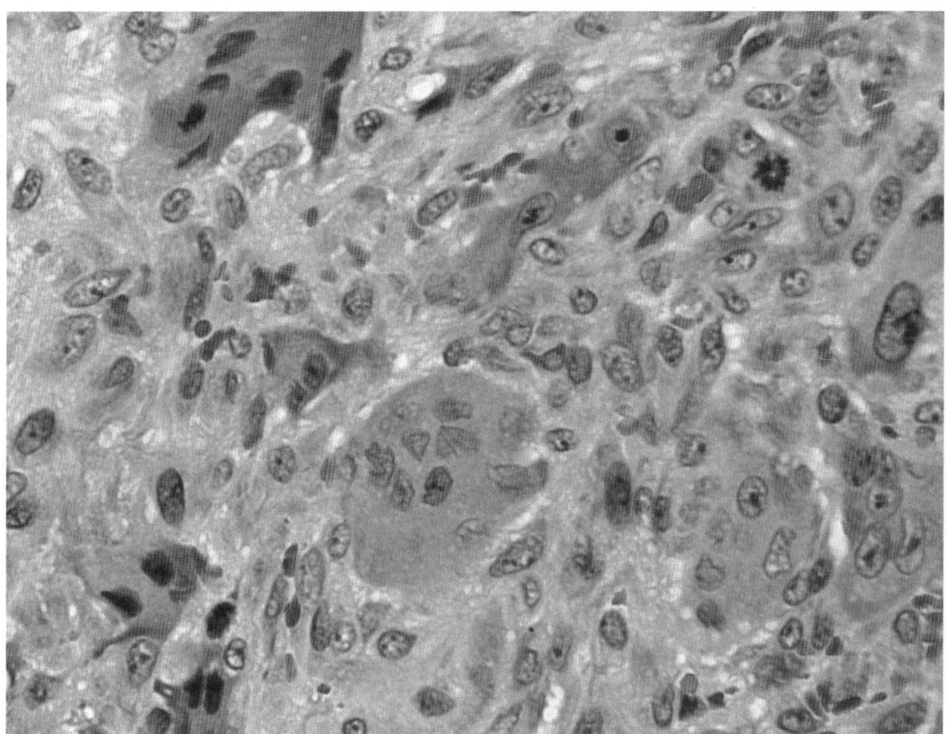

Figure 6.7.2.
Central giant cell granuloma. Giant cells of varying size and shape are surrounded by a cellular, fibrous stroma. Mitotic figures, such as the one at the upper right, are a common finding in this benign, reactive lesion.

6.8 Fibrous Dysplasia

Presentation

Slow-growing, painless expansion of bone causing facial asymmetry. The maxilla is more commonly affected than the mandible. Teenagers and young adults.

Radiographic Appearance

Ground glass or orange peel radiopacity blending subtly into surrounding, normal bone

Microscopic Findings

- Uniform pattern of evenly distributed, variably shaped woven bone trabeculae set in a cellular fibrous stroma.
- New bone appears to be formed by stromal fibroblasts.
- The stromal fibroblasts are plump and devoid of mitotic figures.

Treatment and Prognosis

Observation or surgical recontouring

Additional

Fibrous dysplasia occurs in both monostotic and polyostotic forms; the latter can be associated with endocrine and cutaneous abnormalities.

When fibrous dysplasia affects the maxilla, it usually also involves the neighboring bones of the zygomatic arch and orbit. This is known as *craniofacial fibrous dysplasia.*

In fibrous dysplasia of the jaws, as the lesion matures, the bone becomes increasingly lamellar.

A comparison of the benign fibro-osseous lesions in chart form can be found on page 216.

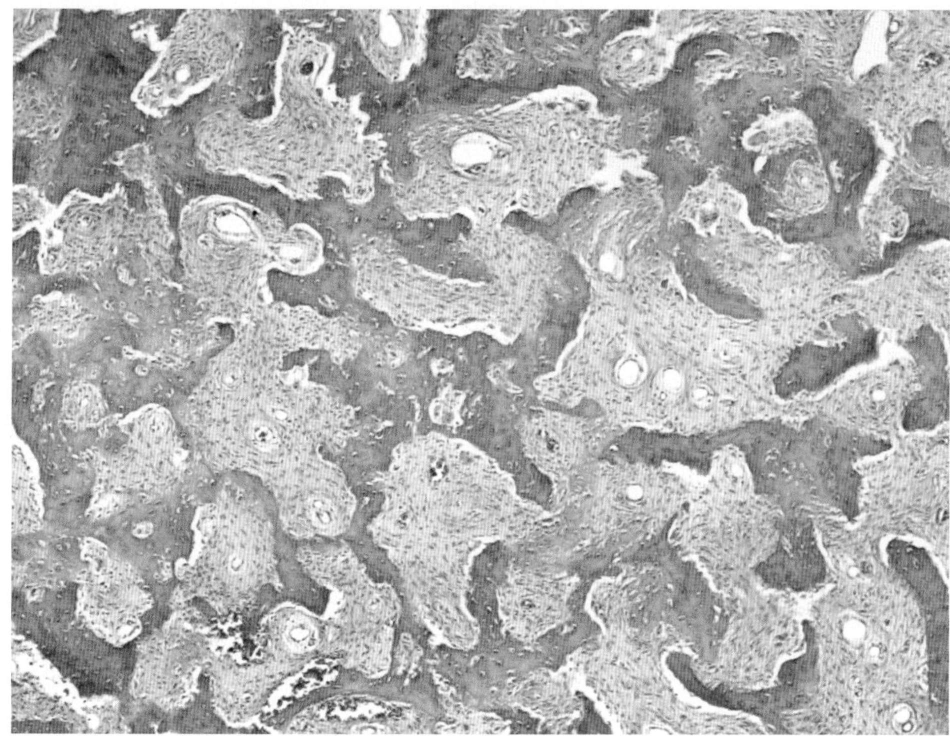

Figure 6.8.1.
Fibrous dysplasia. A uniform pattern of interconnecting woven bone trabeculae resembling Chinese letter characters. The stroma consists of vascular cellular fibrous connective tissue.

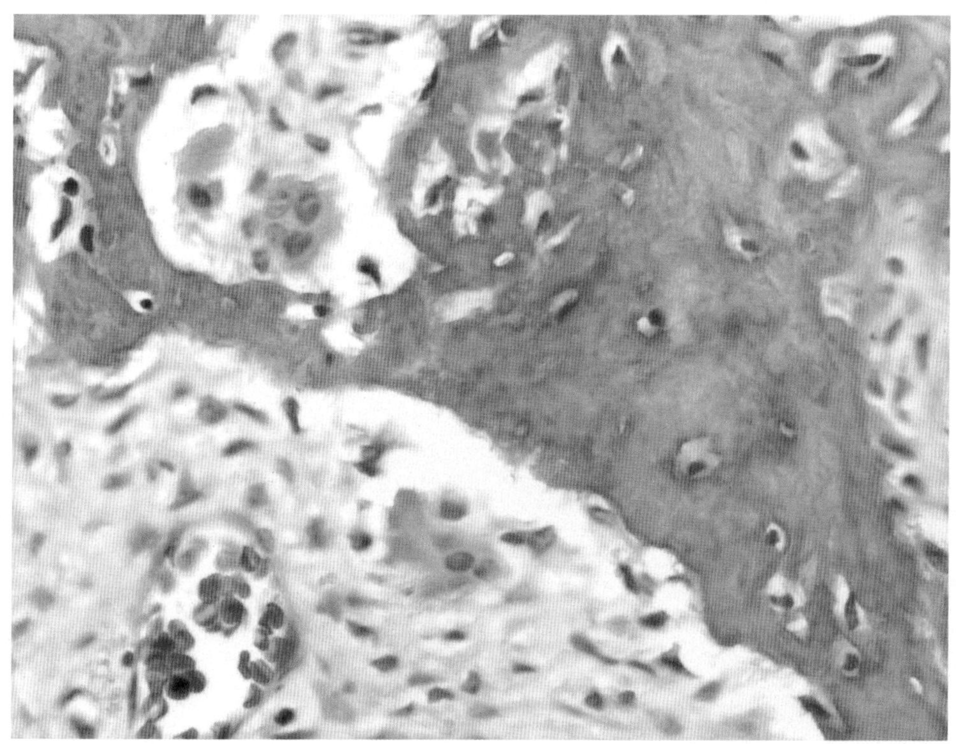

Figure 6.8.2.
Fibrous dysplasia. Metaplastic bony trabeculae set in a loose, fibrous stroma. Occasional osteoclasts are seen.

6.9 Cemento-Osseous Dysplasia

Definition

A nonneoplastic, benign fibro-osseous lesion unique to the tooth-bearing portions of the jaws

Presentation

Generally an asymptomatic, incidental radiographic finding. Pain and fistula formation can result when lesions become infected. The specimen usually consists of granular, gritty fragments.

This condition can present as a localized lesion at the apices of the lower anterior teeth, a solitary radiolucency of the posterior mandible, or as a more generalized process involving two or more quadrants of the jaws. Especially common among black women older than 40 years.

Radiographic Appearance

Mixed radiolucent and radiopaque lesion

Microscopic Findings

- Fibro-collagenous tissue containing variable quantities of cemento-osseous trabeculae
- Retraction artifact of the stroma from the bone trabeculae

Treatment and Prognosis

Unexposed bone requires no treatment. Symptomatic patients with exposed bone may require surgical intervention.

Additional

Simple bone cysts can occur in patients with florid cemento-osseous dysplasia. When biopsied, they are slow to heal.

A comparison of the benign fibro-osseous lesions in chart form can be found on page 216.

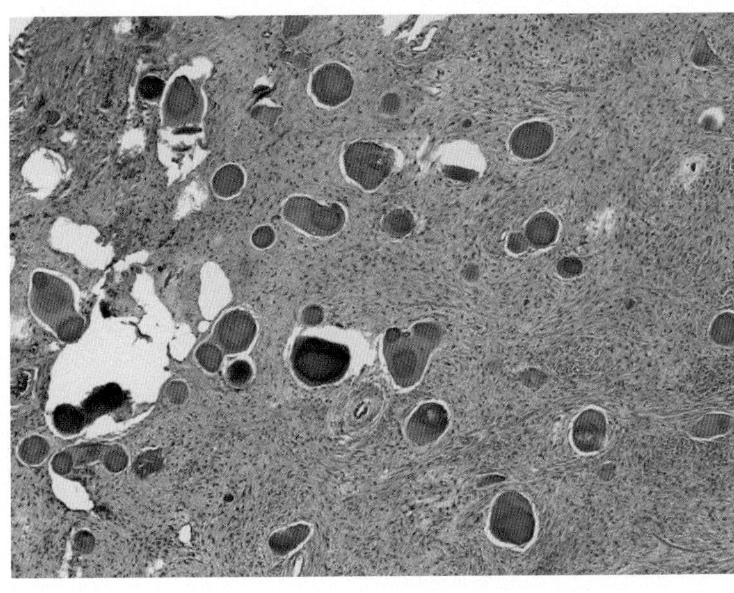

Figure 6.9.1.
Cemento-osseous dysplasia. The calcified material in this case consists of numerous small, spherical, basophilic cementicles. The stroma is cellular, fibrous, and relatively avascular.

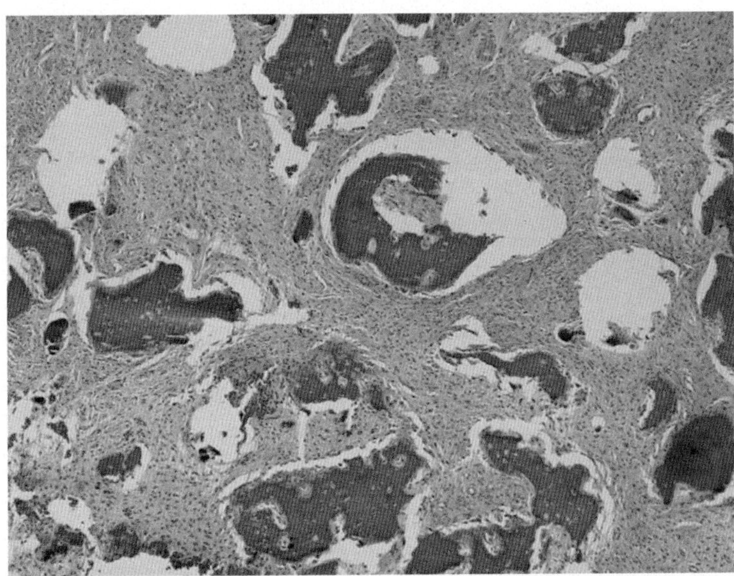

Figure 6.9.2.
Cemento-osseous dysplasia. Variably sized trabeculae of woven bone set in a moderately cellular fibrous connective tissue. Retraction artifact is a common finding. The three disease variants all have a similar histology.

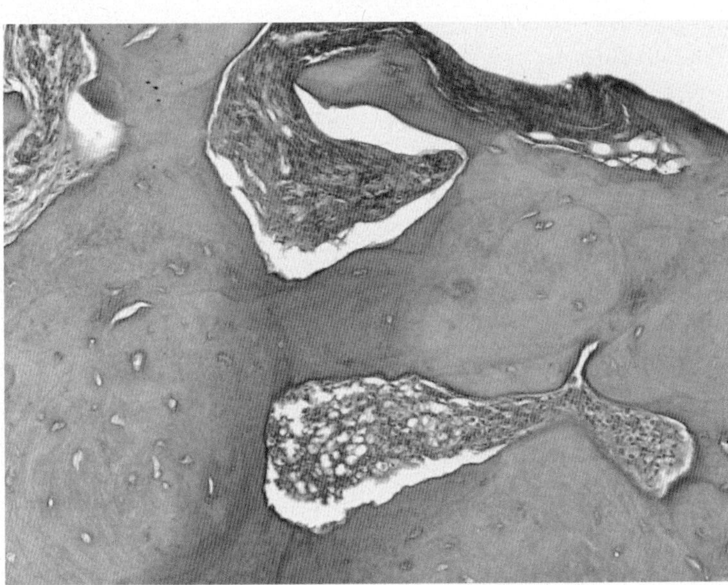

Figure 6.9.3.
Cemento-osseous dysplasia. As the lesion matures, the dysplastic bone trabeculae fuse and form dense necrotic-appearing masses. The stroma is fibrous and avascular.

6.10 Ossifying Fibroma

Definition

This benign fibro-osseous lesion is a true neoplasm and can grow to a large size.

Presentation

Painless swelling, commonly in the mandible, especially the molar area. The tumor, which shells out easily, is usually submitted as a single mass or as a few large pieces. Wide age range, but most often in adults aged 20 to 40 years. More common in females.

Radiographic Appearance

Well-defined, unilocular radiolucency

Microscopic Findings

The tumor is well demarcated and consists of cellular fibrous connective tissue mixed with cemento-osseous trabeculae and calcific spherules of varying size and shape. Woven bone trabeculae are lined by plump osteoblasts.

Treatment and Prognosis

Enucleation. Recurrence is rare.

A comparison of the benign fibro-osseous lesions in chart form can be found below.

Clinicopathologic differential of the benign fibro-osseous lesions

	Fibrous dysplasia	Cemento-osseous dysplasia, focal	Ossifying fibroma	Juvenile trabecular ossifying fibroma
Location	Mostly maxilla	Mandible, posterior	Mandible, esp. posterior	Maxilla
Age	Teenagers and young adults	Over 40 years	Wide age range; mostly adults age 20 to 40	Average age 11 years
Sex predilection	None	Females, esp. African-American	Females more common	Males more common
Rate of growth and nature of expansion	Slow-growing and expansile	Not expansile	Slow-growing and expansile	Rapid, localized expansion
Radiographic appearance	Ground-glass radiopacity blends into adjacent, unaffected bone. Envelops teeth, does not displace them.	Mixed radiolucent-radiopaque lesion	Well-defined radiolucent-radiopaque lesion. Displaces teeth.	Well-defined radiolucent-radiopaque lesion.
Histopathology	• Monotonous pattern of woven bone trabeculae lacking osteoblastic rimming set in a cellular fibrous connective tissue. • Lesion blends into adjacent, normal bone. • As lesion matures, bony trabeculae become more lamellar	• Variable quantities of cemento-osseous tissue set in a cellular fibrous connective stroma. • Calcified material in the form of trabeculae of woven bone or basophilic spherules. • Retraction artifact of bony trabeculae	• Variable quantities of cemento-osseous tissue set in a cellular fibrous connective stroma. • Lesion well-demarcated from adjacent, normal bone. • Woven bone trabeculae are lined by plump osteoblasts.	• Trabeculae of woven bone set in a cellular, well-vascularized, loose fibrous stroma. • Lesion well-demarcated from adjacent, normal bone. • Osteoblastic rimming of tumor bone. Osteoclasts also common. • Foci of hemorrhage may be seen.

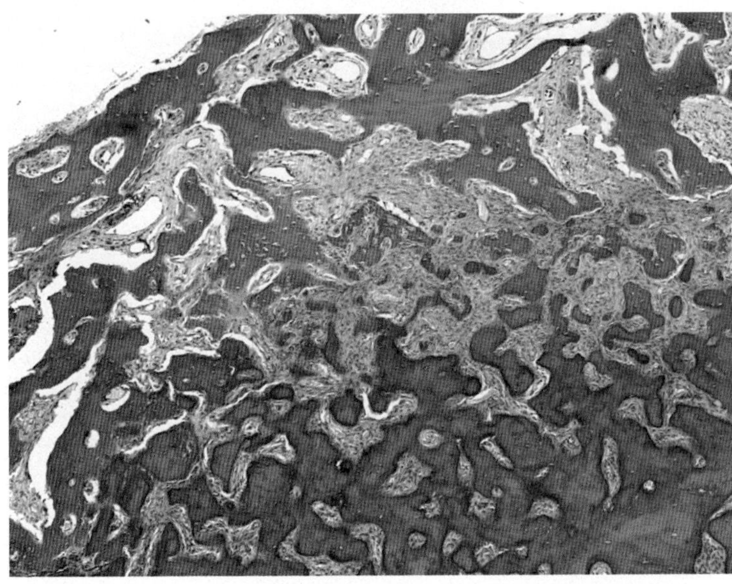

Figure 6.10.1.
Ossifying fibroma. This circumscribed tumor is composed of well-developed, interconnecting cemento-osseous trabeculae.

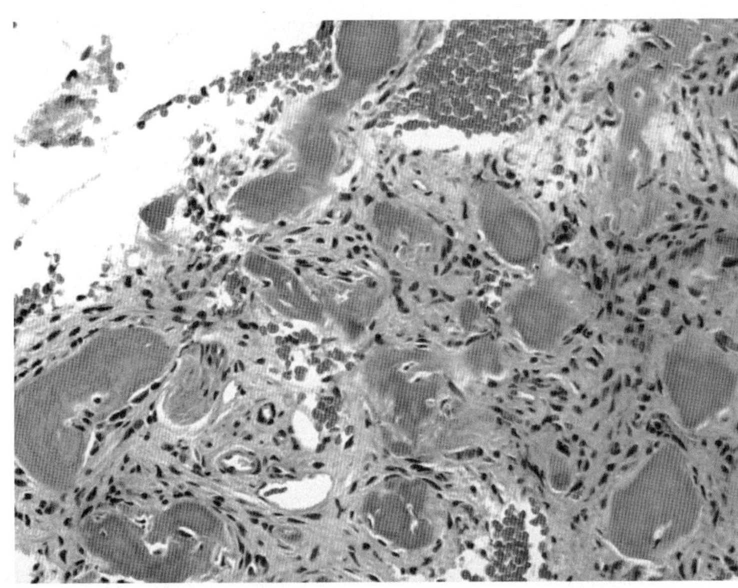

Figure 6.10.2.
Ossifying fibroma. Calcified material in this tumor takes the form of islands of woven bone of variable size and shape. The stroma is cellular, fibrous, and relatively well vascularized. Osteoblasts line some of the woven bone trabeculae.

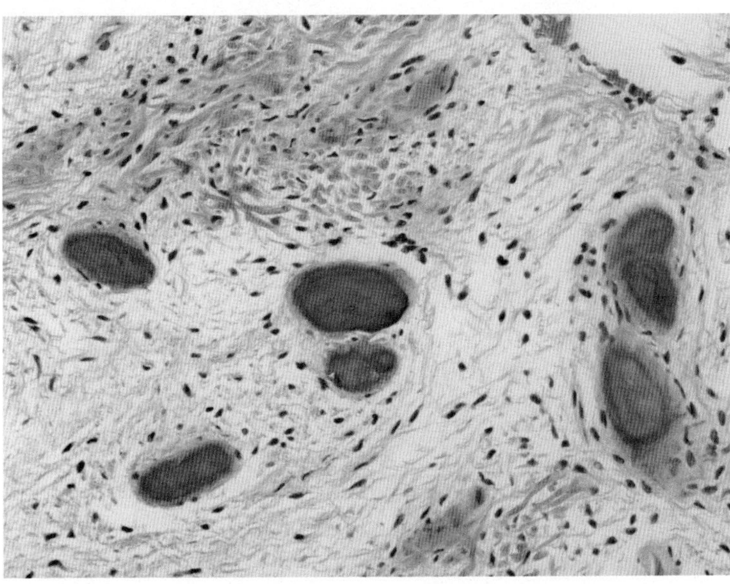

Figure 6.10.3.
Ossifying fibroma. In this example, small cementicles are scattered throughout a loose, fibromyxoid stroma.

6.11 Juvenile Trabecular Ossifying Fibroma

Presentation

Rapid, localized bony expansion. More common in the maxilla. The average age of the patient is 11 years.

Radiographic Appearance

Well defined. Mixed radiolucent and radiopaque lesion.

Microscopic Findings

A well-demarcated tumor composed of trabeculae of woven bone rimmed by plump osteoblasts and osteoclasts. Plump osteocytes are seen within the bony trabeculae. Normal mitoses may be seen.

Treatment and Prognosis

Local excision or resection. These lesions can recur.

Additional

The juvenile psammomatoid ossifying fibroma, a related lesion of the sinonasal bones and orbit, is encountered only infrequently in the maxilla or the mandible.

A comparison of the benign fibro-osseous lesions in chart form can be found on page 216.

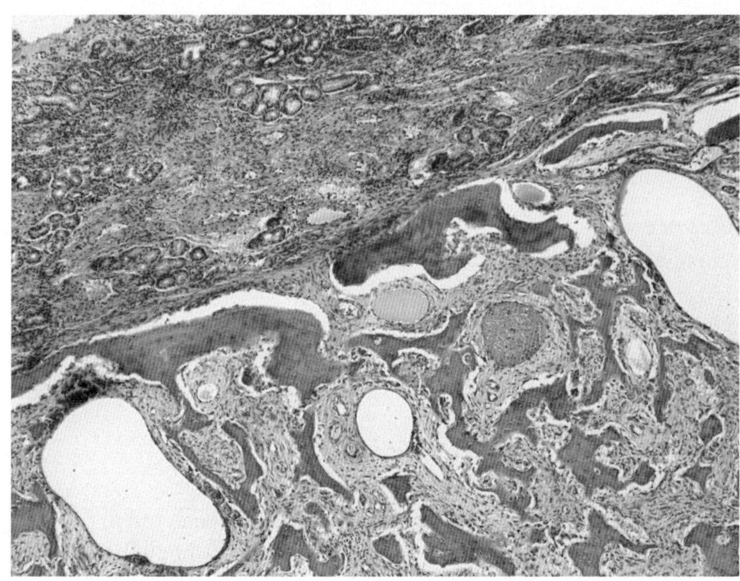

Figure 6.11.1.
Juvenile trabecular ossifying fibroma. A well-circumscribed proliferation of bony trabeculae set in a cellular, vascularized, loose fibrous stroma. Inflamed mucous glands from the mucosa of the maxillary sinus envelop the bony proliferation.

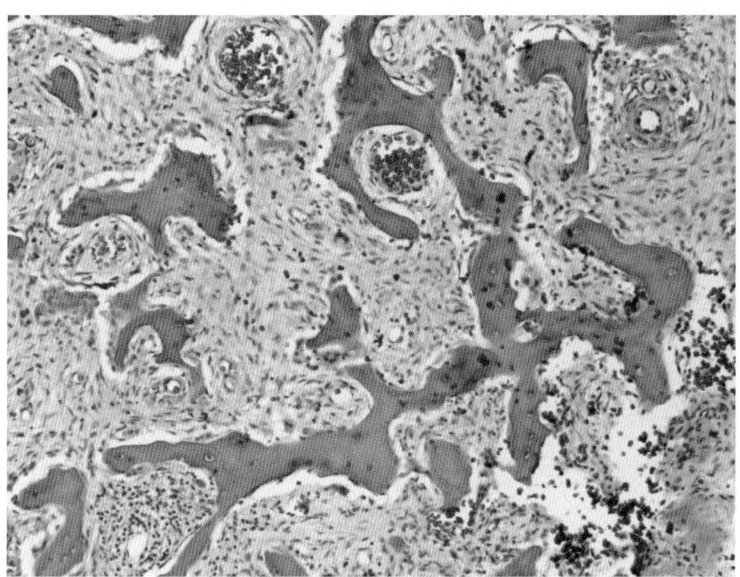

Figure 6.11.2.
Juvenile trabecular ossifying fibroma. Bridging islands of woven bone. The stroma is loose, cellular, and vascular.

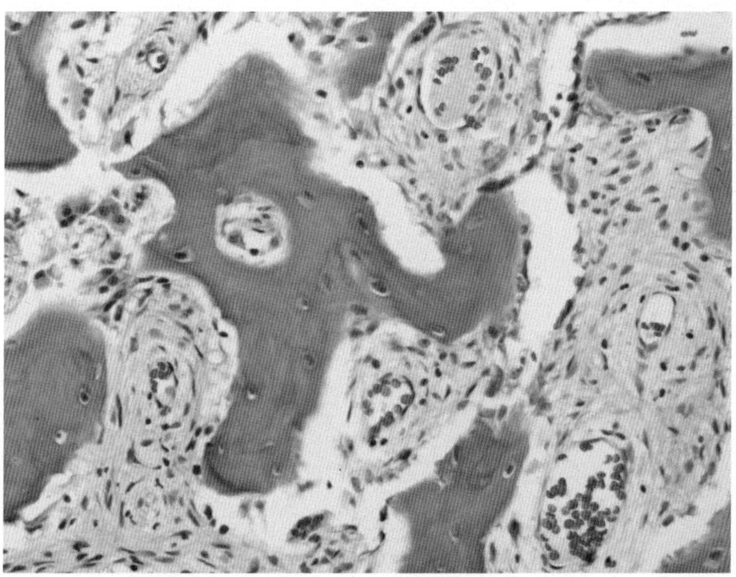

Figure 6.11.3.
Juvenile trabecular ossifying fibroma. Ribbons of osteoblasts, upper right, have been artifactually lifted off the surface of the woven bone. Fibrous stroma is well vascularized.

6.12 Osteoblastoma

Presentation

Painful bony expansion. Most often in the mandible, usually posterior. Patients are usually younger than 30 years. More common in females.

Radiographic Appearance

Mixed radiolucent and radiopaque; circumscribed

Microscopic Findings

- Woven bone trabeculae of uniform width rimmed by clusters of osteoblasts
- Cellular, highly vascular fibrous connective tissue stroma

Histopathologic Differential

- *Cementoblastoma* is attached to the root of a tooth.
- *Osteosarcoma* has a sarcomatous stroma and contains malignant bone and, often, cartilage. Trabeculae of uniform width, osteoblastic rimming, and an abundance of plump, epithelioid osteoblasts in the stroma favor a diagnosis of osteoblastoma.

Treatment and Prognosis

Excision. Prognosis is good.

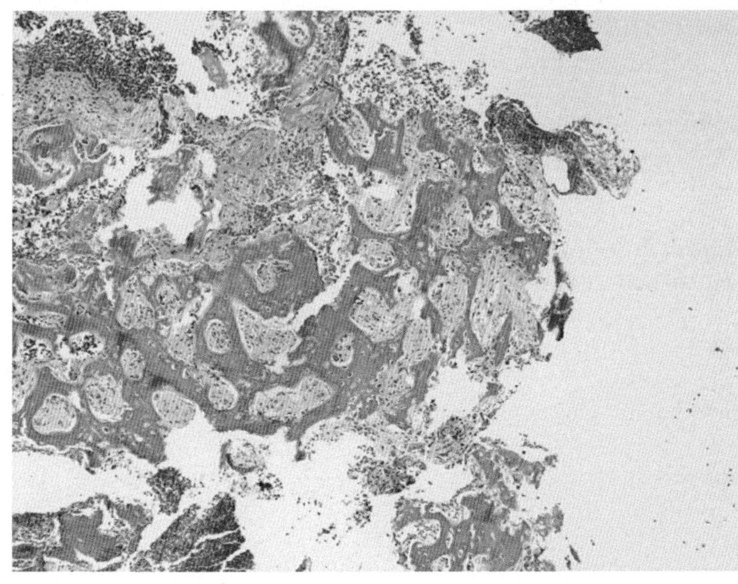

Figure 6.12.1.
Osteoblastoma. The tumor is composed of long, anastamosing, uniform, delicate trabeculae of woven bone set in a well-vascularized fibrous stroma.

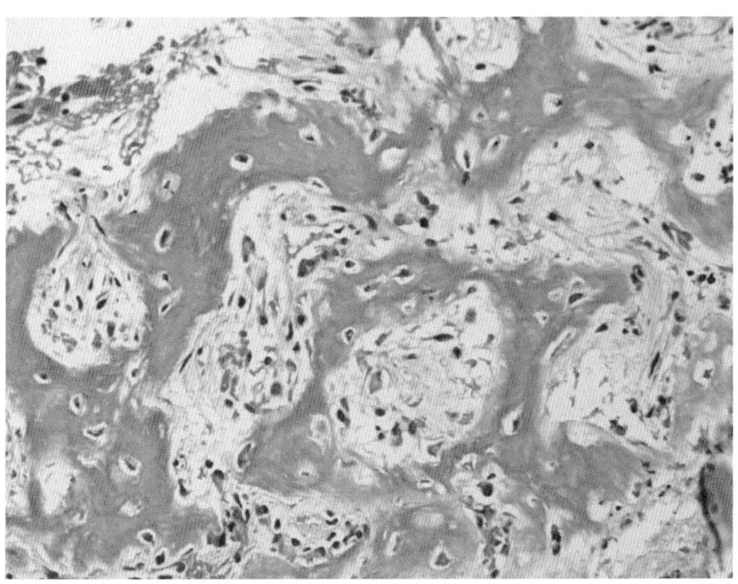

Figure 6.12.2.
Osteoblastoma. Osteoblasts with enlarged nuclei are seen within the woven bone trabeculae and the well-vascularized stroma and line up along the periphery of the bone trabeculae.

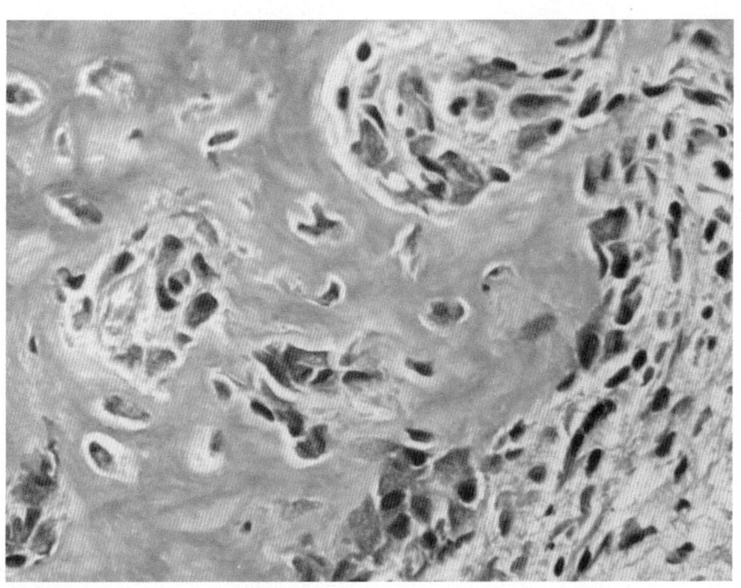

Figure 6.12.3.
Osteoblastoma. Clusters of plump osteoblasts abut the newly formed woven bone trabeculae and are also seen entrapped within the bone and scattered in the stroma. In areas the osteoblasts bridge the bone trabeculae.

6.13 Osteochondroma

Presentation

Slow-growing bony expansion, typically of the mandibular condyle. Difficulty in mouth opening and pain in the area of the temporomandibular joint. The average age of the patient is 40 years. More common in females.

Radiographic Appearance

An osseous protuberance of normal cortical and medullary bone

Microscopic Findings

- Cap of benign hyaline cartilage
- Area resembling endochondral growth plate that blends into mature bone below

Treatment and Prognosis

Excision is curative.

Additional

Osteochondroma is the most common tumor of bone. Its presence in the jaws, however, is extremely rare.

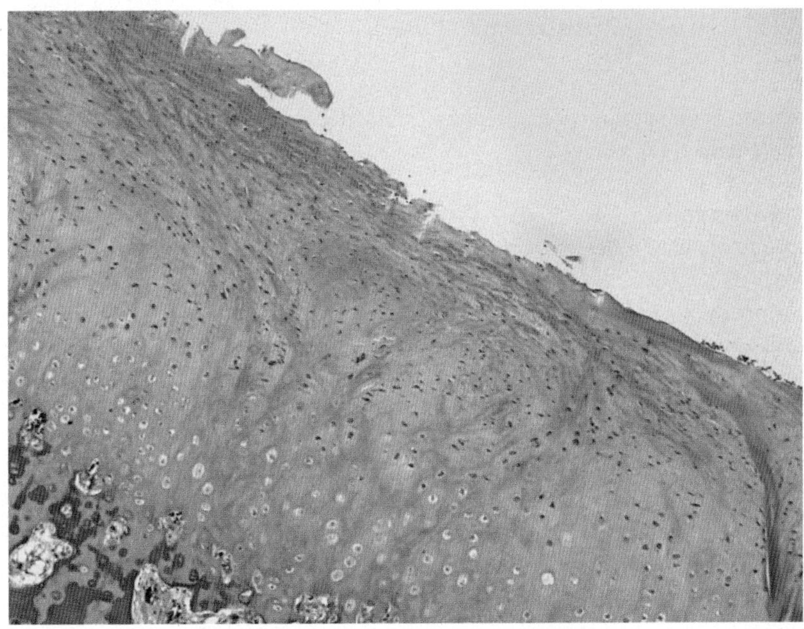

Figure 6.13.1. Osteochondroma. In this example from the mandibular condyle, a surface cap of hyaline cartilage overlies a zone of osteoid spicules that extend into the underlying cancellous bone.

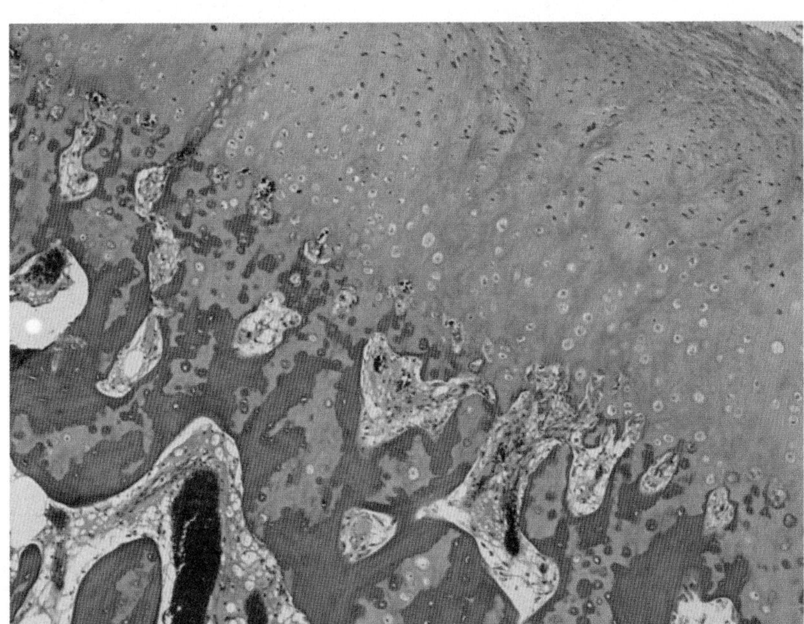

Figure 6.13.2. Osteochondroma. Endochondral woven bone trabeculae are seen below the cartilaginous cap.

6.14 Synovial Chondromatosis

Presentation
Temporomandibular joint dysfunction: swelling, difficulty in mouth opening. Adults; more frequent in females.

Radiographic Appearance
Multiple radiopaque nodules in the temporomandibular joint space (loose bodies)

Microscopic Findings
- Multiple small nodules of hyaline cartilage exhibiting atypical enlarged and binucleate chondrocytes

Histopathologic Differential
A *chondrosarcoma* in the area of the temporomandibular joint is extremely rare. It has invasive features and shows areas of sarcomatous change and necrosis. The cytologic atypia of the cartilage in the nodules of synovial chondromatosis do not connote malignant behavior.

Treatment and Prognosis
Complete excision. Prognosis is excellent.

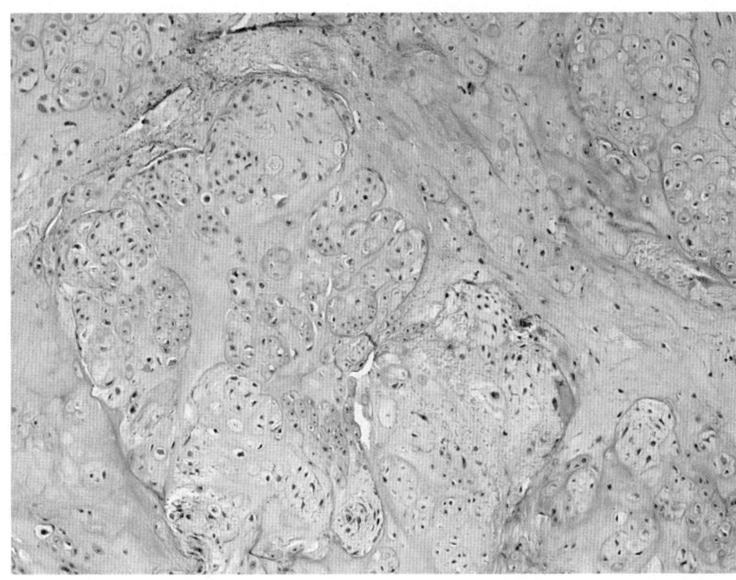

Figure 6.14.1.
Synovial chondromatosis. A nodule of disorganized, highly cellular metaplastic hyaline cartilage.

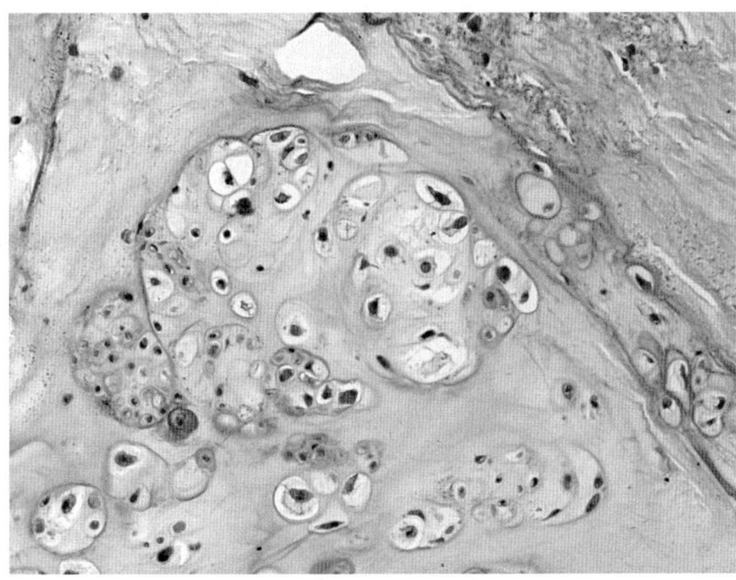

Figure 6.14.2.
Synovial chondromatosis. The chondrocytes are atypical: pleomorphic, hyperchromatic, and multinucleate. Note the similarity of these chondrocytes to those of the chondrosarcoma on page 231.

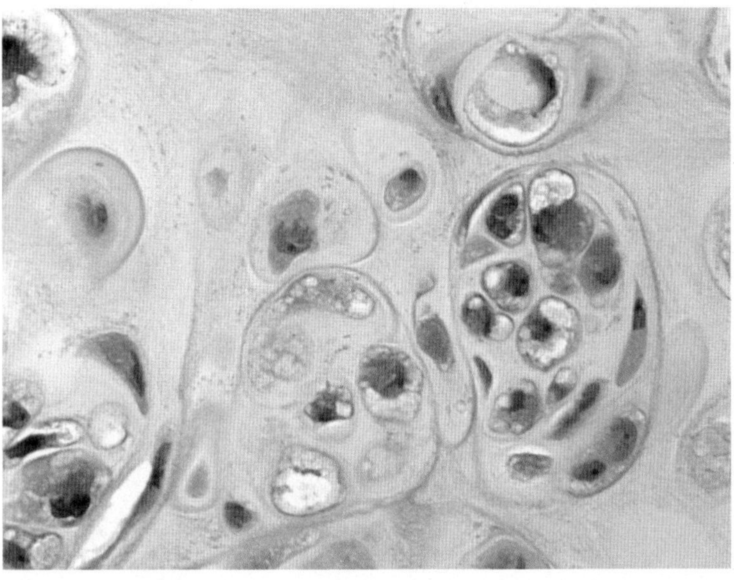

Figure 6.14.3.
Synovial chondromatosis. Note the crowding and anaplasia of chondrocyte nuclei within the lacunae. This should not be interpreted as evidence of a malignant process in this pathologic entity.

6.15 Osteosarcoma

Presentation

Swelling, pain, loosening of teeth, paresthesia of lips and chin (numb chin syndrome). The average age of the patient is 33 years.

Radiographic Appearance

Irregular, destructive mass varying from radiolucent to mixed radiolucent and radiopaque

Microscopic Findings

- Malignant osteoblasts producing atypical bone or cartilage set in a sarcomatous stroma
- The sarcoma cells are plump, hyperchromatic and can show typical and atypical mitoses.
- Deposition of tumor bone on top of residual normal bone can be seen.

Histopathologic Differential

- An *osteoblastoma* lacks sarcomatous stroma and infiltrative features.
- For the differential with *juvenile trabecular ossifying fibroma,* see chart on page 216.

Treatment and Prognosis

Radical surgery with neoadjuvant chemotherapy.

Additional

Osteosarcomas of the jaws are usually of the chondroblastic subtype.

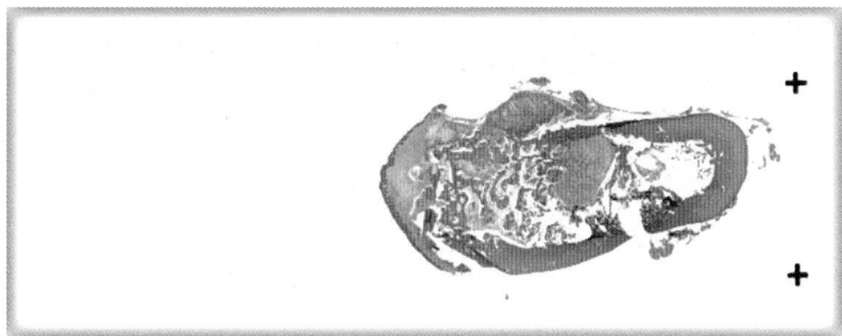

Figure 6.15.1.
Osteosarcoma. Mucosa (at left) overlies a destructive tumor of the mandible, seen in cross section. Tumor can be seen to extend outside of the bone.

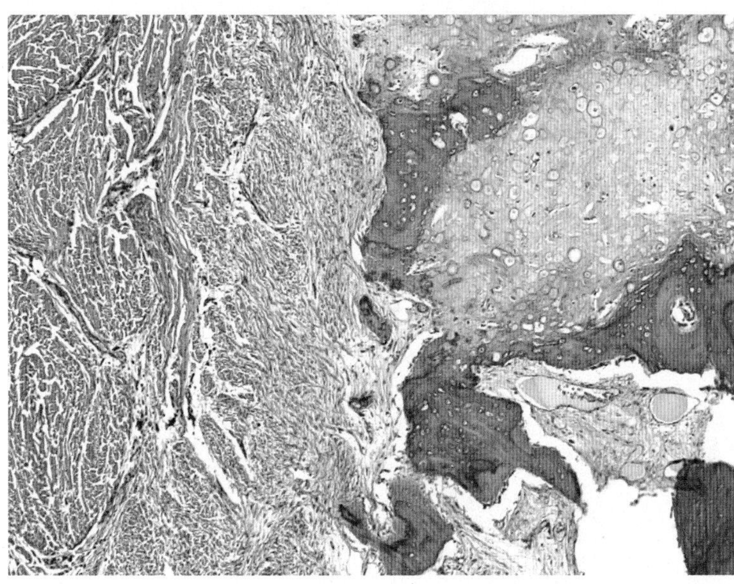

Figure 6.15.2.
Osteosarcoma, chondroblastic type.
A destructive, chondroblastic tumor extends into the thickened periosteum.

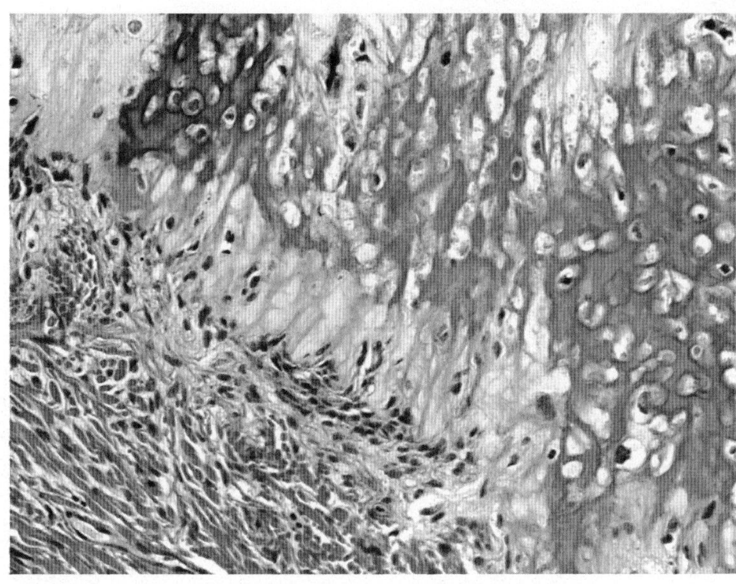

Figure 6.15.3.
Osteosarcoma, chondroblastic type. A front of invasive, atypical tumor bone surfaced by malignant spindle cells.

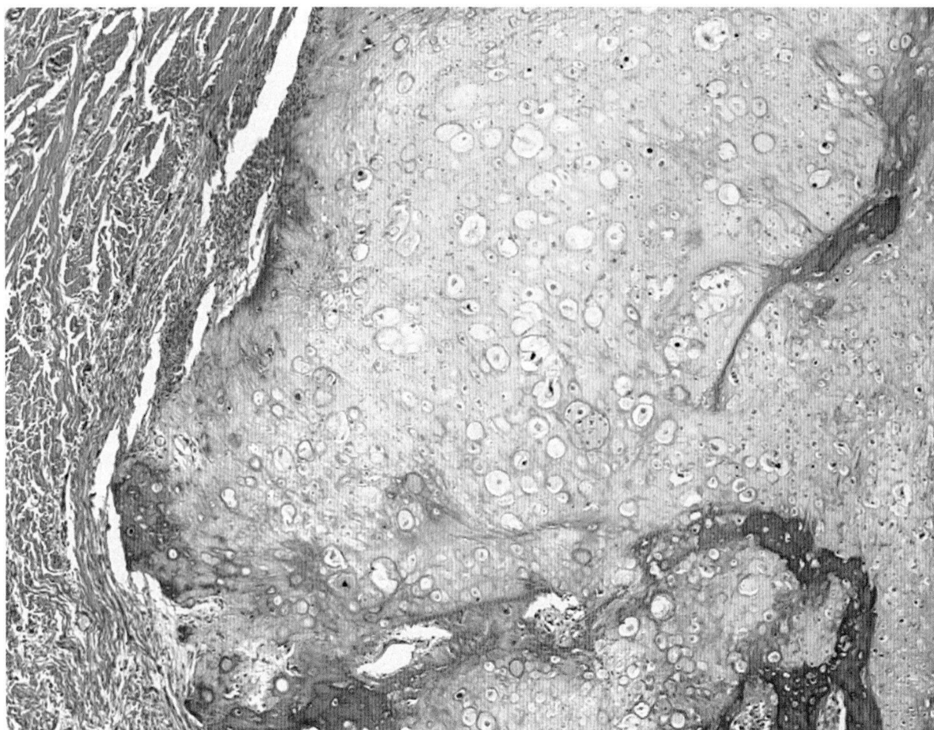

Figure 6.15.4. Osteosarcoma, chondroblastic type. This portion of the tumor consists of an irregular mass of atypical cartilage. The chondroblastic variant is common in the jaws.

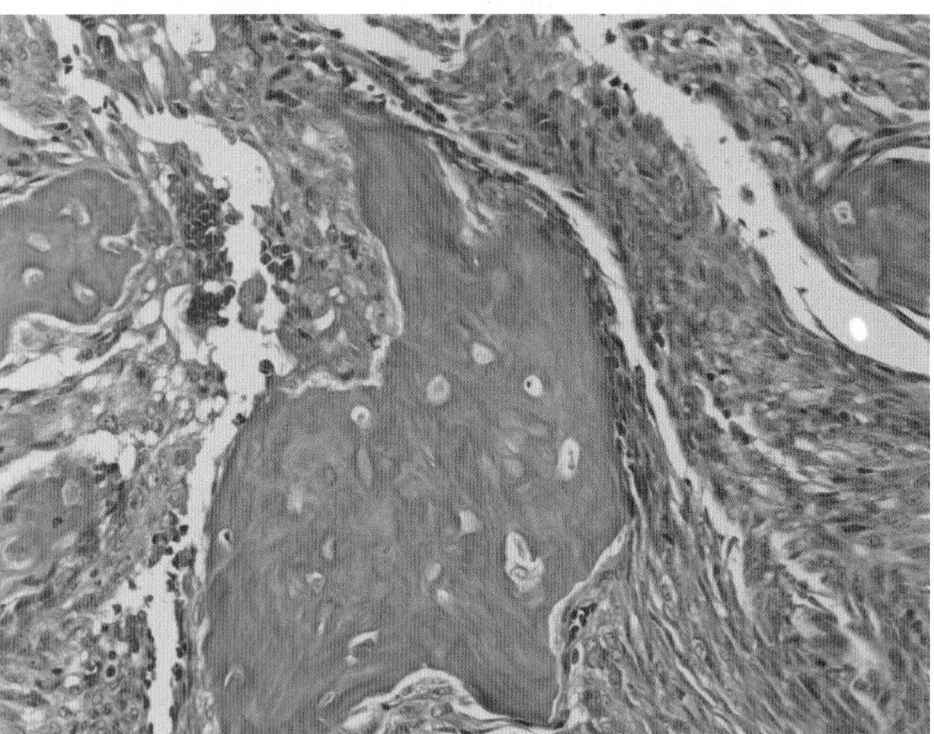

Figure 6.15.5. Osteosarcoma, fibroblastic type. Fragments of residual lamellar bone cortex are surrounded by sarcomatous tissue.

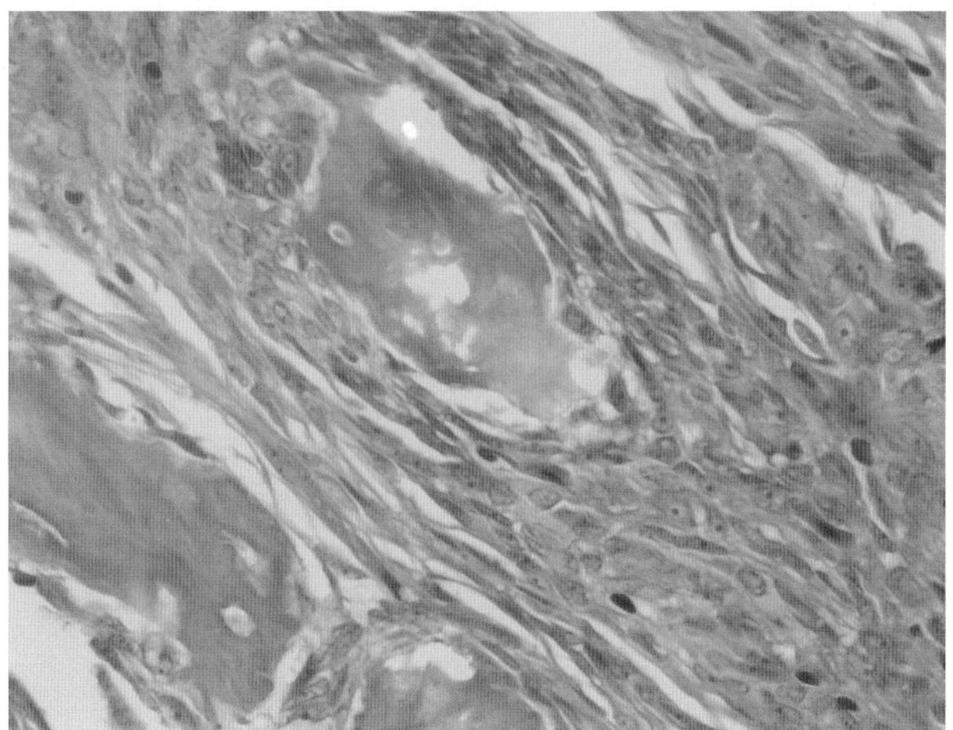

Figure 6.15.6. Osteosarcoma, fibroblastic type. Fascicles of sarcomatous cells and woven tumor bone.

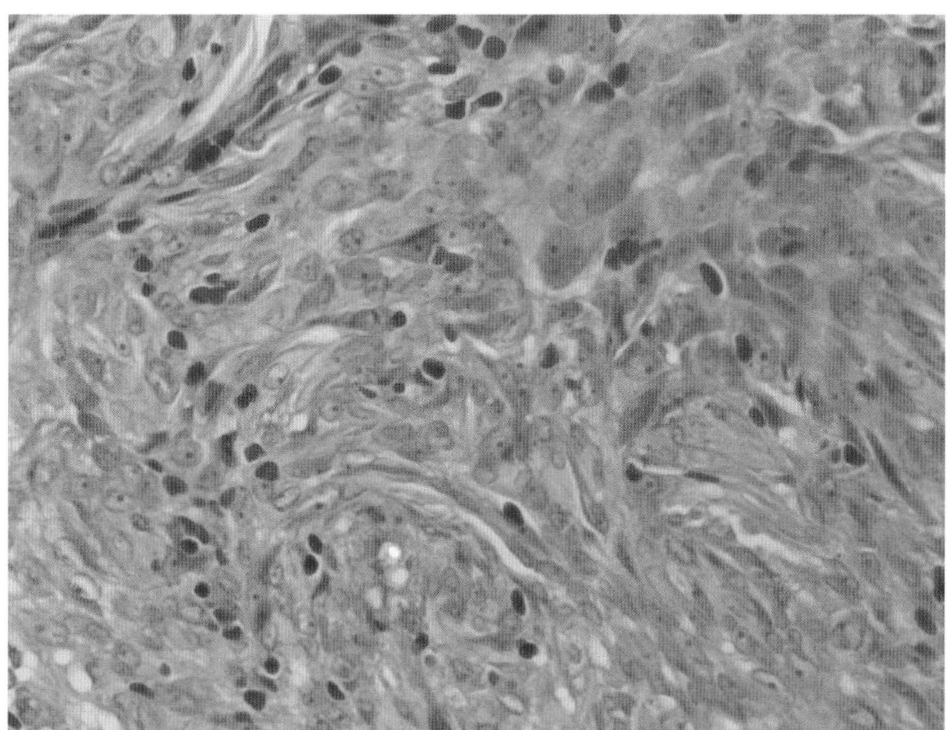

Figure 6.15.7. Osteosarcoma, fibroblastic type. The densely packed tumor cells have both spindle and epithelioid features. The nuclei are enlarged, plump, vesicular and pleomorphic.

6.16 Chondrosarcoma

Presentation

Painless mass; usually maxilla. Generally adults and older adults.

Radiographic Appearance

Radiolucency with irregular, destructive borders. Scattered calcifications are sometimes present.

Microscopic Findings

- Cellular lobules of cartilaginous tissue.
- Nuclei of chondrocytes are enlarged, hyperchromatic, and atypical, often with binucleate forms.
- Myxoid matrix can also be seen.
- Variable number of mitoses, depending on tumor grade, are noted.

Histopathologic Differential

A chondroblastic *osteosarcoma* will have minimal chondroid differentiation and production of malignant woven bone.

Treatment and Prognosis

Radical surgery. Late recurrence common.

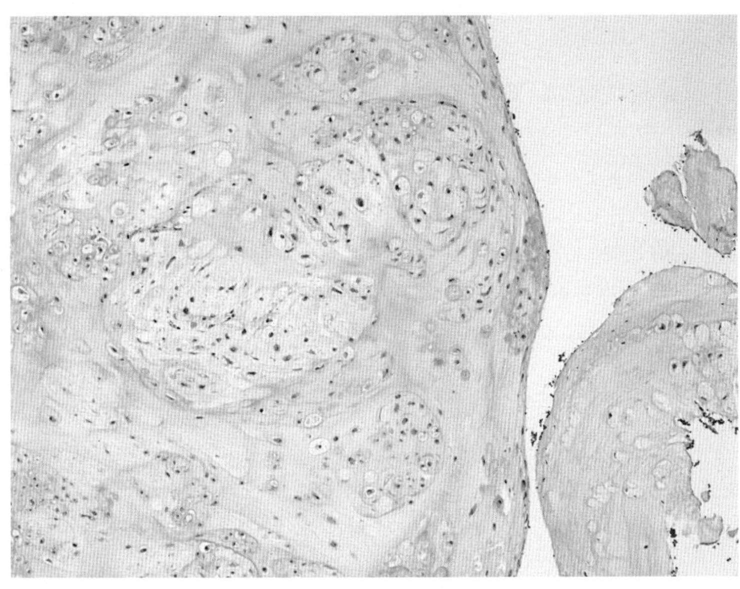

Figure 6.16.1.
Chondrosarcoma. Lobules of atypical hyaline cartilage with increased cellularity.

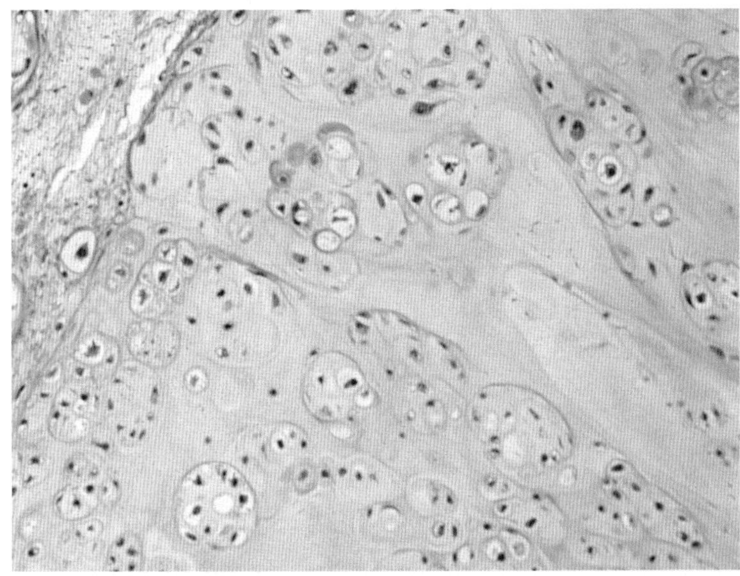

Figure 6.16.2.
Chondrosarcoma. Nests of enlarged chondrocytes, some of which are multinucleated.

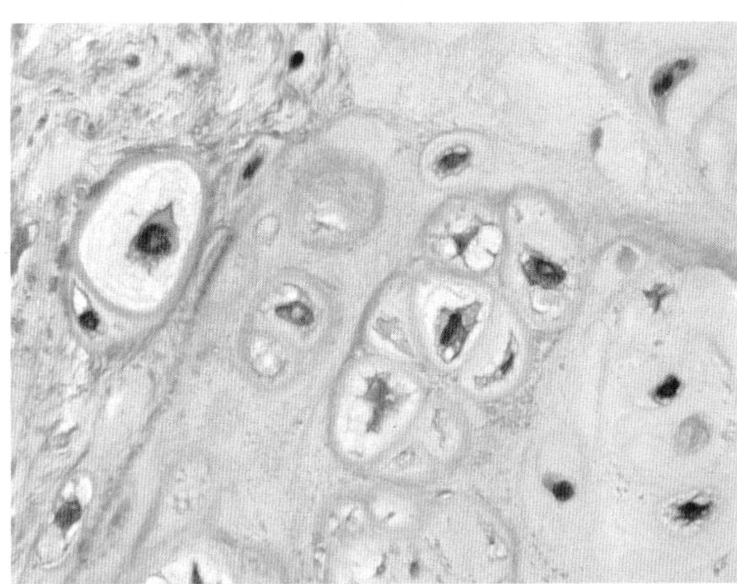

Figure 6.16.3.
Chondrosarcoma. The neoplastic chondrocytes have enlarged, dark-staining nuclei. Occasional bizarre forms are seen.

6.17 Metastatic Tumors

Metastases to the jawbones are relatively rare and, when encountered, are most often found in the molar region of the mandible. The tumors are predominately carcinomas of the breast, lung, prostate, kidney, or colon.

Microscopic Findings

Patients usually present with swelling, pain, and paresthesia of the lips and chin (numb chin syndrome). The radiographic appearance is generally one of a destructive radiolucency.

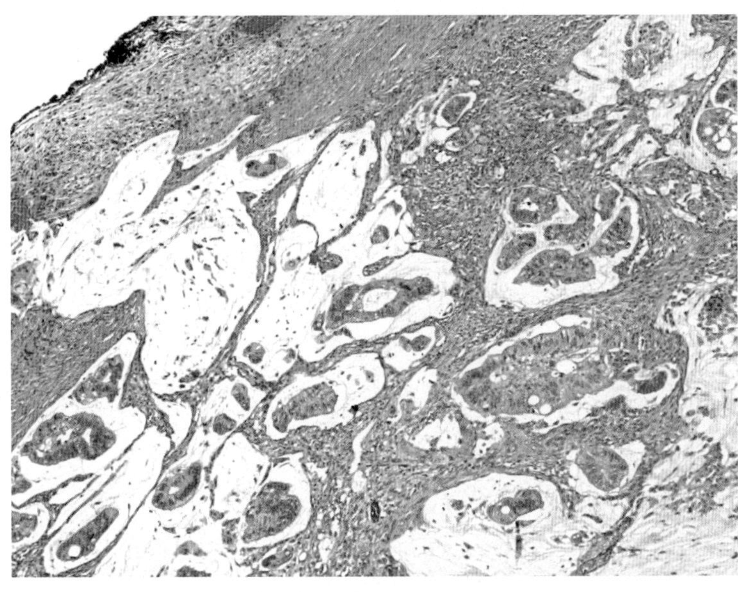

Figure 6.17.1.
Metastatic tumors of the jaws. Mucinous (colloid) carcinoma of the colon. Atypical duct-like structures and tumor cells in a prominent mucinous stroma infiltrate bone.

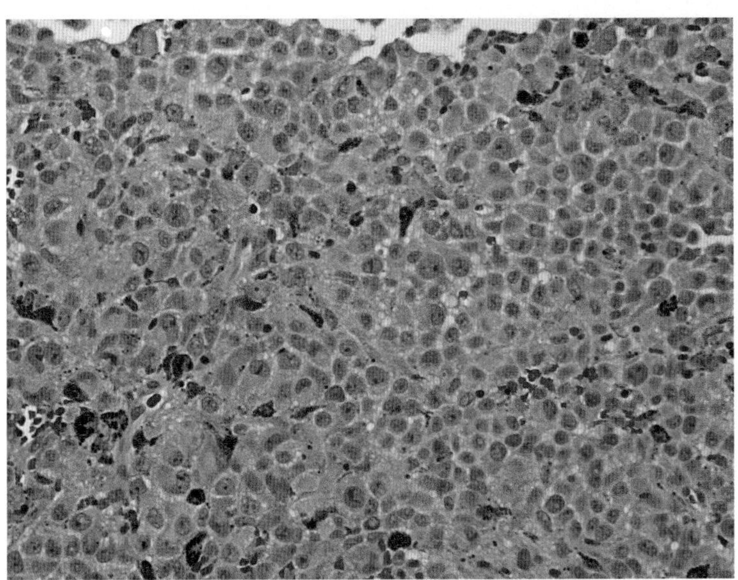

Figure 6.17.2.
Metastatic tumors of the jaws. Melanoma. Sheets of atypical epithelioid melanocytes contains melanin granules.

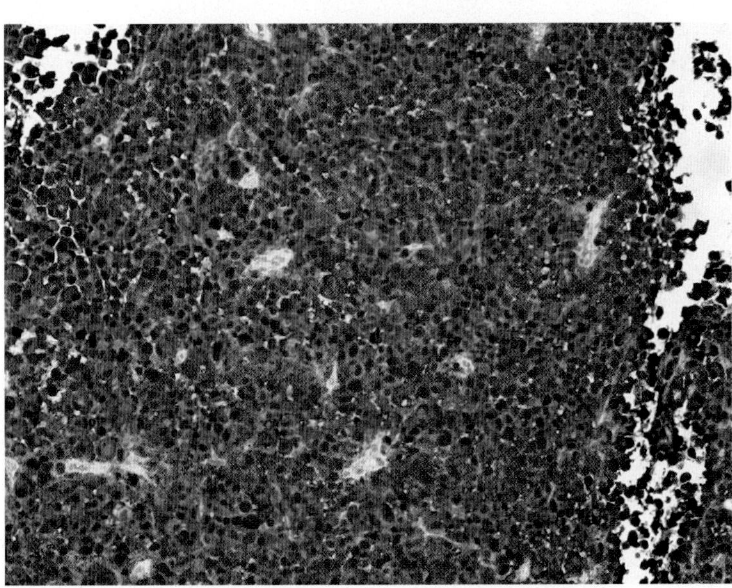

Figure 6.17.3.
Metastatic tumors of the jaws. Melanoma, S100 stain.

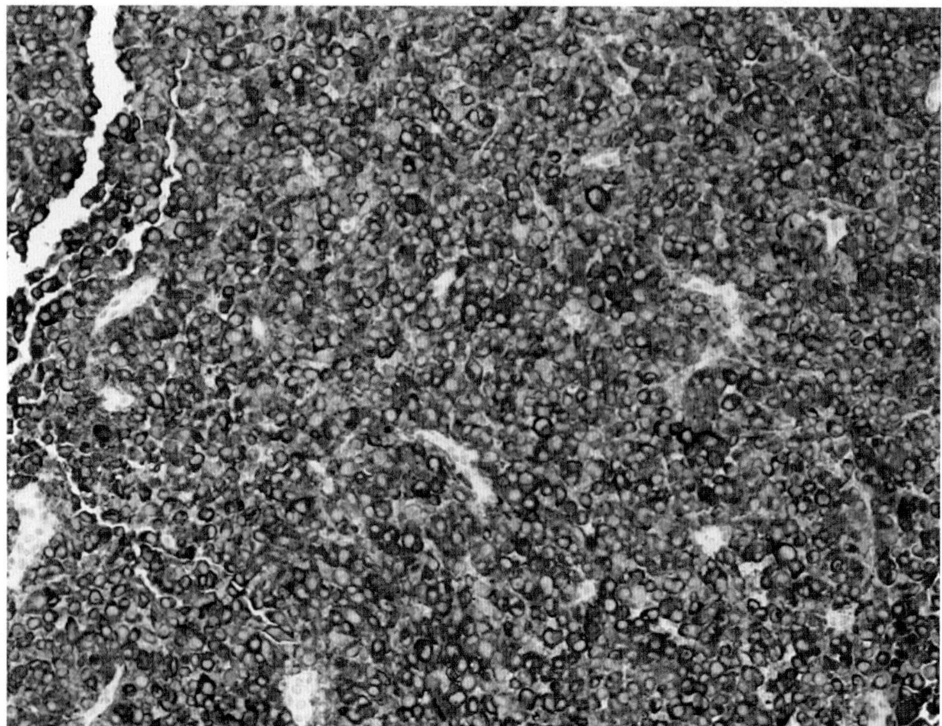

Figure 6.17.4.
Metastatic tumors of the jaws. Melanoma, HMB-45 stain.

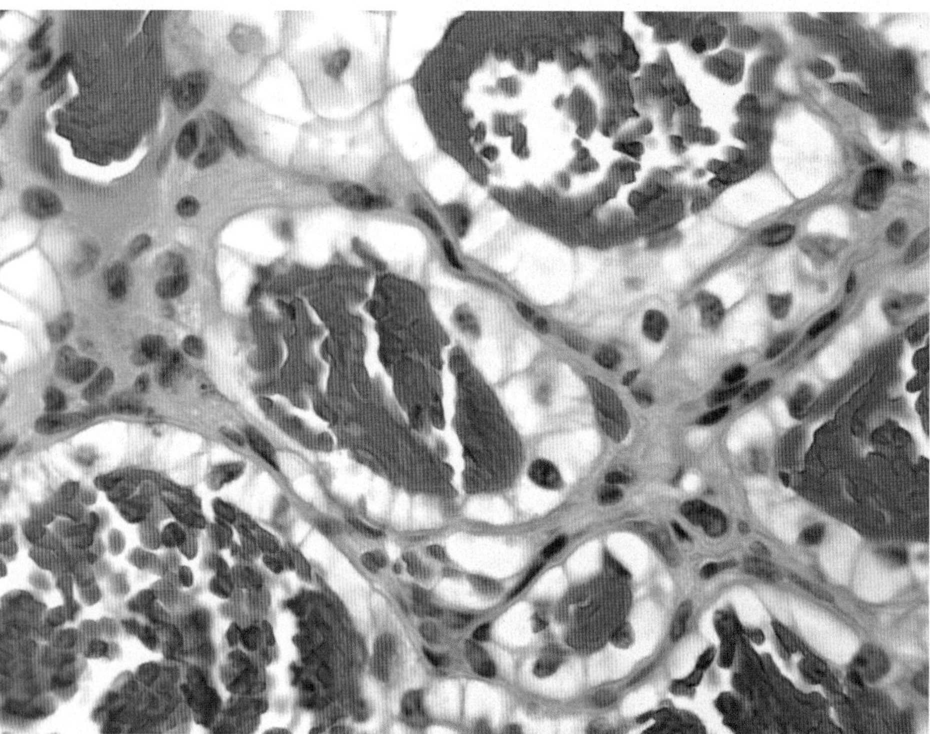

Figure 6.17.5.
Metastatic tumors of the jaws. Renal cell carcinoma. Nests of large clear cells associated with a prominent vascular proliferation.

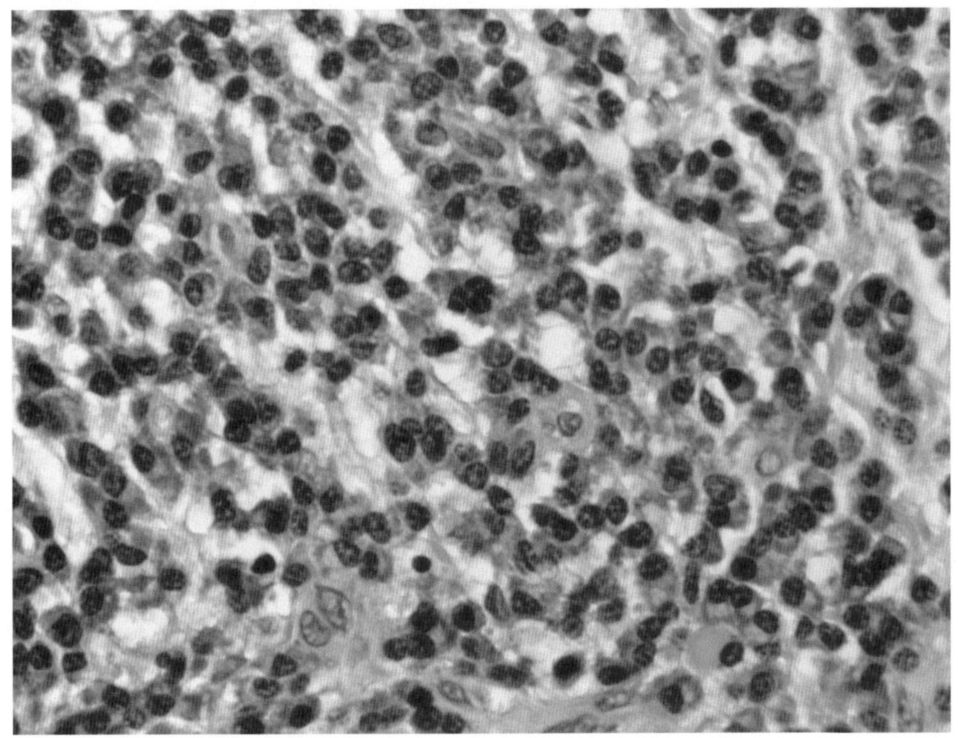

Figure 6.17.6.
Plasmacytoma. Sheets of atypical plasma cells.

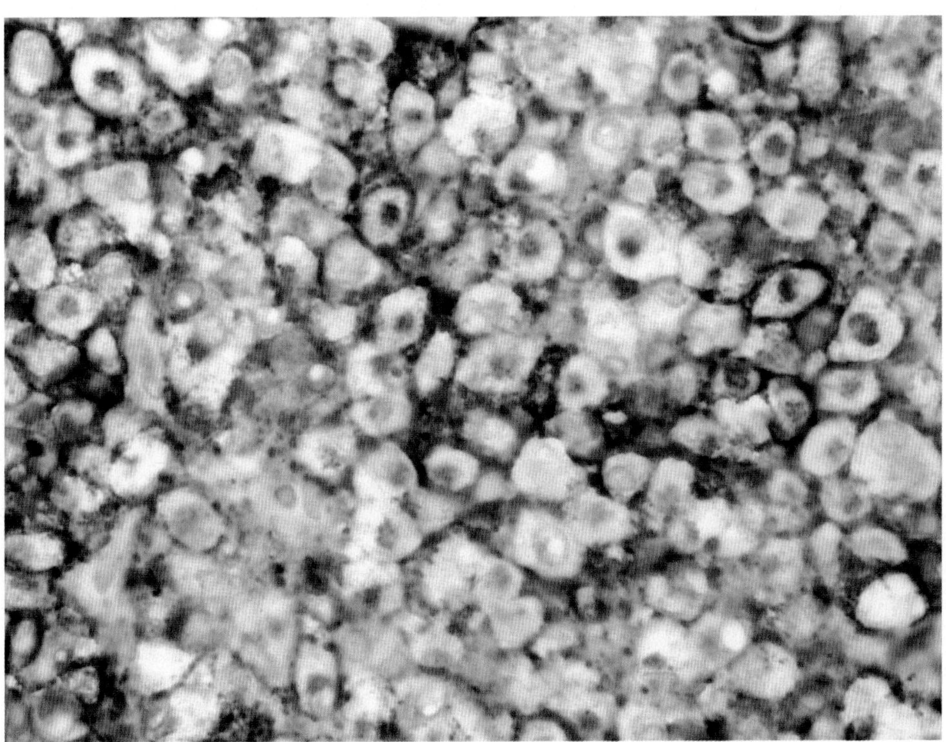

Figure 6.17.7.
Plasmacytoma, CD-138 stain.

Bibliography and Suggested Reading

6.1

Tong AC, Ng IO, Yeung KM. Osteomyelitis with proliferative periostitis: an unusual case. *Oral Surg Oral Med Oral Pathol Oral Radiol Endod.* 2006;102:e14–e19.

6.2

Marx RE, Cillo JE Jr, Ulloa JJ. Oral bisphosphonate-induced osteonecrosis: risk factors, prediction of risk using serum CTX testing, prevention, and treatment. *J Oral Maxillofac Surg.* 2007;65:2397–2410.

Kos M, Kuebler JF, Luczak K, et al. Bisphosphonate-related osteonecrosis of the jaws: a review of 34 cases and evaluation of risk. *Craniomaxillofac Surg.* 2010;38:255–259.

Filleul O, Crompot E, Saussez S. Bisphosphonate-induced osteonecrosis of the jaw: a review of 2,400 patient cases. *J Cancer Res Clin Oncol.* 2010;136:1117–1124.

6.3

Elliot KA. Diagnosis and surgical management of nasopalatine duct cysts. *Laryngoscope.* 2004;114:1336–1340.

6.4

Cano J. Surgical ciliated cyst of the maxilla. *Med Oral Pathol.* 2009;14:e361–e364.

6.5

Perdigão PF, Silva EC, Sakurai E, et al. Idiopathic bone cavity: a clinical, radiographic, and histological study. *Br J Oral Maxillofac Surg.* 2003;41:407–409.

6.6

Breuer C. Mandibular aneurysmal bone cyst in a child. *Eur J Pediatr.* 2010;169:1037–1040.

6.7

Whitaker SB, Waldron CA. Central giant cell lesions of the jaws. A clinical, radiologic, and histopathologic study. *Oral Surg Oral Med Oral Pathol.* 1993;75:199–208.

6.8

Eversole R, Su L, El Mofty S. Benign fibro-osseous lesions of the craniofacial complex: a review. *Head Neck Pathol.* 2008;2:177–202.

6.9

Melrose RJ. The clinico-pathological spectrum of cemento-osseous dysplasia. *Oral Maxillofac Surg Clin North Am.* 1997;9:643–653.

6.10

Su L, Weathers DR, Waldron CA. Distinguishing features of local cemento-osseous dysplasia and cemento-ossifiyng fibromas: a pathologic spectrum of 316 cases. *Oral Med Oral Pathol Oral Surg.* 1997;84:301–309.

6.11

Slootweg PJ, Panders AK, Koopmans R, et al. Juvenile ossifying fibroma: an analysis of 33 cases with emphasis on histopathological aspects. *J Oral Pathol Med.*1994;23:385–388.

6.12

Jones AC, Prihoda TJ, Kacher JE, et al. Osteoblastoma of the maxilla and mandible: a report of 24 cases, review of the literature, and discussion of its relationship to osteoid osteoma of the jaws. *Oral Surg Oral Med Oral Pathol Oral Radiol Endod.* 2006;102:639–650.

6.13

Ord RA. Osteochondroma of the condyle. *Int J Oral Maxillofac Surg.* 2010;39:523–528.

6.14

Von Lindern JJ, Theuerkauf I, Niederhagen B, et al. Synovial chondromatosis of the temporomandibular joint: clinical, diagnostic, and histomorphologic findings. *Oral Surg Oral Med Oral Pathol Oral Radiol Endod.* 2002;94:31–38.

6.15

Patel SG, Meyers P, Huvos AG, et al. Improved outcomes in patients with osteogenic sarcoma of the head and neck. *Cancer.* 2002;95:1495–1503.

6.16

Saito K, Unni KK, Wollan PC, et al. Chondrosarcoma of the jaw and facial bones. *Cancer.* 1995;76:1550–1558.

6.17

D'Silva NJ, Summerlin DJ, Cordell KG, Abdelsayed RA, Tomich CE, Hanks CT, Fear D, Meyrowitz S. Metastatic tumors in the jaws: a retrospective study of 114 cases. *J Am Dent Assoc.* 2006;137(12): 1667–1672.

Hirshberg A, Leibovich P, Buchner A. Metastatic tumors to the jawbones: analysis of 390 cases. *J Oral Pathol Med.* 1994;23(8):337–341.

Muttagi SS, Chaturvedi P, D'Cruz A, Kane S, Chaukar D, Pai P, Singh B, Pawar P. Metastatic tumors to the jaw bones: retrospective analysis from an Indian tertiary referral center. *Indian J Cancer.* 2011;48(2):234–239.

References

Ellis GL, Auclair P. Tumors of the Salivary Glands (AFIP Atlas of Tumor Pathology, Series 4). AFIP, 1996, 2008.

Neville B, Damm DD, Allen CM, Bouquot J. Oral and Maxillofacial Pathology. St Louis: Saunders, an imprint of Elsevier, 2009.

Reichart PA, Philipsen HP. Odontogenic Tumors and Allied Lesions. Hanover Park, IL: Quintessence Books, 2004.

Sciubba JJ, Fantasia JE, Kahn, LB. Tumors and Cysts of the Jaw (AFIP Atlas of Tumor Pathology, Series 3). AFIP, 2001.

Stelow EB, Mills S. Biopsy Interpretation of the Upper Aerodigestive Tract and Ear. Philadelphia: Lippincott, Williams and Wilkins, 2008.

Index

Note: The letters '*f*' and '*t*' following the locators refer to figures and tables respectively.